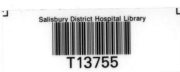
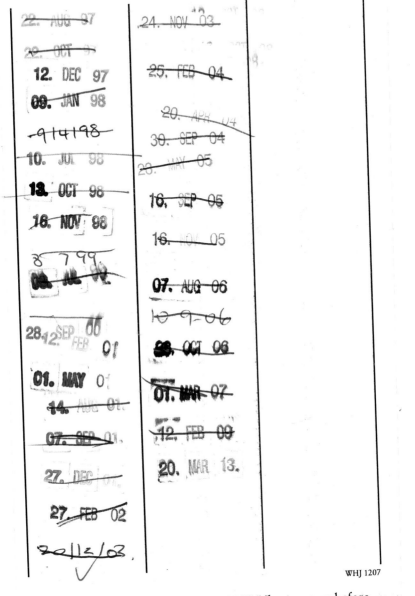

WHJ 1207

Books should be returned to the SDH Library on or before
the date stamped above unless a renewal has been arranged.

Salisbury District Hospital Library

Telephone: Salisbury (01722) 336262 extn. 4432 / 33
Out of hours answer machine in operation

FUNDAMENTALS OF
Plastic Surgery

FUNDAMENTALS OF
Plastic
Surgery

MALCOLM W. MARKS, MD, FACS
Associate Professor of Plastic Surgery
Bowman Gray School of Medicine
Wake Forest University
Winston-Salem, NC

CHARLES MARKS, MD, PhD, FRCP, FRCS, FACS
Professor Emeritus of Surgery
Louisiana State University School of Medicine
New Orleans, LA
Formerly Hunterian Professor
Royal College of Surgeons of England
Executive Medical Director
Florida Department of Corrections
Charlotte, Florida

Foreword by:
LOUIS C. ARGENTA, MD
Professor and Chairman, Department of Plastic Surgery
Bowman Gray School of Medicine
Wake Forest University
Winston-Salem, NC

Illustrations by:
ANNEMARIE JOHNSON, CMI
Biomedical Communications
Bowman Gray School of Medicine
Wake Forest University
Winston-Salem, NC

W.B. SAUNDERS COMPANY
A Division of Harcourt Brace & Company
Philadelphia London Toronto Montreal Sydney Tokyo

W.B. SAUNDERS COMPANY
A Division of Harcourt Brace & Company

The Curtis Center
Independence Square West
Philadelphia, Pennsylvania 19106

Library of Congress Cataloging-in-Publication Data

Marks, Malcolm W.
Fundamentals of plastic surgery / Malcolm W. Marks, Charles Marks; foreword by Louis C.
Argenta; artist, Annemarie Johnson.

    p.   cm.

ISBN 0–7216–6449–0

1. Surgery, Plastic.   I. Marks, Charles.   II. Title.   [DNLM: 1. Surgery, Plastic—methods.
    WO 600 M346f 1997]

RD118.M377 1997   617.9′5—dc20

DNLM/DLC   96–8868

FUNDAMENTALS OF PLASTIC SURGERY   ISBN 0–7216–6449–0

Printed in the United States of America.

Last digit is the print number: 9   8   7   6   5   4   3   2   1

Foreword

This book responds to two important problems facing plastic and reconstructive surgery as we enter the twenty-first century. The first is the need for an organized presentation of the exponentially enlarging field of plastic and reconstructive surgery for medical students and trainee surgical residents. There is a fine line between the provision of an inadequate amount of information that fails to stimulate and inform the neophyte surgical student on the one hand and an excessive amount of information that overwhelms, discourages, and confuses on the other. As medical training continues on its course of fragmentation into ever-smaller subspecialties, the amount of time available to transmit the information within the expanding horizons of plastic and reconstructive surgery becomes progressively curtailed.

This book summarizes the fundamental body of knowledge pertaining to the field of plastic and reconstructive surgery into a "digestible form" that can be read with immediate comprehension within a brief period. Accordingly, residents rotating through their plastic surgery training during a 1- to 2-month period can be "gavaged" with information that will be useful to them no matter in which surgical subspecialty they may ultimately become engaged. Medical students and physician assistant students will also be rapidly exposed to the scope and depth of the plastic and reconstructive surgery arena, and, it is hoped, the desire of bright aspirants to enter into and expand the field will be stimulated.

The second problem that is addressed concerns the need to provide a rapid infusion of a fundamental core of knowledge of the specialty to new residents commencing their plastic and reconstructive surgical training. The book provides an opportunity for the first-year resident to be introduced in depth to the substance of the specialty within the first month of residency. After reading this book, the neophyte surgeon will develop a basic, yet broad, comprehension of the problems that may arise in the emergency room, clinic, or operating room. Mastery of this information, instilled at the outset of training, should stimulate the trainee to delve deeper into larger texts and more stratified literature.

The authors are to be commended. Few individuals in the field have demonstrated the dedication and wisdom to undertake a non–multiauthored book. This volume represents a prodigious amount of work in an era in which faculty are already overwhelmed by the pressure of their duties. This book is destined to provide a classic reference to the broad details of plastic and reconstructive surgery and will, it is hoped, plant the seeds of progress for a new generation of plastic surgeons entering the twenty-first century.

Louis C. Argenta, MD
Professor and Chairman
Department of Plastic Surgery
Bowman Gray School of Medicine
Wake Forest University
Winston-Salem, NC

Preface

Fundamentals of Plastic Surgery provides an overview of the entire field of plastic and reconstructive surgery so structured in length and format that it can be reviewed in a short time. Intended primarily for residents undergoing training in plastic surgery, it is especially suitable for surgical house staff and students on a plastic surgery service, as well as nurses and physician assistants concerned with the treatment of plastic surgery patients. The text provides a significant amount of core information that is the basis of the specialty without overwhelming the reader. Two authors have shared in the writing and editorial responsibilities. Malcolm Marks is a board-certified plastic surgeon who has been involved in the training of plastic surgery residents, rotating house officers, and students for 13 years. Charles Marks is a thoracic and vascular surgeon with a PhD in anatomy who has also been involved full-time in a university teaching environment for more than 30 years.

We wish to express our appreciation to those who have worked toward the completion of this book. We thank Tori Faust, Linda Fowler, Kelly Matthews, and Kara Shinault who typed the manuscript and its multiple revisions. The excellent illustrations reflect the hard work of Annemarie Johnson.

We are especially grateful to the residents, students, and hospital staff with whom we have worked and who have inspired the writing of *Fundamentals of Plastic Surgery*. We thank our families for their patience during the long hours of preparation of the manuscript.

Contents

CHAPTER 1

Wound Management 1

Wound Healing and Management 3

Suture Techniques 10

Excision of Lesions 13

Management of Scars 14

CHAPTER 2

Skin Lesions 19

Benign Cystic Lesions 21

Epidermal Lesions 21

Benign Pigmented Skin Lesions 22

Tumors of Epidermal Appendages 25

Fibrous Lesions 26

Lesions of Neural Origin 27

Vascular Lesions 27

Lymphatic Malformations 30

Malignant Vascular Tumors 30

Miscellaneous Lesions 31

Miscellaneous Infectious Conditions 31

Malignant Tumors of the Skin 32

CHAPTER 3

Laser Therapy 41

Laser Physics 43

Major Lasers Used Surgically 44

Laser Hazards 46

CHAPTER 4

Burns 49

The Burn Wound 51

Medical Treatment 55

Operative Management of Burn Wounds 58

Electrical Burns 60

Chemical Burns 61

Cold Injury 61

Burn Rehabilitation 62

CHAPTER 5

Grafts and Implants 65

Skin Grafts 67

Cartilage Grafts 73

Bone Grafts 73

Collagen 75

Alloplastic Material 75

CHAPTER 6

Flaps 79

Definition 81

Skin Flaps 81

Composite Flaps 87

Muscle and Musculocutaneous Flaps 90

Fasciocutaneous Flaps 97

CHAPTER 7

Tissue Expansion 101

Tissue Response to Expansion 105

Regional Expansion 105

CHAPTER 8

Microvascular Surgery 113

Microsurgical Technique 115

Replantation 118

Free Tissue Transfer 121

Microneural Repair 126

Nerve Grafting 129

CHAPTER 9

Craniofacial Surgery 131

The Skull 133

Anomalies of Craniofacial Development 135

Craniosynostosis 139

Management of Craniofacial Malformations 142

Correction of Facial Skeletal Deformities 151

CHAPTER 10

Cleft Lip and Palate 153

The Cleft Deformity 155

Principles of Cleft Lip Repairs 157

Clefts of the Secondary Palate 163

Repair of the Palate 165

Secondary Palatal Problems 169

CHAPTER 11

Head and Neck 175

Oromandibular Disorders 177

Oral and Oropharyngeal Carcinoma 180

Maxillary Carcinoma 184

Primary Salivary Gland Tumors 186

The Neck 191

Tumors of the Thyroid Gland 196

Radical Neck Dissection 197

CHAPTER 12

Maxillofacial Trauma 201

Soft Tissue Injury 203

Facial Fractures 211

Temporomandibular Joint 226

CHAPTER 13

Reconstructive Procedures of the Face 229

Periorbital Reconstruction 231

Lip Reconstruction 240

The Ear 243

Ear Reconstruction 244

Reconstruction of Nasal Defects 246

Facial Paralysis 249

CHAPTER 14

Aesthetic Facial Surgery 255

The Nose 257

Rhytidectomy 264

Forehead-Brow Lift 270

Blepharoplasty 271

Ancillary Aesthetic Procedures 275

Hair Replacement 277

CHAPTER 15
Breast and Chest Wall: Breast and Developmental Chest Wall Pathology 283

The Breast 285

Breast Cancer and Reconstruction 294

Congenital Malformations of the Chest Wall 302

CHAPTER 16
Trunk and Lower Extremity 307

Acquired Chest Wall Defects 309

Back 311

Abdominal Wall Deformities 313

Lower Extremity 314

The Pressure Sore 320

Body Contouring 325

CHAPTER 17
Genitourinary System 333

Development of the Urogenital System 335

Hypospadias 337

Epispadias 339

Exstrophy of the Bladder 340

Injuries to the Male Genitalia 340

Penile Implants for Impotence 341

Sex Identification 342

Reconstruction of the Vagina 343

CHAPTER 18
The Hand and Upper Limb 347

The Wrist 349

The Hand 351

Nerve Compression Syndromes 371

Tendon Transfer for Muscle Paralysis 373

The Arthritic Hand 376

Hand Tumors 379

Congenital Hand Anomalies 380

Index 385

CHAPTER 1

Wound Management

The English word *surgery* is derived from the older form "chirurgery," which is, in turn, related to the French "chirurere" and Latin "chiruraia." The common denominator in each of these terms is the Greek "Kheirourgia" with its two roots, *keir* (hand) and *ergon* (work). Thus, surgery represents "handwork" and the surgeon is accordingly a handworker. The word *plastic* is derived from the Latin "plasticus" and the Greek "plastikos," which mean to create, to shape, and to mold. In his monograph on nasal surgery in 1818, von Graefe first used the term *Rhinoplastik*, and within half a century the semantic connotation of plastic surgery was well established.

Reconstructive surgery has reference as long ago as 700 B.C. in the Sushruta Samhita, with descriptions of nose reconstruction using forehead flaps. The need to replace parts of the body destroyed or deformed by trauma or disease acted as a stimulus to technical developments in this field. As the flow of surgical knowledge from India and the Middle East entered the cultures of Egypt, Greece, and Rome, the Latin translations of the Indian, Arabic, and Greek manuscripts found their way to the universities of Europe and established the basis of modern plastic and reconstructive surgery.

From the sixteenth to the nineteenth century, Paré, Tagliacozzi, von Graefe, Dieffenbach, Reverdin, Ollier, Thiersch, Wolfe, and Krause, among many others, established a strong foundation for this newest branch of surgery. The twentieth century has seen spectacular advances in the understanding of wound healing, tissue metabolism, circulation, and antibiosis. Complemented by advanced instrumentation and computerization, the specialty of plastic and reconstructive surgery now embraces the areas of congenital deformities, burns, head and neck tumors, maxillofacial trauma, hand surgery, cosmetic surgery, and microvascular techniques.

Unlike the general surgeon, whose operative procedures are essentially excisional and thus destructive, the reconstructive role of the plastic surgeon imposes certain added responsibilities. In addition to an education and training that has depth as well as breadth, the results of one's operative procedures depend upon an understanding of the patient's psyche and personality as well as an appreciation of the patient's defects and disabilities.

WOUND HEALING AND MANAGEMENT

The management of unhealed and improperly healed wounds represents the most common indication for the application of reconstructive techniques. Primary skin closure, wound débridement, skin grafting, tissue transfer, scar revision, and Z-plasty are the most frequently used techniques. The success of any of these procedures requires understanding of the process of wound healing, the factors that impair the process, and the microanatomy of all tissues.

Normal Skin

The skin is composed of two layers, the epidermis and dermis, with an underlying subcutaneous layer (Fig. 1–1).

Epidermis. The epidermis establishes the vital barrier between the external

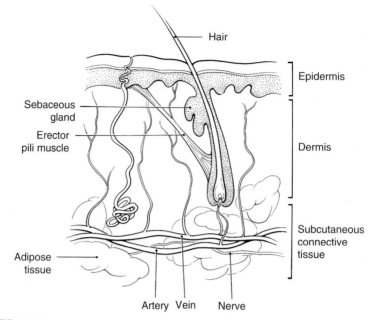

FIGURE 1–1. The skin is composed of two layers, the epidermis and the dermis, with an underlying subcutaneous layer.

and internal environment of the body. It prevents invasion by bacteria and other unabsorbable noxious substances and protects the deeper layers from trauma. It is a stratified squamous epithelium composed of the superficial stratum corneum (a dead desquamating layer) and the deeper malpighian stratum. The malpighian stratum is composed variably of the stratum lucidum, stratum granulosum, and stratum spinosum and consistently of the stratum germinativum or basal layer. The basal layer of cells undergoes continuous multiplication, thereby maintaining a stratified epithelial layer.

Dermis. The dermis consists of a superficial layer, the papillary dermis, and a deep layer, the reticular dermis. The dermis is made up of collagen, which is the basic protein that provides the framework for all tissues and organs. The papillary dermal collagen is finer, whereas the reticular dermal collagen is dense. The strength of the collagen fibers, whether part of dermis, tendon, or ligamentous tissue, depends on the linkages within and between its molecules, which are made up of three peptide chains twisted in a right-handed helix. The amino acid glycine is present in every third position. Amino acids unique to collagen are hydroxyproline and hydroxylysine. Collagen is synthesized in the endoplasmic reticulum of fibroblasts, where ascorbic acid (vitamin C) is required to hydroxylate proline to hydroxyproline. Lack of ascorbic acid impedes collagen production, with poor wound healing as an expression of occult scurvy.

The Schiff base is an amino group of hydroxylysine that bonds with an aldehyde group of another hydroxylysine, determining the strength of the collagen fibers. Seven distinct types of collagen have been identified, with types I and III the prevalent components of skin.

The dermis is separated from the epidermis by a connective tissue layer (the basement membrane). Adnexal structures including sebaceous glands, sweat glands, and hair follicles are found throughout the dermis, with hair follicles and sweat glands extending into the subcutaneous connective tissues.

Subcutaneous Layer. The subcutaneous layer is composed of fat lobules and connective tissue. Connective tissue is a continuous fabric of fibrous tissue, composing about 30 per cent of body weight, that extends throughout the entire body. It consists of collagen, reticulum, and elastin within the ground substance of mucopolysaccharides and mucoproteins. Scattered throughout the fibers are fat cells, fibroblasts, histiocytes, mast cells, and plasma cells.

Wound Healing

A cleanly incised wound through the epidermis, dermis, and subcutaneous tissue undergoes a series of concurrent dynamic changes that can be categorized as inflammatory, catabolic, and fibroplastic (Fig. 1–2). Immediately after injury, the wound fills with blood that clots. The inflammatory reaction leads to epithelialization of the wound, and scar tissue gradually develops and is remodeled so as to firmly appose the wound edges. This represents healing by first intention. Healing by second intention occurs in a wound in which tissue is lost and the wound edges are not apposed. The development of granulation tissue and wound contraction then form a base for advancing epithelium or for a skin graft.

Inflammation. Immediately after injury, local vasoconstriction stops the bleeding and the wound clots. Within 10 minutes, local vasodilatation occurs as a result of the release of intracellular materials such as histamine and serotonin into the extracellular compartment of the injured tissue. This vascular response lasts about 30 minutes. Continued vasodilatation and vascular permeability are due to the effects of prostaglandin E_1 and E_2. Plasma leaks into the surrounding tissues with migration of polymorphonuclear leukocytes and monocytes. The inflammatory reaction is localized first by fibrin obstruction of the lymphatics and later by the local accumulation of the glycoprotein fibronectin, which localizes the reaction by producing local adhesion of fibroblasts, fibrin, and collagen.

The polymorphonuclear leukocytes exert their early phagocytic activity with their débridement of injured and damaged cells and of blood clot. As the inflammatory reaction proceeds, the mononuclear cells become more prominent and active in collecting the debris not digested by the polymorphonuclear leukocytes.

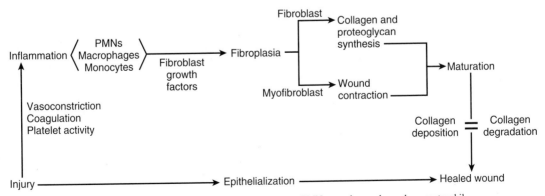

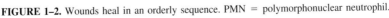

FIGURE 1–2. Wounds heal in an orderly sequence. PMN = polymorphonuclear neutrophil.

In chronic inflammation the mononuclear cells become the dominant phagocytic agent and conjoin to become giant cells, as seen in foreign body reaction or tuberculosis. Platelet-derived growth factor (PDGF) attracts polymorphs and mononuclear cells to the area of injury and affects their replication in the repair process. Later in the repair process, PDGF attracts fibroblasts to the repair site. The macrophage plays an essential role in attracting and stimulating fibroblast activity with the secretion of fibroblast growth factors. This phase of wound healing is evident clinically by the cardinal signs of inflammation—redness (rubor), heat (calor), pain (dolor), and loss of function (functio laesa).

Fibroplasia. Within 72 hours, with the elimination of devitalized tissue and foreign bodies, the wound progresses to the fibroplastic or proliferative stage of healing. Collagen and ground substances are laid down by fibroblasts. The tensile strength of the wound increases, reaching its maximum by the 21st day as collagen cross-linking progresses.

Epithelialization. Within 48 hours, a layer of fine epithelium covers a sutured clean wound as a result of the mitotic activity of the epidermal basal cells, followed by a sheetlike migration of the epithelium along the wound edges and across the incision. Contact inhibition of growth occurs as soon as the expanding epithelium comes in contact with other epithelial cells. As the wound matures, the epithelium thickens but never develops the rete pegs or other components of normal epithelium.

Granulation. An open wound fills with clot, with the development of a fibrin network. Phagocytes and monocytes proceed with their local débridement while capillary buds and fibroblasts proliferate into the clot. The capillary buds secrete lytic enzymes that fragment the fibrin. Vascular arcades develop after canalization of the capillary buds, with provision of nutrients, oxygen, and phagocytic cells for the removal of dead tissue and clot. Proliferating fibroblasts accompany the vessels and deposit collagen so that within 6 days healthy pink granulation tissue is present. Cross-linking of collagen and atrophy of blood vessels result in healing of the wound by an epithelialized white scar.

Contraction. Contraction of a wound appears to be mediated by the myofibroblast, which is a fibroblast with many characteristics of a smooth muscle cell. These cells have features that suggest a specialization for contractility and are found in granulation tissue and tendons. They have also been identified in breast capsules and in abnormal palmar and plantar tissues in patients with Dupuytren's contracture.

Maturation. Maturation or the remodeling phase of wound healing begins late in the proliferative phase and continues for 1 to 2 years or longer in children. During this stage an equilibrium in collagen deposition and degradation occurs as collagen bundles are remodeled and reoriented.

Impairment of Wound Healing

GENERAL FACTORS

1. Nutrition
   A. Ascorbic acid (vitamin C) deficiency impairs collagen secretion by fibroblasts through impaired hydroxylation of proline and lysine.

B. Protein deficiency in the form of hypoalbuminemia leads to edema of wounds as well as deficiency of essential amino acids.
C. Zinc is an important enzyme component, and deficiency may detrimentally affect healing after trauma or burns.
2. Systemic disease: Diabetes mellitus and anemia deter healing by compromise of tissue oxygenation.
3. Steroids: Suppression of the inflammatory response and collagen lysis may impair healing during the early days after injury. The inhibiting effects of corticosteroids can be reversed with oral vitamin A.
4. Sepsis: Systemic sepsis retards the healing process.
5. Cytotoxic drugs: 5-fluorouracil, methotrexate, and cyclophosphamide impair wound healing by suppression of collagen synthesis and fibroblast replication.

LOCAL FACTORS

1. Blood suppply: Well-vascularized, well-oxygenated areas heal well. Patients with local vessel disease attributable to atherosclerosis or diabetic arteriopathy heal poorly. Impaired vascularity due to post-irradiation fibrosis impairs healing.

2. Hematoma or seroma in a wound separates the wound edges and impairs healing.

3. Sepsis and retained foreign body, which perpetuates the local inflammatory reaction, retard the healing process.

4. Miscellaneous conditions: Underlying malignancy or granulomatous disease, such as tuberculosis, luetic disease, and mycoses, impairs healing.

Disorders of Collagen Synthesis and Maturation

1. *Impedance to Molecular Cross-Linkage*
   A. Lathyrism: Animals eating sweet-pea seeds develop loss of tissue tensile strength, with vascular aneurysms and skeletal deformities. Certain drugs such as β-aminoproprionitrite induce lathyrism by inhibiting enzymes mediating intramolecular and intermolecular cross-linking of collagen.
   B. Penicillamine: This drug blocks molecular cross-linkage by reacting with aldehyde groups.
2. *Clinical Syndromes Associated With Collagen Disorders*
   A. Ehlers-Danlos syndrome: This is a genetically determined disorder in which abnormal collagen maturation and tissue fragility cause hyperextensibility and laxity of skin and ligamentous tissues. Purpura may cause hemorrhage after surgical procedures. Delayed and prolonged healing leads to the development of darkly pigmented or hypertrophic telangiectatic scars. Aortic defects and aortic dissection may occur.
   B. Pseudoxanthoma elasticum: This condition is the result of variable inheritance patterns. It is characterized by skin of "plucked chicken" appearance due to degeneration of elastic fibers and premature skin laxity. Peripheral arterial and coronary artery insuffïciency is often present.
   C. Cutis laxa: Marked gravitational skin laxity is attributable to a decrease in number or size of dermal elastin fibers. Associated abnormalities include pulmonary disease, heart disease, and aneurysms of the great vessels.

D. Progeria: This inherited autosomal recessive disorder is characterized by a facial appearance of premature aging. Growth retardation, atherosclerotic cardiovascular disease, and a shortened life span are constant features.

E. Werner syndrome: Owing to autosomal recessive inheritance, this rare condition is characterized by skin changes similar to those of scleroderma and associated microangiopathy.

F. Marfan syndrome: Arachnodactyly, subluxation of the ocular lens, and aortic medial defect are usually associated with laxity of ligaments, hypermobility of joints, and scoliosis.

Aging of Skin

Flattening of the dermal-epidermal junction, diminution in the amount of collagen, loss of elastic fibers, and a decrease in the cellular components such as melanocytes and Langhans cells occur with age. These microscopic changes are reflected clinically by thinning and atrophy of the skin, decreased elasticity, greater vulnerability to shearing forces and ultraviolet light, and increased susceptibility to cutaneous malignancy. As the degree of skin atrophy progresses, it becomes lax, so that gravity causes the skin to hang from sites of firm, deep attachments. The associated atrophy of the underlying musculoaponeurotic and osseous structures aggravates the sagging of the cutaneous layer.

Keloid and Hypertrophic Scar

Pigmented races such as Africans and Asians are more likely than whites to develop keloids. An abnormal scar results from either the production of defective collagen or an abnormal deposition and degradation of collagen. The ear lobe, shoulder, sternum, and back are areas especially prone to develop hypertrophic scars or keloids. Hypertrophic scar is characterized by excessive scar tissue within the confines of the original wound or scar, whereas a keloid is scar tissue that invades adjacent previously uninvolved tissues (Fig. 1–3). Keloid and hypertrophic scars are characterized by disorganization of collagen bundles and whorls of collagen instead of discrete bundle formation. Excessive amounts of fibronectin are found in hypertrophic and keloid scars. Microvascular occlusion by endothelial hyperplasia and corresponding hypoxia may be a significant factor in the pathogenesis of these lesions. A profusion of perivascular myofibroblasts may also play a role in the vascular occlusion process.

The intralesional injection of corticosteroids combined with pressure dressings reduces hypertrophic scars by inhibiting inflammatory fibroplasia and increasing collagenolytic activity. Triamcinolone, 10 mg/mL, is infiltrated into the lesion with a 25- or 27-gauge needle. A treatment course of three or four injections 3 to 4 weeks apart is usually required. Care must be taken not to infiltrate surrounding tissues because of the risk of subcutaneous tissue atrophy and hypopigmentation. Cortisone injections result in a widening of the scar as it flattens. It also induces telangiectasia, which can be treated later with the tunable dye laser. The clinical use of β-aminoproprionitrite and colchicine has been of minimal benefit. Radiation therapy is helpful in controlling keloid formation: 500 to 600 rads delivered in two or three divided doses within several days of excision.

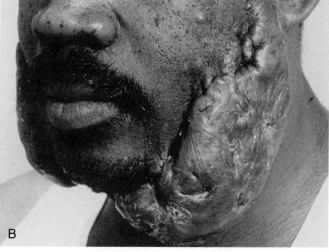

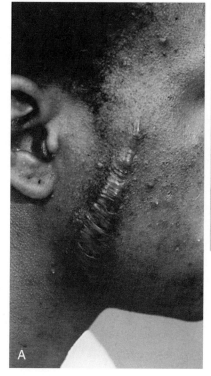

FIGURE 1–3. *A*, Hypertrophic scar results from an overabundance of collagen within the confines of the original wound. *B*, A keloid results from an overabundance of collagen extending from the original wound into adjacent skin and subcutaneous tissue.

Wound Care

Primary Closure. A wound may be defined as traumatized if the wound edges have been appreciably damaged and as nontraumatized if it is a cleanly incised wound. Within the first 6 hours of wounding, the lesion may be considered contaminated; after 6 to 8 hours, the wound must be considered potentially infected. After the wound is gently débrided and cleansed with saline irrigation, any visible foreign material should be removed. If the wound is contaminated with debris, pulsatile saline irrigation can be done with a mechanical pump. The wound margins should be carefully excised without causing functional or cosmetic deformity. Adequate hemostasis is accomplished by clamp and ligature or electrocautery. The wound margins are handled carefully with skin hooks or fine-toothed forceps. Absorbable suture material should be used for ligature and for subcutaneous suture. Polyglycolic acid sutures (e.g., Dexon [Davis & Geck, Manuti, Puerto Rico] or Vicryl [Ethicon Inc, Somerville, NJ]) are preferable to catgut, which causes a greater inflammatory reaction. The wound margins should be apposed without tension. Reduction of tension may be achieved by wound undermining and precise approximation of the wound edges by subcuticular sutures that evert the skin edges.

Skin Sutures. The quality of skin healing is determined not only by the tension across a suture line but by avoiding shearing stress across the healing dermis. Eversion of the skin edges is necessary for good healing, and sutures should not be tied tightly to avoid strangulation of the wound edges. Sutures are removed early, facilitated by a secure dermal closure with absorbable suture. Steri-Strips (3M, St. Paul, MN) are used to maintain skin apposition after removal of skin sutures. As a general rule, facial sutures are removed in 4 to 5 days, scalp sutures in 7 to 10 days, and trunk and extremity sutures in 10 to 14 days.

Choice of Skin Sutures. Although skin sutures are a matter of personal preference, each type of material has its advantages and disadvantages. Suture material may be made from naturally occurring substances (silk, cotton, catgut, and stainless steel) or may be synthetic (Dacron, nylon, and polypropylene). They may be absorbable (catgut, polyglycolic acid, and polydioxanone (PDS) or nonabsorbable (nylon, Dacron, polypropylene, silk, cotton, and stainless steel). Sutures may be nonfilamentous or have multiple filaments that are braided or twisted. Ideal skin sutures are monofilament nylon or prolene on a curved needle with an atraumatic cutting edge. The suture material is swaged into the haft.

SUTURE TECHNIQUES

Subcutaneous sutures should be placed so as to eliminate any dead space, to reduce tension across the wound margin prior to inserting the skin sutures, and to approximate and evert the wound margins. Dermal sutures are placed so that the knot, when tied, lies in the depths of the wound rather than against the superficial dermis and epidermis (Fig. 1–4).

Skin sutures are of several types:

1. Interrupted: A simple series of loop sutures knotted on one side of the wound is used to approximate the skin edges with absolute alignment and no overlapping of margins. The suture should include the whole dermis, and the needle should take an equal bite on each side (Fig. 1–5).

2. Vertical mattress suture: This is used to ensure eversion of the skin edges (Fig. 1–6).

3. Horizontal mattress suture: Although it provides close approximation and eversion of the skin edges, it may cause some skin ischemia (Fig. 1–7).

4. Subcuticular (intradermal) continuous suture: This is a good method of skin closure. Use of a polypropylene suture is preferred for easy removal. This technique avoids the risk of any skin suture marks (Fig. 1–8).

5. Continuous over-and-over suture: Rapidly performed and hemostatic, it

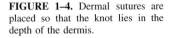
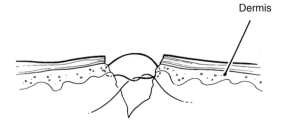

FIGURE 1–4. Dermal sutures are placed so that the knot lies in the depth of the dermis.

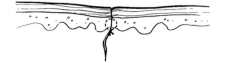

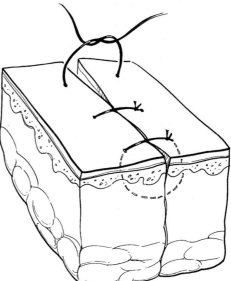

FIGURE 1–5. Simple interrupted skin suture.

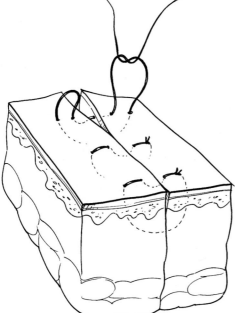

FIGURE 1–6. Vertical mattress suture.

FIGURE 1–7. Horizontal mattress suture.

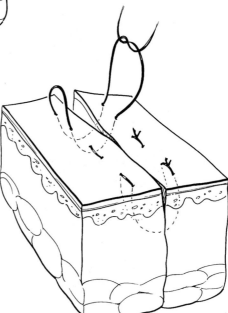

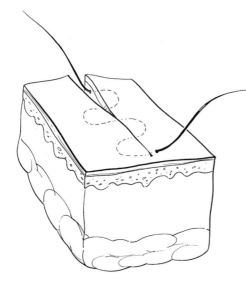

FIGURE 1–8. Running subcuticular suture.

has the disadvantage of leaving suture marks and is thus not used in visible areas (Fig. 1–9).

6. Skin staples and skin clips: Closure of skin is quick and time-saving. Early removal is essential in visible areas to avoid permanent staple marks on the skin.

7. Tissue adhesive: Methyl-2-cyanoacrylate and isobutyl-2-cyanoacrylate are capable of acting as tissue adhesives.

Delayed Primary Closure. Wounds with high bacterial contamination, crushing injuries, and serious risk of infection are best treated by early débridement and left open and dressed for 4 to 5 days with appropriate antibiotic coverage. After this lapse of time, granulation tissue is well formed and the wound is amenable to secondary suture or skin grafting.

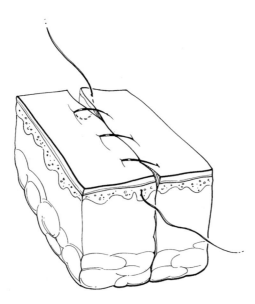

FIGURE 1–9. Running simple suture.

EXCISION OF LESIONS

Preparation. Shaving hair is usually unnecessary and always avoided in aesthetically important areas such as eyebrows, hairline, and moustache. The skin is prepared with an antiseptic such as povidone-iodine or Hibiclens (Stuart Pharmaceutical, Wilmington, DE). Skin incisions are planned and marked with methylene blue. Ideally the final scar lies in a skin crease or wrinkle or parallel to the lines of relaxed tension (Fig. 1–10).

Anesthesia. Anesthesia is achieved with infiltration of a local anesthetic, using a 27- or 30-gauge needle. Lidocaine, 0.5 to 1.0 per cent, provides 1 to 1.5 hours of anesthesia, whereas bupivacaine (Marcaine), 0.5 to 1.0 per cent, provides 6 to 8 hours of anesthesia and aids in postoperative comfort. A mixture that includes epinephrine in concentrations of 1:400,000 to 1:100,000 is used for local hemostasis. Five minutes is allowed to achieve hemostasis and is evident by blanching of the infiltrated skin. Sodium bicarbonate, 8.4 per cent, added to the local anesthetic (1 part sodium bicarbonate to 10 parts anesthetic) minimizes the burning sensation on infiltration. The application of topical EMLA cream (2.5 per cent lidocaine and 2.5 per cent prilocaine in a fatty acid ester [Astra Pharmaceutical, Westborough, MA]) 40 minutes prior to injection minimizes the needle stick.

Excision. The skin is incised perpendicular to its surface, and the incision carried down the appropriate layer. The lesion is excised either circumferentially or elliptically. Circular excision minimizes the amount of tissue excised and allows tension lines to orient the axis of closure. Redundant tissue (dog ears) is removed as needed.

An elliptical excision must be carefully oriented preoperatively so that the final scar lies in the desired direction. The length of an elliptical incision should be about four times the width of the lesion to neatly taper the excision and minimize dog ears.

Lesions involving free margins of the lip, nose, ear, and eyelids may be

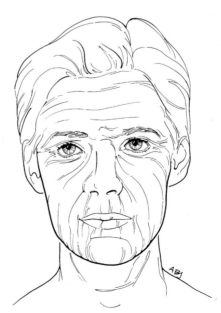

FIGURE 1–10. Lines of relaxed tension run perpendicular to the long axis of the facial muscles. These lines of expression evolve into the wrinkles of aging.

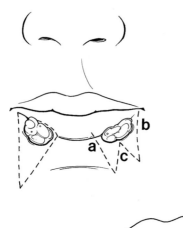

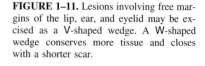

FIGURE 1–11. Lesions involving free margins of the lip, ear, and eyelid may be excised as a V-shaped wedge. A W-shaped wedge conserves more tissue and closes with a shorter scar.

excised as a wedge. A V-shaped wedge closes as a straight line, whereas a W-shaped wedge conserves more tissue and closes with a shorter scar (Fig. 1–11).

MANAGEMENT OF SCARS

Scars, whether attributable to sutured incisions or lacerations or subsequent to secondary healing of unsutured wounds, are at first raised, red, and hard owing to increased vascularity. Over the ensuing 6 to 12 months, the scar gradually becomes pale, flat, and soft. Any plans for scar revision should generally be delayed for at least 6 months and generally for 12 months. Revision surgery of a scar may be necessary as a result of limitation of function, irritation or pain, or unsightly appearance.

LIMITATION OF FUNCTION

Contraction of a scar occurs in both length and depth. A linear scar is more likely to contract if it is at right angles to Langer lines (lines of tension) or to flexure lines. The associated fixation of the skin to the underlying tissue aggravates the effects of fibrosis and contracture, especially over fingers and joints.

IRRITABLE AND PAINFUL SCARS

Pain may be due to involvement of nerves in deep scar tissue or adherence of the scar to a neuroma.

UNSIGHTLY APPEARANCE

A *hypertrophic scar* is generally confined to the scar area and is more likely to occur in children and adolescents. It is more likely to develop in a wound that has suffered prolonged infection. *Depressed scars* are usually due to loss of subcutaneous tissue. *Dirt-ingrained scars* result from road particles buried in the depths of the wound.

A single band or a wide sheet causing contracture across a flexor surface may be treated by making an incision across the contracture. It is deepened and undermined, with division of all bands of scar tissue, and the tissues in the area are opened to overcome any foreshortening. Undermined unhealthy scar tissue may require excision. The defect is then covered with a split-thickness skin graft and the joint immobilized in the corrected position for several weeks.

A linear scar with normal surrounding skin may be completely relieved by a Z-plasty. Broad contractures are best excised with incorporation of Z-plasties. Z-plasty limbs can then be transposed to reduce the defect, and the remainder of the skin defect can be grafted.

Wounds with superficial tattooing of debris should be acutely dermabraded. If particles are incorporated into the healed wound, the wound should be excised and repaired. Hypertrophic scars may respond to the application of pressure by taping or splinting over the scar. Silicone elastomer works well as a splint and may have to be maintained for 6 months or longer. Intralesional cortisone in conjunction with a pressure garment may flatten the hypertrophic scar. Scar revision in conjunction with these modalities may be necessary, although attempt at conservative management is indicated prior to surgery in most instances.

Depressed scars require either excision or preferably de-epithelialization. The adjacent skin and subcutaneous tissues are then undermined and advanced and the layers carefully approximated.

THE Z-PLASTY

The Z-plasty is a technique whereby two interdigitating triangular flaps are transposed or interchanged, one for the other. The three limbs of the design, when drawn out on the skin, are Z-shaped. The limbs of the Z should be equal in length to the central figure and extend outward at an angle of 60 degrees (Fig. 1–12).

Transposition of the Z results in gain in length along the direction of the common limb of the Z, and a change in direction of the common limb of the Z. Z-plasties may be designed in a serial fashion along the course of a wound

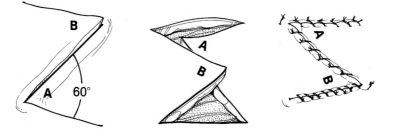

FIGURE 1–12. The Z-plasty: Two interdigitating triangular flaps are transposed, changing the direction and increasing the length of the common limb of the triangular flaps. The greater the angle of the triangle, the greater the length gained up to an angle of about 60 degrees.

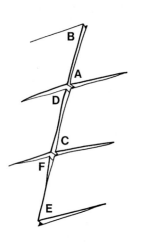

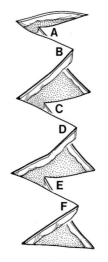

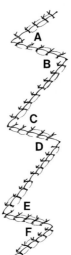

FIGURE 1–13. Multiple Z-plasties may be designed in sequence to break up scars and release contractures.

FIGURE 1–14. Four-flap Z-plasty: Two opposing flaps of about 90 degrees are each bisected into two flaps. The flaps are interposed, providing more lengthening than a single Z-plasty.

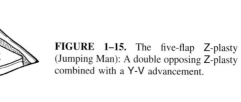

FIGURE 1–15. The five-flap Z-plasty (Jumping Man): A double opposing Z-plasty combined with a Y-V advancement.

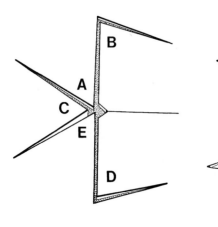

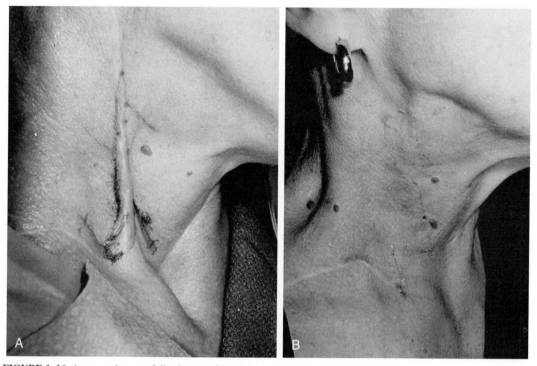

FIGURE 1–16. A contracting scar following carotid endarterectomy *(A)* is effectively released by excision of the hypertrophic scar with a closure incorporating two Z-plasties *(B)*.

(Fig. 1–13) or as multiple Z-plasties, such as the four-flap (Fig. 1–14) or five-flap (Fig. 1–15) Z-plasty.

Indications for the Z-plasty include treatment of linear contractions (Fig. 1–16) and management of facial scars: As the common limb changes direction, a series of multiple Z-plasties converts a prominent facial scar to an imperceptible one. It is particularly effective in releasing U-shaped scars with heaped-up tissue in the middle of the U; and deepening of web spaces.

THE W-PLASTY

After scar excision in which the long axis of the wound lies across the skin tension lines, small isosceles triangles 5 to 6 mm in length with apical angles of 50 to 60 degrees are cut out on each wound margin so that they interdigitate when approximated. A combination of W-plasty with several Z-plasties may be necessary in the management of complex scars. These techniques must be used very selectively and carefully. Injudicious application can lead to W- and Z-shaped scars that are more unsightly than the original scar.

Suggested Readings

Borges AF, Alexander JE: Relaxed and skin tension lines, Z-plasties on scars, and fusiform excision of lesions. Br J Plast Surg 15:242, 1962

Hunt TK, Knighton DR, Thakrol KK, et al: Studies on inflammation and wound healing. Angiogenesis and collagen synthesis stimulated in vitro by resident and activated wound macrophages. Surgery 96:148, 1984

McGregor IA: The theoretical basis of the Z-plasty. Br J Plast Surg 9:256, 1957

Peacock EE: Symposium on biological control of scar tissue. Plast Reconstr Surg 41:8, 1968

Peacock EE, Madden JW, Trier WC: Biologic basis for the treatment of keloids and hypertrophic scars. South Med J 63:775, 1970

Proctor DJ, Kivirikko KI, Tuderman L, et al: The biosynthesis of collagen and its disorders. N Engl J Med 301:13, 1979

Ryan GB, Cliff WJ, Gabbiani G, et al: Myofibroblasts in human granulation tissue. Human Pathol 5:55, 1974

CHAPTER 2

Skin Lesions

BENIGN CYSTIC LESIONS

Epidermal Inclusion Cyst

These are common, painless, slow-growing keratinizing cysts that are caused by a penetrating injury, often overlooked, that embeds keratin-producing epithelium into the subcutaneous tissues. They are frequently found in the finger pulp and are firm and mobile. Complete excision is the treatment of choice.

Milia are epidermal inclusion cysts 1 to 2 mm in diameter commonly occurring on the face. They are smooth white papules and respond to unroofing.

Sebaceous Cyst

These cysts are most frequently found in the scalp and other hair-bearing areas. They may be single or multiple. The cyst is located within the skin, moving with it, and a punctum is visible over it.

Complications include infection progressing to suppuration and abscess formation, ulceration and the development of a chronic granuloma resembling a squamous epithelioma, and a sebaceous horn, which represents keratinization of a sebaceous cyst.

A sebaceous cyst can be removed by an elliptical incision around the punctum and, with careful dissection, separation of the cyst wall from the surrounding tissues and intact removal. The wound is then closed in two layers, with obliteration of the cavity. Alternatively, the cyst may be incised, its "cheesy" contents evacuated, and the lining dissected out. The contents are composed of squamous debris and not sebaceous material. "Sebaceous cyst" is therefore a misnomer; *keratinous cyst* would be a more appropriate term.

Dermoid Cyst

These develop at the sites of embryologic fusion and are generally found near the anterior and posterior fontanelles, at the root of the nose, and near the occiput and aural and temporal regions. The most common site is above the lateral aspect of the eyebrow, and the lesion is referred to as an external angular dermoid (Fig. 2–1). Although these lesions are congenital in nature, they may not appear until several years after birth. They enlarge slowly and occasionally become infected. They are free from the overlying skin but may be firmly adherent to the underlying bone. Occasionally a pedicle may connect such a dermoid through a defect in the skull to the dura. Radiographic examination of the area is essential to define the latter category. A dermoid cyst at the root of the nose may similarly have an intranasal extension, requiring that the nasal bones be split through a midline incision. The external angular dermoid is approached through an incision along the upper border of the eyebrow, leaving an inconspicuous scar.

Pathologic study of the dermoid reveals a stratified squamous epithelial lining containing hair follicles and sebaceous and sweat glands.

EPIDERMAL LESIONS

1. Seborrheic keratosis: Cauliflower-like papillary masses affecting the face, trunk, and arms of older individuals. They have a stuck-on appearance and

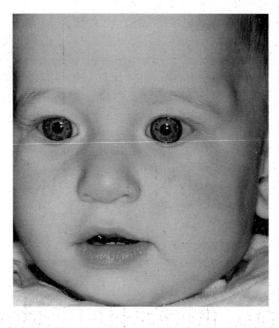

FIGURE 2–1. A dermoid cyst of the lateral brow. These cysts are composed of a squamous epithelial lining containing hair follicles and sebaceous and sweat glands. They occur at sites of embryologic fusion.

consist of basal cells and keratinous material. They are benign and are managed by shaving.

2. Keratosis follicularis (Darier disease): A hereditary keratinization leading to formation of warty masses with a distinct unpleasant odor on the face, neck, chest, axilla, and inguinal area. Vitamin A acid cream, salicylic acid in propylene gel, and isotretinoin have been palliative.

3. Keratosis palmaris et plantaris. A condition characterized by thickening of the soles and palms. Fissures may develop in the thickened skin, requiring excision and grafting.

4. Nevus verrucosus: A papillary tan keratotic plaque that may be linear or patchy. It is evident at birth or early in childhood. The dermis is involved in the development of the lesion, and removal requires full-thickness skin excision. They are benign lesions, and removal is for aesthetic considerations (Fig. 2–2).

5. Actinic (solar) keratosis: Flat discrete lesions occurring on the exposed surfaces of older people, with underlying erythema and superficial hyperkeratosis. They are noninvasive, situated above the basement membrane. Actinic keratoses are premalignant lesions and may progress to squamous cell carcinoma. They are best treated by cryotherapy, curettage, and electrodesiccation, or 5-fluorouracil (5-FU).

6. Keratoacanthoma: A benign cutaneous neoplasm occurring on exposed hairy skin. The lesion is dome-shaped with a central keratinous plug (Fig. 2–3). They grow rapidly over a 6-week period and slowly regress over 2 to 6 months. Because of the slow nature of regression and the risk of confusion with a squamous cell carcinoma, they are best excised.

BENIGN PIGMENTED SKIN LESIONS

The epidermis contains several heterogeneous cells within its several layers of keratinocytes. These include melanocytes and Langhans cells. Nerve processes extend focally into the epidermis.

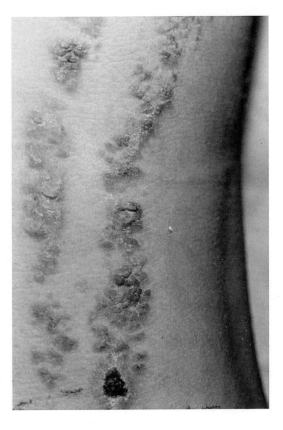

FIGURE 2–2. Nevus verrucosus: A papillary keratotic plaque involving the epidermis and dermis. Removal requires full-thickness skin excision and is done for aesthetic reasons.

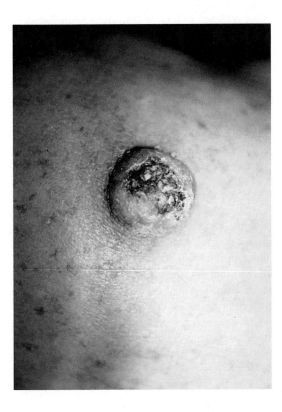

FIGURE 2–3. Keratoacanthoma: These are dome-shaped lesions with a central keratinous plug. They grow rapidly over a 6-week period and regress over 2 to 6 months. There is a risk of confusion with squamous cell carcinoma, and excision is indicated.

Pigmented nevi are benign tumors of melanocytes and/or nevus cells. Derived from migratory neuroectodermal components, these nevi are present in all individuals to a variable degree. Although they may present at birth, they usually appear during adolescence and increase in number during middle age. They are usually called a nevocellular nevus, a pigmented nevus, or colloquially a mole.

Types of pigmented nevi are as follows:

Intradermal nevus: Nevus cells are confined to the dermis. The lesion presents as a mound, often with hair growth. The pigment may disappear in later life. Although it may enlarge and become inflamed and painful because of an associated epidermoid cyst or after plucking the hairs, it does not develop malignant propensity. It may present as a pigmented patch in infancy, with a growth of long, coarse hair. Malignant transformation is unusual except in the very large congenital nevus, which is occasionally associated with the development of malignant melanoma.

Compound nevus: Delayed maturation of the nevus cells with their presence in the epidermis and the dermis results in a mole that is present from childhood and is characteristically raised and reddish brown and has a warty appearance.

Junctional nevus: This type is characterized by the accumulation and arrangement of cells at the dermal-epidermal interface. The cells become pleomorphic and may be difficult to distinguish from malignant cells on occasion. It presents as a flat brown lesion up to 1 cm in diameter.

Dysplastic nevus: This is an acquired pigmented lesion of the skin. Presenting usually in sun-exposed areas, they may be multiple, 6 mm in diameter or larger, with irregular borders and a variable mix of color. They may have a familial basis or may present sporadically without a family history. These lesions have a high propensity for developing into malignant melanoma. Careful observation of these lesions is essential, and excision should be done if any suspicious changes occur.

Giant pigmented nevus: This presents as a large congenital, pigmented, hairy, soft verrucous lesion that extends along a dermatomal distribution, usually on the head, trunk, pelvic area, and extremities. Malignant transformation, although infrequent, may develop in childhood or adolescence, especially in the highly pigmented lesions. These lesions are best managed by excision. Large lesions may require multiple serial excisions and sophisticated reconstructive techniques, including tissue expansion, flap rotation, and skin grafting (Fig. 2–4).

Lentigo maligna (the melanotic freckle of Hutchinson): This flat brown lesion most commonly occurs on the face. However, it may also present on the neck, back, or elsewhere on the body. Although the 1- to 2-cm lesion at first resembles a junctional nevus, it grows slowly but progressively to become a spreading irregular confluence of varying pigmentation until it becomes a superficial malignant melanoma. Removal of the melanotic freckle is recommended before invasive melanoma develops.

Blue nevus: This presents as a firm, well-defined blue intradermal nodule that consists of a grouping of normal dermal melanocytes.

Nevus of Ota: Predominating in females, the blue-gray lesion affects the periorbital area, cheeks, and forehead and is usually present at birth or soon after. It may resemble a melanoma, requiring excision for differentiation.

Lentigo senilis: These lesions develop in older people in areas exposed to actinic rays, such as face, neck, arms, and dorsal surfaces of the hand. The smooth dark brown patches, about 1.5 cm in diameter, consist of increased numbers of mature melanocytes.

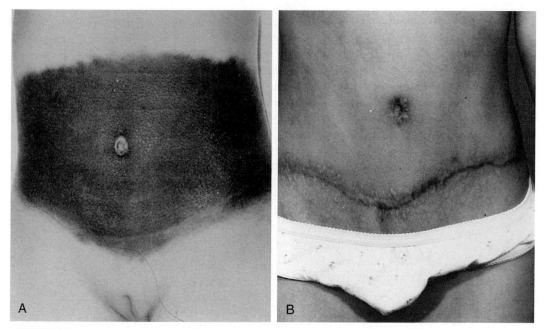

FIGURE 2–4. A giant pigmented nevus *(A)* excised by serial excision, with secondary reconstruction of the umbilicus *(B)*.

Ephelis (freckle): Brown lesions resulting from melanocytic overproduction of melanin.

TUMORS OF EPIDERMAL APPENDAGES

Epidermal appendages include hair follicles, eccrine and apocrine glands, and sebaceous glands. Tumors of the epidermal appendages differentiate toward one of these structures and are classified accordingly.

Syringoma: 2- to 3-mm multiple papules, occurring more commonly in adult women, usually located in the lower eyelids. They may also develop on the lower face, neck, and trunk. They are easily removed by cryotherapy, electrodesiccation, or laser coagulation. They are of eccrine origin.

Poroma: Benign reddish nodule, on palmar or plantar skin, in a shallow depression surrounded by a hyperkeratotic ridge. They are of eccrine origin.

Spiradenoma: A solitary, painful subcutaneous tumor of eccrine origin located on the ventral torso in young adults.

Cylindroma (turban tumor): Occurs on the scalp or forehead. They may be solitary or multiple, presenting as smooth nodules of variable size. They may be so numerous as to coalesce, giving a turban appearance. They differentiate toward an apocrine structure.

Cystadenoma: A small benign nevoid nodule that is often translucent, containing brownish fluid that gives the nodule a pigmented hue. It is usually located on the face and is of apocrine origin.

Papillary syringocystadenoma: A verrucose lesion of apocrine origin, usually located on the scalp. It may become bullous, exuding fluid. Histologically there may be foci of basal cell epithelioma, and it may be part of a nevus sebaceus.

Tricholemmoma: A benign tumor of the scalp composed of cells with nuclear palisading of hair follicle sheaths.

Trichoepithelioma: Occurs as a solitary lesion in childhood or as multiple lesions in adolescence. When multiple, it is usually an inherited condition involving the central face. It is of hair follicle origin.

Calcifying epithelioma of Malherbe (pilomatrixoma): A single, hard nodule 1 to 2 cm in size covered by normal skin. It differentiates toward hair structure, occurring in children and young adults on the face and arms. This benign lesion consists of an encapsulated mass of epidermoid cells.

Nevus sebaceus (Jadassohn tumor): A finely nodular, raised, hairless, yellowish plaque occurring in the scalp area and occasionally on the face and neck. There is risk of developing a malignant basal cell carcinoma, so removal prior to puberty is advisable (Fig. 2–5).

Senile sebaceous hyperplasia: Occurs on the face and nose as firm to soft lesions with telangiectatic rims, requiring histologic examination for differentiation.

Sebaceous adenoma: Pedunculated nodular lesion involving the scalp or face. These small lesions can be readily excised.

Rhinophyma: A severe form of acne rosaceae characterized by bulbous, red thickening of the nasal skin. Histology demonstrates sebaceous gland hyperplasia and dermal vascular proliferation. It is managed by excision and grafting, shaving to the deeper dermis using a "hot knife" or dermabrasion (Fig. 2–6).

FIBROUS LESIONS

Dermatofibroma. This presents as a hard nodule, most frequently on an extremity. It is usually less than 1 cm and a purple-brown color. It is slow growing

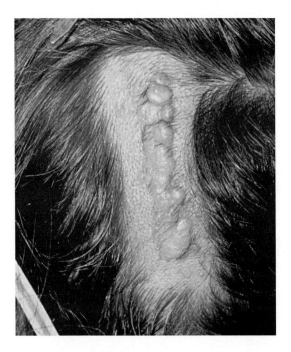

FIGURE 2–5. A nevus sebaceus (Jadassohn tumor), a nodular raised yellowish plaque usually involving the scalp or face. Excision is recommended by puberty because of risk of skin carcinoma.

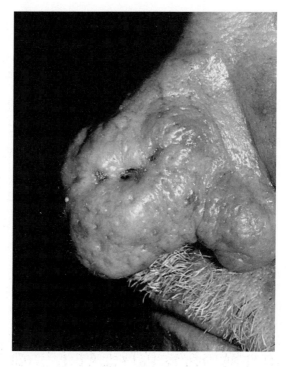

FIGURE 2–6. Rhinophyma: Sebaceous gland hyperplasia and dermal vascular proliferation of the nasal skin causes a red, thickened, bulbous nose.

and benign. Histologically it is loaded with spindle-shaped cells, with variable presence of histiocytes and fibroblasts.

Dermatofibrosarcoma protuberans. Occurring predominantly on the trunk and thighs, the slowly growing, hard, nodular mass may become complicated by ulceration and infection as well as scarring and contracture. Wide excision is essential to prevent local recurrence. Microscopic examination of the lesion reveals the characteristic "cartwheel" arrangement of the hypercellular, nonencapsulated fibrous whorls, with numerous mitoses and finger-like extensions into adjacent cutis and fascia.

LESIONS OF NEURAL ORIGIN

Neurilemoma. This is a benign neoplasm of Schwann cells which arises from the nerve sheath.

Neurofibroma. This is a benign neoplasm of Schwann cells and endoneural fibroblasts. It may be a solitary lesion or multiple, as part of von Recklinghausen disease. This hereditary condition is characterized by multiple neurofibroblasts, café-au-lait spots, and axillary pigmentation. Sarcomatous degeneration yields a highly aggressive spindle-cell neoplasm.

VASCULAR LESIONS

Vascular lesions result from either cellular proliferation of vascular elements (hemangioma) or structural anomalies of blood vessels with abnormal hemodynamics (vascular malformations).

Hemangioma

Hemangiomas are the most common vascular lesions. They occur in 4 to 5 of every 100 live births and are present at birth or within the first weeks of life. They evolve by a combination of endothelial proliferation and development of circulation.

The *strawberry hemangioma* begins as a small spot or blemish at birth. It rapidly enlarges to become a raised, red vascular tumor composed of thick endothelium-lined capillaries with small lumina, which can be emptied by compression. Progressive fibrosis leads to spontaneous disappearance of the lesion by the age of 5 to 7 years, leaving a pale patch within an area of baggy skin (Fig. 2–7). If the subcutaneous tissues are involved, they present as a soft blue compressible mass *(cavernous hemangioma)* composed of large, thin-walled venous endothelium-lined channels. Cavernous hemangiomas are preformed and, although not always visible at birth, later canalize and rapidly fill with blood, providing the illusion of rapid enlargement. Cavernous hemangiomas may develop in any organ in the body but most commonly occur in subcutaneous tissues, with the overlying skin involved in a capillary hood, providing a mixed or capillary-cavernous hemangioma.

Spontaneous regression usually commences by 2 years of age with thrombosis of the cavernous tissue. The majority of strawberry hemangiomas require only expectant treatment unless there is a complication or failure to involute by 6 to 7 years of age.

Complications of hemangiomas are primarily the following:

Hemorrhage: Surface abrasion may cause profuse hemorrhage that is readily controlled by pressure or ligation of the bleeding site.
Infection: The lesion may develop superficial necrosis as it involutes. This requires local wound care with dressing changes and topical antibiotics. If the child is ill or there is surrounding cellulitis, systemic antibiotics may be necessary.
Involvement of adjacent structures: Hemangiomas around the lips and mouth may interfere with feeding or cause dental distortion. Expanding lesions near the eye may occlude vision. This requires immediate treatment or the eye may be permanently impaired by amblyopia. Amblyopia is a nonseeing eye resulting from the brain's inability to incorporate the eye's stimuli. It can occur

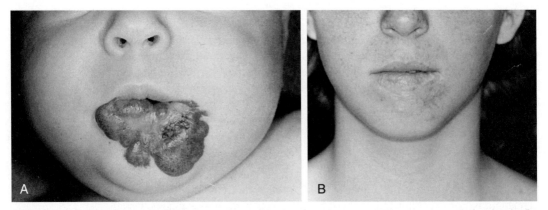

FIGURE 2–7. Capillary hemangiomas *(A)* may enlarge rapidly for 10 to 12 months and then spontaneously involute by 5 to 7 years, leaving a patch of baggy skin *(B)*.

after an eye is obstructed for as little as 6 to 7 days in children less than 1 year of age.

Kasabach-Merritt syndrome: This syndrome is seen in giant hemangiomas associated with intravascular coagulopathy caused by sequestration of platelets within the tumor.

Methods of treatment, when indicated, include pressure and systemic corticosteroids, injection of steroids or sclerosing agents to induce thrombosis, laser photocoagulation, and surgical excision with appropriate local reconstruction.

Vascular Malformation

These lesions, although present at birth, may not manifest themselves for several months. They develop by hemodynamic phenomena and may be low-flow capillary or venous malformations or high-flow arteriovenous malformations.

CAPILLARY MALFORMATION

Port Wine Stain. This congenital lesion presents at birth as a flat dark to red patch of variable extent that, in later life, may become nodular. The dilated capillaries involve the entire thickness of the skin. The use of local irradiation or systemic corticosteroids has no role in the management of these lesions. They are effectively treated with the tunable dye laser. They are not to be confused with a salmon patch, which is a pink discoloration of the skin noted over the occiput and back of the neck soon after birth. Usually 2 or 3 cm in diameter, it fades with time and requires no active treatment.

The Spider or Arachnoid Nevus. This is an acquired lesion characterized by a small central vessel surrounded by fine radiating capillaries. It may occur in crops and may fade spontaneously. Its induction by circulating estrogen causes its frequent appearance during pregnancy or in association with acquired liver disease. It is occasionally associated with telangiectases of the mucosa of the gastrointestinal tract. These lesions may be treated by injection of sclerosing agents or laser photocoagulation.

VENOUS MALFORMATION

This is a spongy lesion with a blue discoloration. It becomes more prominent with crying or the Valsalva maneuver. It is generally a benign lesion requiring management only for aesthetic purposes. Localized lesions may be resectable, although they commonly involve local vital structures. Sclerotherapy with appropriate agents may be effective.

ARTERIAL MALFORMATION

This is an unstable high-flow lesion. It may expand slowly or at an alarmingly rapid rate de novo or after trauma, change in hormonal status, or previous incomplete excision. Resection of a large arteriovenous malformation should be preceded by selective embolization of feeding vessels.

Vascular Malformation Syndromes

Sturge-Weber syndrome: Port wine stain in the distribution of the trigeminal nerve with vascular malformation of the leptomeninges. These patients usually have seizure disorders.

Klippel-Trenaunay syndrome: Port wine stain with underlying lymphatic and venous malformations. There is often gross skeletal hypertrophy.

Rendu-Osler-Weber syndrome: Malformed ectatic vessels in skin, viscera, and mucous membranes. Hemorrhage is often a presenting symptom.

Von Hippel–Lindau syndrome: Vascular tumors involve the cerebellum and retina.

Maffucci syndrome: Vascular malformations with skeletal deformities, enchondromas, and visceral vascular malformations. Patients may develop chondrosarcomas.

LYMPHATIC MALFORMATIONS

Lymphangiomas are thin-walled lymph spaces that infiltrate and become adherent to surrounding structures. They result from congenital malformation of the lymphatic vessels and present as tumors in infancy. The lesions enlarge as the child grows and are prone to rapid enlargement concomitant with injection.

Capillary lymphangioma consists of a mass of capillary-sized lymphatic channels. Superficial lesions, especially those involving mucous membranes, may be controlled by photocoagulation.

Cavernous lymphangioma is a mass consisting of dilated lymphatic vessels.

Cystic lymphangioma (cystic hygroma) consists of endothelium-lined cysts. The lesion may occur anywhere in the body but is most commonly found in the neck or axilla. Cervical cystic hygromas may become large and cause symptoms by compressing adjacent structures. Surgical excision with preservation of adjacent vital structures is recommended by 3 years of age to minimize iatrogenic injury.

MALIGNANT VASCULAR TUMORS

Angiosarcoma. This is a malignant tumor of endothelial cells affecting the myocardium in children and the head and neck of elderly people. It occasionally occurs elsewhere and must be excised if possible. It is a highly malignant lesion with early hematogenous spread.

Lymphangiosarcoma. An uncommon lesion, it was often seen as a complication of lymphedema in the ipsilateral arm after radical mastectomy.

Kaposi Sarcoma. A clinicopathologic subtype of the malignant vascular tumor. There are two major types: (1) A slowly progressive disease of middle-aged or older men affecting the lower limbs. The nodular lesions, composed of vascular and spindle components, enlarge and coalesce. They progress slowly but over a decade disseminate to regional lymph nodes and internal organs. Radiation therapy to the peripheral lesions is the treatment of choice. (2) Acquired immune deficiency syndrome (AIDS): Patients with overt AIDS present with either an opportunistic infection or Kaposi sarcoma. The disease progresses rapidly, with metastases and death within 2 years.

MISCELLANEOUS LESIONS

Xanthomas are characterized by focal accumulations of lipid-laden histiocytes and giant cells and foamy cytoplasm. *Xanthelasma palpebrarum* are elongated, slightly raised plaques near the inner canthus of the eyelids. They are clues to the possible association of hyperlipoproteinemia and atherosclerotic cardiovascular disease. *Xanthoma planum* is characterized by more extensive involvement of neck, axillae, palmar creases, and other parts of the body. Disseminated xanthelasma may be associated with Hand-Schüller-Christian disease or liver disease. Cosmetic treatment of isolated foci may consist of excision, electrodesiccation, or topical application of trichloracetic acid.

Granular cell myoblastoma is a hard, usually solitary, flesh-colored nodular tumor that may undergo ulceration and most commonly affects the tongue. It may also affect internal organs. Growing slowly, the lesion is composed of non–lipid-containing cells with a granular cytoplasm. Wide excision is necessary to prevent local recurrence.

Pyogenic granuloma is a red polypoid growth, usually on the extremities or face. The cause is unclear, but histologically these lesions are similar to a proliferating hemangioma. They are treated by excision.

Glomus tumor is a benign vascular lesion derived from normal arteriovenous communications. It most commonly presents subungually on the hands and feet. The associated throbbing pain is relieved by excision of the tumor.

Hair follicle nevus occurs on the face or scalp as a small papule with a central pore that carries wispy hairs.

Epithelioma adenoides cysticum is a benign lesion of the face and scalp. It develops as an inherited disorder in young females at or soon after puberty. The papular lesion consists of keratotic basal cells.

MISCELLANEOUS INFECTIOUS CONDITIONS

Hydradenitis Suppurativa. Chronic suppuration of the apocrine glands of the axilla and genitoanal area presents with red, tender, nodular areas that lead to the development of abscesses with discharging sinuses. The lesions remain superficial to the deep fascia. The acute stages are generally well controlled by systemic and topical antibiotic therapy, but the persistence of chronic discharging sinuses is best treated surgically. The affected tissue is excised down to the deep fascia. Primary suture repair is usually possible in the axilla, but in the groin and perianal area a thin split-thickness skin graft needs to be applied. Alternatively, the area is allowed to close by contraction and epithelialization, with whirlpool and frequent dressing changes.

Pilonidal Sinus. This is a hair-bearing sinus or abscess occurring predominantly in young male adults and is situated in the upper part of the anal cleft, overlying the sacrococcygeal area. It may cause a persistent discharge at the base of the spine, associated with recurrent episodes of pain and tenderness as the sinus orifice becomes blocked, causing the formation of an abscess. At one time thought to be congenital, it is now considered to be acquired as a result of sitting for long periods, which causes implantation of hairs into and under the skin in this area. The condition is best treated by total excision of the main and any associated tracts. The residual defect is obliterated by deep sutures, with primary suture of the skin. If the lesion is severely contaminated, the residual cavity may be marsupialized and permitted to granulate from the base, healing taking about 6 weeks to occur.

MALIGNANT TUMORS OF THE SKIN

The common varieties of dermal malignancy are basal cell carcinoma, squamous cell carcinoma, and malignant melanoma.

Although topical 5-FU may have a limited role in the treatment of dermal malignancy, surgery, radiation therapy, or a combination of the two remains the cornerstone of optional therapy. To ensure surgical cure of a malignant lesion, the excision should be carried beyond the limits of the tumor, with confirmation by pathologic examination that all tumor has been removed. With cure of the disease assured, repair or reconstruction of the residual structural defect should, ideally, be done at the same operation.

Prevention of skin cancer requires prompt attention to the following areas:

Solar (actinic) keratoses: The sun-damaged skin may demonstrate focal areas of scaling, crusting, or ulceration. These lesions are controlled with freezing. The development of subjacent induration suggests the development of an early squamous cell carcinoma that requires excision.

Bowen disease (intraepidermal carcinoma): A red scaly patch with a slightly raised edge and associated induration of the epidermis usually presents on the trunk or limbs. When such a lesion develops on the penis, it is defined as erythroplasia of Queyrat. The lesion is slowly growing, noninvasive, and nonmetastasizing. It may progress to become an invasive squamous cell carcinoma if left untreated.

Xeroderma pigmentosum: This is an inherited hypersensitivity to actinic rays in which areas of keratosis and spotty pigmentation affect exposed surfaces of the body. The development of premalignant areas heralds the need for treatment with topical 5-FU, dermabrasion, or excision before one of the three major forms of dermal cancer develops.

Cutaneous T-cell lymphoma (mycosis fungoides): This cutaneous form of lymphoma causes the development of dermal plaques, nodules, ulcers, and pruritic erythematous scaly patches. Appropriate histologic diagnosis requires systemic drug therapy for lymphoma by an oncologist.

Basal Cell Carcinoma

Basal cell carcinoma is the most common malignant tumor of the skin, occurring most often on the head and neck. Its occurrence is directly related to sun exposure, arising from the basal layer of skin epithelium or from the external root sheath of the hair follicle. Less common causes include x-irradiation exposure, human papillomavirus infection, and immunosuppression in transplant and immunocompromised patients. It is a locally aggressive tumor that rarely metastasizes. It usually presents on the face and head, commencing as a pearly gray papule with a telangiectatic rim or an indurated plaque or nodule that ulcerates. The ulcer may scale over many times, with extension of the ulcerative process. These lesions are common on the eyelid and inner canthus, where a high concentration of pilosebaceous follicles exists.

CLINICAL VARIETIES

Nodular ulcerative type: This, the most common variety, usually involves the face. Commencing as a firm papule with telangiectasia, it grows slowly before ulceration extends to cause much tissue destruction (rodent ulcer) (Fig. 2–8).

Superficial basal cell types: Frequently multiple, these lesions are usually found on the trunk, presenting as lightly pigmented, erythematous patches.

Morphea-like basal cell carcinoma: A sclerosing yellow-white patch with ill-defined borders. These tumors consist of small nests of tumor cells with a dense sclerotic stroma (Fig. 2–9).

Pigmented variety: Similar to the nodular ulcerative type, the lesions demonstrate deep brownish black pigmentation.

Basal cell nevus syndrome (Gorlin syndrome): This is a rare, autosomal dominant disorder characterized by the development of numerous basal cell lesions in childhood. Associated other anomalies of bone, skin, eyes, and nervous and reproductive systems include skin pits of palms and soles, cysts of the jaw, splayed or bifid ribs, ectopic dural calcification, and mental retardation. The lesions remain quiescent until after puberty, when malignant transformation develops.

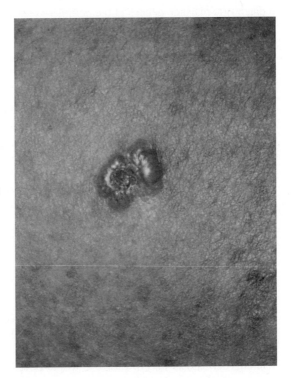

FIGURE 2–8. A nodular basal cell carcinoma.

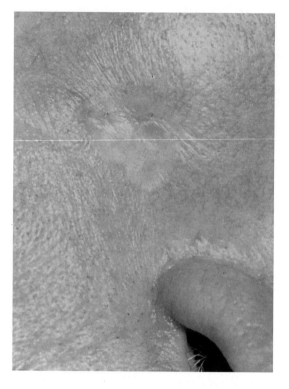

FIGURE 2–9. A morphea basal cell carcinoma presenting as a sclerosing patch with ill-defined borders.

HISTOLOGIC IDENTIFICATION

The lesion demonstrates tumor cells arranged to form nests, cords, and islands within the dermis. The small cells resemble the normal epidermal basal cells with a diagnostic palisade pattern at the periphery of the nests. Mitotic figures are rarely present. A mass of fibrovascular mucinous tissue surrounds the tumor nests.

TREATMENT

In several areas on the face, growth may penetrate deeply with minimal external evidence: the inner canthus of the eye, with growth spreading along the medial orbital wall with early involvement of the ethmoid cells, and at the alar base, where spread occurs along the nasal wall. An infiltrating basal cell carcinoma of the ear rim rapidly involves the underlying cartilage. Basal cell carcinomas are best managed by surgical excision with a conservative margin guided by histologic control.

Squamous Cell Carcinoma

Squamous cell carcinoma tends to occur in older patients exposed to solar radiation. It may develop at sites of chronic inflammation, such as chronic osteomyelitis, long-standing discharging sinuses, radiation or thermal injury, and exposure to organic hydrocarbons, tobacco, and betel. Immunosuppressive drugs and long-standing dermatosis may predispose to the development of this rapidly growing neoplasm that has the capacity to spread by direct infiltration and to metastasize by lymphatic and hematogenous routes.

The lesion presents as a sharply defined plaque or as a single painless, firm, red nodule with keratotic scales. The development of a shallow ulcer with rolled everted edges is typical of the condition (Fig. 2–10).

Histologic examination of a biopsy specimen reveals atypical squamous cells that are well differentiated with the development of epithelial pearls—concentric layers of squamous cells with central keratinization. Dermal lymphocytic and plasma cell infiltrations are also found beneath the tumor.

Regional lymph nodes may be involved and clinically palpable. Treatment requires a two-fold strategy. The primary lesion can be successfully treated by excisional surgery or radiation therapy in selected cases. Lymph node involvement is best treated surgically by block dissection. In the absence of lymph node involvement, the area should be kept under regular observation.

MOHS EXCISION

Recurrent skin cancers, skin cancers in anatomically sensitive areas such as the nasal tip and medial canthus, and sclerosing cancers may require excision by Mohs technique. The lesion is excised, and frozen sections of the tangentially sectioned deep margins are read by the surgeon. Positive areas are identified and excised, and tangential deep margins are re-evaluated until the area is clear of all microscopic tumor (Fig. 2–11). Mohs technique provides the highest rate of cure, maximal preservation of uninvolved tissue, and the advantage of immediate reconstruction.

MERKEL CELL TUMOR

This presents as a single epidermal, dermal, or subcutaneous nodule that grows aggressively and metastasizes to lymph nodes, viscera, and bones. The

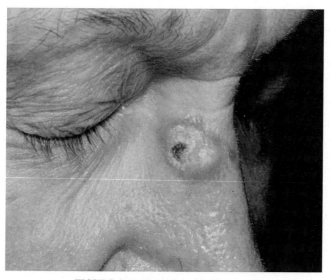

FIGURE 2–10. Squamous cell carcinoma.

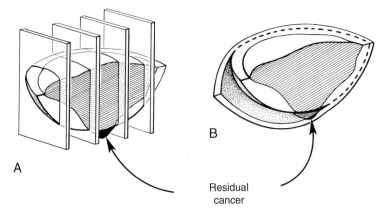

Residual
cancer

FIGURE 2–11. *A,* In a standard frozen histologic specimen, the specimen is sectioned vertically, which risks missing a small focus of cancer between the vertical sections. *B,* In the Mohs technique, the deep margin is sectioned tangentially. Foci of cancer in the tangential section are mapped, the corresponding areas in the resection wound are re-excised, and deep margins are again evaluated by tangential section. This process is repeated until the area is cleared of all microscopic tumor.

tumor cells arise from neuroendocrine cells of neural crest origin and contain granules similar to the neurosecretory granules of the epidermal Merkel cells. Microscopy reveals the basophilic cells to be arranged in a rosette pattern, with an irregularly arranged trabecular pattern.

Malignant Melanoma

Melanoma is a malignant tumor of the pigment cells of the skin. It is particularly common in fair-skinned individuals who are exposed to equatorial sunlight but is increasing in many parts of the world. Although uncommon in blacks, it may occur in blacks in the subungual and plantar aspects of the hands and feet.

A genetic predisposition is suggested by the occurrence of multiple melanomas within members of a family. It is unusual for the condition to affect children before puberty.

Although the primary growth may remain small, rapid spread to lymph nodes and widespread hematogenous dissemination may occur at an early stage.

Although most melanomas arise de novo, some may commence with malignant change in a junctional nevus that persists after puberty. Repeated trauma of such lesions may predispose them to malignant transformation. All cellular nevi exposed to frictional trauma should thus be excised prophylactically.

Suspicious changes in a pigmented lesion should be assumed to be a harbinger of malignant change: alteration in physical character, irritation or pruritus, increase in size, increase in pigmentation or spread of pigment beyond the margin of the lesion, and bleeding and scab formation.

VARIETIES OF MELANOMA

Lentigo malignant melanoma: Occurring on sun-exposed surfaces, this variety accounts for half of the head and neck melanomas. It is the least aggressive melanoma, arising in a pre-existing lentigo maligna (Hutchinson's freckle).

Superficial spreading melanoma: This variety constitutes more than 60 per cent of melanomas in Caucasians and this is the most common variety. It tends to occur on the trunk of males and the back of women's legs, although any body

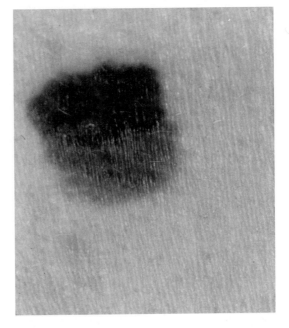

FIGURE 2–12. A superficial spreading melanoma presenting as a flat, irregularly pigmented lesion with irregular borders.

surface may be involved. The melanoma presents as a slightly raised or flat, irregularly pigmented lesion (Fig. 2–12). As vertical growth commences, a prominent nodularity with surface ulceration develops. Histologic examination of the lesion shows proliferation of uniformly atypical melanocytes singly and in nests throughout the epidermis. Extension of these cells into the papillary layer of the dermis may occur.

Nodular melanoma: Occurring at any age, this lesion invades the dermis rapidly and aggressively, predominantly affecting the head, neck, and trunk. Histologic examination reveals the dermal penetration, and the epidermal melanocytes extend radially from the site of invasion through rete ridges (Fig. 2–13).

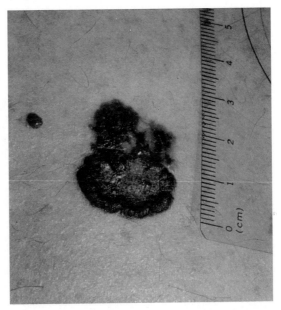

FIGURE 2–13. A raised nodular melanoma with irregular pigment and border.

Acral lentiginous melanoma: Representing less than 2 per cent of cases among Caucasians, this type is found in about 50 per cent of cases among blacks, Asians, and Hispanics. It occurs on the palms, soles, mucous membranes (e.g., lip), or mucocutaneous junctions (e.g., anus). An aggressive tumor, it metastasizes rapidly. Histologically the large, atypical melanocytes develop within a thickened epidermis and spread radially along the dermoepidermoid junction.

If there is any suspicion that a lesion is a melanoma, removal is accomplished as an excisional biopsy.

PROGNOSIS

In the absence of lymph node involvement or hematogenous dissemination, prognosis is determined by the histologic extent of invasion.

Clark Levels of Invasion (Fig. 2–14)

Level 1: Intra-epidermal: Cells superficial to the basement membrane.
Level 2: Papillary dermal: Cells extend through the basement membrane to papillary dermis.
Level 3: Papillary reticular interface: Cells begin to accumulate at the interface between papillary and reticular dermis.
Level 4: Reticular dermal: Cells extend between bundles of reticular dermis collagen.
Level 5: Invasion of subcutaneous tissue.

The superficial spreading melanoma is usually composed of levels 1 and 2. The nodular invasive type is usually level 3 to 5. Associated ulceration is indicative of poor prognosis. The more deeply penetrating lesions have a greater prospect of regional lymph node metastases and a poorer prognosis.

Five-year survival by Clark level of invasion has been found to be level 3, 70 per cent; level 4, 55 per cent; and level 5, 20 per cent.

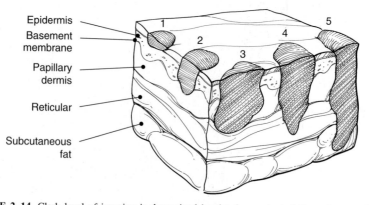

FIGURE 2–14. Clark level of invasion is determined by the deep extent of the melanoma. Level 1 involves growth superficial to the basement membrane. Level 2 involves extension of tumor through the basement membrane into the papillary dermis. Level 3 involves growth to the interface between the papillary and reticular dermis. Level 4 involves extension into the reticular dermis. Level 5 reflects invasion into the subcutaneous tissues.

Breslow's Classification

An oculomicrometer is used to measure the thickness of the melanoma on the histologic slide. The depth of penetration correlates well with the overall survival.

1. Melanoma less than 0.75 mm thick: Good prognosis
2. Melanoma penetrating 0.76 to 1.5 mm: Increasing metastatic potential
3. Melanoma greater than 1.5 mm thick: Highest incidence of regional lymph node involvement and poorest overall survival

Regional lymph node status relative to 5-year survival has been found to be (1) no regional lymph node metastases—75 per cent, and (2) four or more nodes involved—25 per cent or less.

MANAGEMENT

Careful examination of the lesion, including biopsy and scrutinization for regional lymph node involvement, is essential. Search for a second primary is important.

Melanomas of the head and neck metastasize to parotid and cervical lymph nodes. Lesions of the upper extremity spread to axillary nodes and those of the lower extremity to the superficial and deep inguinal nodes. Trunk melanomas may spread to the ipsilateral axillary and/or inguinal nodes, and if the lesion is in the midline it may spread bilaterally to nodal areas. Lymph node enlargement may present after previous excision of a pigmented lesion with no evidence of residual melanoma under the well-healed scar.

Chest radiography, complete blood count, and liver function studies are carried out routinely, and urinalysis for melanois is done in disseminated melanomatous disease. In selected patients with regional lymph node involvement, liver and brain scans may be appropriate.

TREATMENT

Surgical Excision. Once a histologic diagnosis of melanoma has been made, a wide local excision is accomplished so that no residual melanoma cells are left, thereby providing assurance that local recurrence is unlikely. For tumors less than 1 mm thick, a resection margin of 1 cm from the lesion suffices. If the thickness is more than 1 mm or invasiveness is beyond level 2, a margin of 2.5 to 3 cm is recommended.

Because deep fascia acts as a barrier to continued lymphatic spread, excision of deep fascia is not necessary.

With the adequate removal of the primary lesion, the wound is closed by suture, if possible, or by either split-thickness skin graft or local flap rotation.

Regional Lymph Nodes. If the regional lymph nodes are clinically involved, a radical lymphadenectomy should be done. Pathologic involvement of one node reduces the prospect of 10-year survival to 40 per cent. Involvement of two or more nodes reduces the survival prognosis greatly.

The problem of whether to perform lymphadenectomy prophylactically in the absence of apparent involvement is a highly contentious one. In general, if one takes into account the patient's age, the state of general health, and the patient's preference, it appears reasonable to recommend prophylactic lymphadenectomy when the lesion thickness is greater than 1.5 mm and in patients with Clark level 4 melanomas.

Metastatic Disease. Resection of localized pulmonary metastasis or a solitary cerebral deposit requires assurance that the primary tumor has been controlled and no other visceral metastases are present.

Chemotherapy

Systemic. Unfortunately, melanomatous tumors are essentially unresponsive to systemic chemotherapy. Although dacarbazine (DTIC) may be the best single agent, a combination of vincristine, bleomycin, nitrosoureas, and dacarbazine may be better. *cis*-Platinum has also been used. Although adjuvant chemotherapy, immunotherapy, and bacille Calmette-Guérin have not been helpful, recent use of interleukin-2 and LAK cells has provided a basis for optimism.

Regional Melphalan or Nitrogen Mustard. Perfusion of peripheral limb melanomas with these drugs using extracorporal circulation has been successful in reducing the size of large melanomas. Hepatic artery perfusion may be helpful in the management of hepatic metastases.

Suggested Readings

Balch CM, Soong S-J, Milton GW, et al: A comparison of prognostic factors and surgical results in 1786 patients with localized (stage I) melanoma treated in Alabama, USA, and New South Wales, Australia. Ann Surg 196:677, 1982

Balch CM, Soong S-J, Murad TM, et al: A multifactorial analysis of melanoma: III. Prognostic factors in melanoma patients with lymph node metastases (stage II). Ann Surg 193:377, 1981

Breslow A: Thickness, cross-sectional areas and depth of invasion in the prognosis of cutaneous melanoma. Ann Surg 172:902, 1970

Clark WH Jr: A classification of malignant melanoma in man correlated with histogenesis and biologic behavior. *In* Montagana W, Hu F (eds): Advances in Biology of the Skin. London, Pergamon Press 1967, p 621

Edgerton MT: The treatment of hemangiomas: With special reference to the role of steroid therapy. Ann Surg 183:517, 1976

Grabb WC, Dingman RO, O'Neal RM, et al: Facial hamartomas in children: Neurofibroma, lymphangioma, and hemangioma. Plast Reconstr Surg 66:509, 1980

Milton GW: Clinical diagnosis of malignant melanoma. Br J Surg 55:755, 1968

Mohs FE: Mohs micrographic surgery: A historical perspective. Derm Clin 7:609–612, 1989

Mulliken JB, Glowacki J: Hemangiomas and vascular malformations in infants and children: A classification based on endothelial characteristics. Plast Reconstr Surg 69:412, 1982

Pinkus H, Mehregan AH: Premalignant skin lesions. Clin Plast Surg 7:289, 1980

Taylor GA, Barisoni D: Ten years' experience in the surgical treatment of basal cell carcinoma. A study of factors associated with recurrence. Br J Surg 60:522, 1973

CHAPTER **3**

Laser Therapy

LASER PHYSICS

Light amplification by stimulated emission of radiation (laser) demonstrates precision in its ability to affect tissue at a distance with minimal surrounding trauma. The application of laser therapy in the treatment of many cutaneous disorders requires an analysis of its mode of action and of the varieties of lasers that are appropriate to specific conditions.

Lasers were introduced as surgical tools in the 1960s with the introduction of a ruby crystal that produced its intense deep red beam. This was followed by the helium neon gas laser and then by the carbon dioxide (CO_2) gas laser. Subsequent to the introduction of the neodymium yttrium aluminum garnet (Nd:YAG) laser came the argon (AR^+) laser. Myriad substances have been used to produce laser energy, the latest experimental laser using titanium sapphire.

The Laser Effect

In contrast to the scalpel, which uses a mechanical force to cut, or the electrocautery, which uses electrical energy to cut and coagulate tissue, the laser uses photons or light energy to cut, coagulate, and vaporize tissue.

The laser produces a stream of photons, and its application for surgical use is based on three qualities possessed by the photons:

Single color: Light is that portion of the electromagnetic spectrum that is visible, and color represents a wavelength of visible light, so when a light source produces a single color or wavelength it is defined as being *monochromatic*. Each tissue type reacts differently to different colors of laser energy.

Single direction: With all the photons traveling in one direction, it is possible to deliver high doses of energy accurately to the selected tissue. Ordinary light scatters its medley of random wavelengths or colors, whereas laser light is directed into a very narrow cone in one direction without divergence *(collimation)*.

Precise correlation to frequency and wavelength: This precision is measured by *coherence* and enables pinpoint focusing.

Conversion of Light to Heat Energy

When photons strike the target tissue, internal reflection of the photons by the various components of the tissue creates the phenomenon of scatter. The scatter continues until all the photons are converted to heat or leave the tissues. When light is reflected from the tissue, it is termed *backscatter* and is a source of ocular danger to the user of the laser system if protective eyewear is not worn. The shorter wavelengths produce greater scatter and therefore less penetration. It is the absorbed light that is clinically effective as it is converted to heat. The heat produced in the tissue at the site of laser impact raises the tissue temperature, which then produces the biologic effect.

As some of the heat is dissipated by spread through the tissues, the volume of tissue affected is larger than that indicated by the size of the laser energy impact spot.

As the temperature of the tissue is raised, it passes through several stages, including denaturation, coagulation, vacuolization, vaporization, carbonization, and incandescence. Coagulation and vaporization are the most clinically significant, coagulation occurring at about 60°C and vaporization at 100°C.

Tissue light absorption is variable and is determined by light-absorbing chromophores such as melanin, oxyhemoglobin, and hemoglobin. Knowledge of the absorption spectrum of a target tissue dictates the ideal wavelength of laser light. Knowledge of a tissue's *thermal relaxation time* determines the time of exposure to laser light that results in damage to the target area without conduction to and damage of adjacent areas. The extent of damage is also a function of dose and time.

Dosage

There are three components to the amount of energy delivered by the laser: (1) *power* is the measurement of laser light expressed in watts, that is, a measurement of heat. (2) *time*: The product of power and time (i.e., power × time) represents energy measure in joules. (3) *area*: Energy delivered over a given surgical area or spot size represents energy density, which is equivalent to dosage.

The low dosage of laser light produces coagulation effects, and high dosage produces either vaporization or cutting, depending on the area exposed to the energy.

The dosage equation can be amended by altering either time, power, or spot size. Safety around vulnerable structures is best achieved by reducing the length of exposure rather than the power. Also, with constant power and time settings, the surgical dosage can be varied by changing the spot size.

$$\text{Energy density} = \frac{\text{Power} \times \text{Time}}{\text{Area (spot size)}}$$

Thermal injury to tissue is represented by three zones: central zone of vaporization, outer zone of tissue necrosis, and peripheral zone of thermal conductivity and repair.

MAJOR LASERS USED SURGICALLY

Lasers are classified by the wavelength (color) of light produced and by the source of the light. The light produced is either a continuous wave or a pulsed laser light. Lasers can also be modified, as in Q-switched lasers, to a higher peak power with even shorter pulse duration (Table 3–1).

Continuous-Wave Infrared Lasers

CO₂ LASER

The CO_2 laser may be used for cutting or vaporization. Infrared light with a spectrum of 10,600 nm causes an instantaneous conversion of the intracellular and

TABLE 3–1. Classification of Lasers by Source of Light

Type of Laser	Color of Light	Wavelength (nm)	Responsive Lesions
Continuous-wave lasers			
CO_2	Invisible (infrared)	10,600	Excision or vaporization of multiple lesions
Nd:YAG	Invisible (infrared)	1064	Vascular lesions, pigmented lesions
Argon	Blue-green	488–514	Vascular lesions
Krypton	Green	521, 530	Pigmented lesions
Krypton	Yellow	568	Vascular lesions
Pulsed lasers			
Copper vapor	Green	511	Superficial pigmented lesions
Copper vapor	Yellow	578	Vascular lesions
Flash lamp–pumped organic dye (vascular)	Yellow	577, 585	Vascular lesions
Flash lamp–pumped organic dye (pigmented)	Green	510	Pigmented lesions
Q-switched lasers			
Alexandrite	Red	755	Pigmented lesions, tattoos
Ruby	Red	694	Pigmented lesions, tattoos
Nd:YAG (frequency doubled)	Green	532	Pigmented lesions, tattoos, vascular lesions

extracellular H_2O from a liquid to gas state. A beam focused to a spot of less than 2 mm allows precision cutting with hemostasis as vessels are sealed. By defocusing the beam and decreasing power, the laser can be used to vaporize water in the tissue, causing the carbon component to become char. The char shields tissues from further laser exposure and must be removed as the lesion is treated layer by layer. A multitude of conditions, including warts, tattoos, vascular lesions, and superficial benign and malignant skin lesions, have been effectively treated with this laser.

NEODYMIUM:YAG LASER

The Nd:YAG laser produces near infrared light at a wavelength of 1064 nm. The extent of thermal injury is difficult to control because of depth of penetration, and safer lasers are available for treating vascular lesions.

Continuous-Wave Visible Light Lasers

ARGON LASER

The argon laser, which produces blue-green light at wavelengths of 488 to 514 nm, has been used successfully in treating vascular lesions because hemoglobin absorbs light in the 500-nm range. The laser is associated with collateral thermal injury and, although effective in treating the target vascular lesions, has caused unpredictable scarring and hypopigmentation, especially in children. It is better reserved for treating the dark, thicker port wine stains in adults.

KRYPTON LASERS

These lasers produce light in several wavelengths, including 568 nm (yellow light) and 521 nm or 530 nm (both green light). The yellow light is effective in treating vascular lesions, and the green light is effective in treating pigmented lesions. As with any laser producing long light pulses, risk of scarring is higher.

Pulsed Lasers

COPPER VAPOR LASERS

Copper vapor lasers are used to produce light at wavelengths of 578 nm (yellow light) and 511 nm (green light). The yellow light is effective in treatment of vascular lesions, and the green light is used for treatment of benign pigmented lesions.

FLASH LAMP–PUMPED PULSED DYE LASERS

These lasers produce very short pulses of light. Because the pulse is timed to match the thermal relaxation of the target lesion vessels, heat destruction of adjacent uninvolved tissues is minimal and risk of scarring is low compared with that for other lasers. The laser produces yellow light at wavelengths of 585 nm or 577 nm as the flash lamp pumps a solution containing organic dye. The yellow light is effective in treating vascular lesions and is the state-of-the-art laser in dealing with port wine stains (Fig. 3–1). Complications are minimal, although treatment results in significant purpura (Fig. 3–2), which resolves in 2 to 14 days. Lesions are treated at 6-week intervals; generally multiple treatments are required to ablate a port wine stain.

A newer flash lamp pulsed laser is available which produces green light at a wavelength of 510 nm. This laser, like other green light lasers, is effective in treatment of benign pigmented lesions.

Q-Switched Lasers

The Q-switched lasers include the alexandrite, ruby, and Q-switched Nd:YAG laser. The alexandrite laser produces red light at a wavelength of 755 nm, and early experience demonstrates efficacy in treating benign pigmented lesions and tattoos. The ruby laser also produces red light at a wavelength of 694 nm and is used in treatment of benign pigmented lesions and tattoos. The Q-switched Nd:YAG laser pulses the infrared light through potassium titanyl phosphate. This produces a green light with a wavelength of 532 nm and is effective in treating tattoos, benign pigmented lesions, and vascular lesions.

LASER HAZARDS

Accidental exposure of anything other than the target tissue can lead to potential tissue damage, with the eye and skin the most likely sites for such mishaps. Exposure may be direct, from the delivery device, or indirect, in the form of reflection from some object in the path of the laser beam.

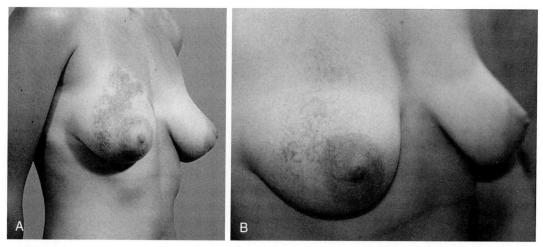

FIGURE 3–1. Preoperative *(A)* and postoperative *(B)* views of a port wine stain after three treatments with the flash lamp–pumped pulsed dye laser.

It is important to use nonflammable anesthetic agents, and flammable drapes should not be exposed to the beam near the target tissue, as the production of heat may reach a critical temperature with an ensuing fire.

Protective measures must include protective eyeglasses for the operating room personnel when the laser is in use, as well as for the patient.

The laser unit must be properly installed and regularly checked. The area should be well-ventilated with provision for the evacuation of smoke and fumes generated during the laser procedure. Warning signs should be posted at all entrances to the unit when the laser is in use. Surgeons using the laser should be trained and certified in its use.

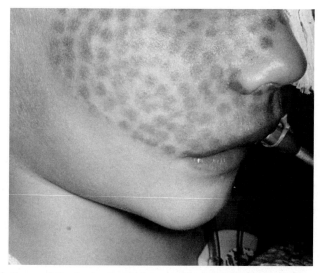

FIGURE 3–2. Purpura following treatment of a port wine stain with the flash lamp–pumped pulsed dye laser.

Suggested Readings

Apfelberg DB (ed): Cutaneous laser surgery—clinical and laboratory investigations. Lasers Surg Med (Special issue) 6:2–99, 1986

Tan OT, Sherwood K, Gilchrest BA: Treatment of children with port wine stains using the flashlamp-pulsed tunable dye laser. N Engl J Med 320:416–421, 1989

Wheeland RG: Clinical uses of lasers in dermatology. Lasers Surg Med 16:2–23, 1995

CHAPTER 4

Burns

THE BURN WOUND

A burn represents tissue damage due to dry heat. Tissue damage due to moist heat is called a scald. The pathologic effects and modes of management are identical for both. Because of the characteristic increase in capillary permeability in the zone of tissue damage, fluid, electrolytes, and protein are lost from the intravascular compartment into the interstitial tissues. If the loss of fluid is large, a state of hypovolemic shock ensues. The degree of shock can be anticipated because the amount of fluid lost is directly proportional to the surface area of the burn.

There are essentially four stages in the acute management of burns: (1) anticipation and treatment of shock, (2) prevention of infection, (3) proper management of the burned tissue with early grafting of full-thickness skin loss, and (4) prevention of complications with adequate nutritional support.

After evaluating the burn victim for any associated injuries, respiratory insufficiency, or other life-threatening circumstances and appropriately dealing with them, the extent of the burn is assessed.

Extent of the Burn

After removal of the patient's clothing, the extent of the burn can be determined using established formulas:

1. Wallace rule of nines: This can be used to provide an estimate of the per cent of adult body surface area (BSA) burned. The front of the torso, the back, and each lower limb represents 18 per cent of BSA. Each upper limb and the head and neck represent 9 per cent each, and the perineum represents 1 per cent (Fig. 4–1). A more accurate assessment of burn BSA is depicted in Figure 4–2.

2. Lund and Browder chart: Because the percentage of BSA changes with

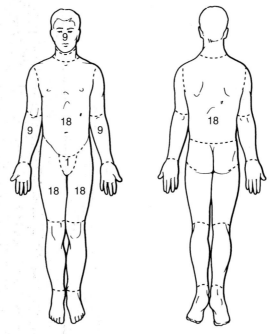

FIGURE 4–1. The body surface area of a burn may be estimated by Wallace's rule of nine's.

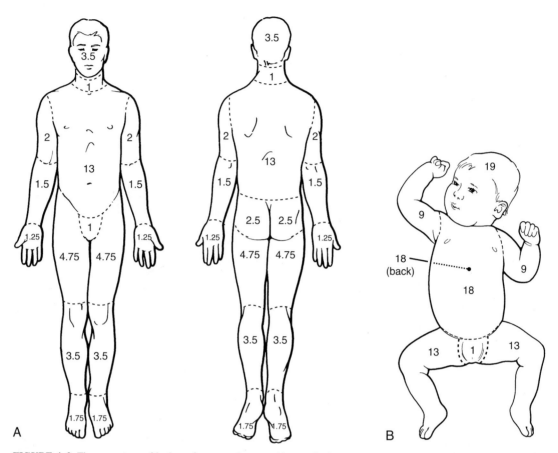

FIGURE 4–2. The percentage of body surface area changes with growth. A more accurate assessment of burn surface area is represented by these diagrams depicting the Lund-Browder chart estimate of burn surface area for adults *(A)* and infants *(B)*.

growth, a more accurate assessment can be made in children as well as adults by use of this chart (Table 4–1).

3. A rapid assessment of small area burns can be made by the fact that the palmar surface of the examining hand represents about 1 per cent of BSA.

TABLE 4–1. Lund–Browder Chart Estimating Per Cent of Burn Surface Area

Area	Infant	1–4 Years	5–9 Years	10–14 Years	15 Years	Adult
Head	19	17	13	11	9	7
Neck	2	2	2	2	2	2
Anterior trunk	13	13	13	13	13	13
Posterior trunk	13	13	13	13	13	13
Right buttock	2.5	2.5	2.5	2.5	2.5	2.5
Left buttock	2.5	2.5	2.5	2.5	2.5	2.5
Genitalia	1	1	1	1	1	1
Right upper arm	4	4	4	4	4	4
Left upper arm	4	4	4	4	4	4
Right lower arm	3	3	3	3	3	3
Left lower arm	3	3	3	3	3	3
Right hand	2.5	2.5	2.5	2.5	2.5	2.5
Left hand	2.5	2.5	2.5	2.5	2.5	2.5
Right thigh	5.5	6.5	8	8.5	9	9.5
Left thigh	5.5	6.5	8	8.5	9	9.5
Right leg	5	5	5.5	6	6.5	7
Left leg	5	5	5.5	6	6.5	7
Right foot	3.5	3.5	3.5	3.5	3.5	3.5
Left foot	3.5	3.5	3.5	3.5	3.5	3.5

Depth of the Burn

The coagulative necrosis of tissue caused by burn injury may be categorized as full or partial thickness.

1. Full-thickness burn: The tissue destruction includes the deepest hair follicles and sweat glands. Healing, if the wound is small, may occur by contraction and epithelialization from the healthy wound edge. If a large area is affected, skin grafting will be necessary.

2. Partial-thickness burn: The deep dermis is preserved, and epithelialization of the wound develops from the surviving hair follicles and sweat glands within 3 weeks.

Fresh burns may be conveniently categorized by degree:

1. First-degree burns: The area appears red, erythematous, and raised from the surrounding normal skin. There are stinging pain and mild edema but no blistering. First-degree burns should not be included in the estimate of burned area for purposes of calculating intravenous fluid therapy. Healing is usually total within a week.

2. Second-degree burns: Blistering of the skin is accompanied by painful erythema and subcutaneous edema. If the blisters rupture, the wound weeps serum. In deeper second-degree burns, after the blisters have burst, the wound becomes blanched and dry and has diminished sensation to touch or pinprick, making it difficult to differentiate from third-degree burn.

3. Third-degree burns: Full-thickness skin to or into the subcutaneous tissue (Fig. 4–3).

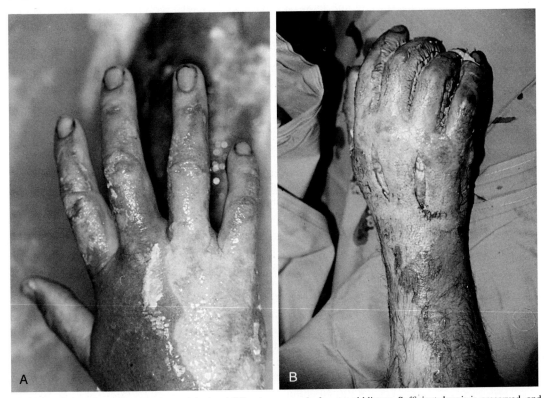

FIGURE 4–3. *A,* Partial-thickness burn of the hand following removal of ruptured blisters. Sufficient dermis is preserved, and epithelialization will occur from surviving hair follicles and sweat glands. *B,* A full-thickness burn with destruction of all layers of the dermis. Escharotomies have been performed to ensure blood flow to the digits.

TABLE 4–2. Severity of Burn

Depth of Burn	Mild		Moderate		Severe	
	Adult	*Child/Infirm*	*Adult*	*Child/Infirm*	*Adult*	*Child/Infirm*
Second degree	< 15%	< 10%	15–25%	10–15%	> 25%	> 20%
Third degree	< 2%	< 2%	2–10%	2–10%	> 10%	> 10%

Severity of Burn

The severity of a burn is determined by burn BSA, depth of burn, and age of patient. Severity of the burn injury provides a guideline to need for hospitalization, specialized burn unit, and extent of monitoring and treatment of the patient. Smoke inhalation renders any burn severe, and burns of the face, hands, perineum, and soles of the feet may provide challenging wound problems that must be dealt with individually. Minor burns can generally be treated on an outpatient basis, whereas moderate burns require nonintensive hospital care. Severe burns require treatment in a specialized unit (Table 4–2).

Pathophysiology of Burns

Local Effects. Tissue injury depends on the nature of the burn, the source and intensity of the burn, and the temporal relationship to the source. Thermal injury exerts its effects by direct conduction of heat or by electromagnetic radiation. Nerves and vessels are most vulnerable to heat conduction, whereas bone is most resistant. Electromagnetic irradiation from ultraviolet rays or infrared waves exerts injury either thermally or by microwave effect, whereas x-rays cause tissue ionization.

The burn wound suffers a central zone of tissue coagulative necrosis. At its edge is a zone of vascular stasis where cells suffer reversible anoxia with the potential for recovery. Peripheral to this is a zone of hyperemia where total cellular recovery is usual.

Systemic Effects. In burns affecting more than 30 per cent of the BSA, the massive transudation of fluid and proteins into the extravascular space leads to a decrease in circulating blood volume, with reduced cardiac output, increased peripheral resistance, and development of hypoproteinemia and elevated liver enzymes. With the reduction in circulating blood volume and cardiac output, oliguria with impaired renal function ensues. Impaired pulmonary function can be aggravated by smoke-inhalation effects.

Leukocytosis develops early and persists for some time. A sudden drop in the white cell count may indicate the commencement of sepsis. Abnormal forms of red cells are noted in the blood within a few hours of the burn. Hemolysis of red cells occurs and may lead to hemoglobinuria. There is increased secretion of pituitary adrenocorticotropic hormone.

After 48 hours, as capillaries regain their tone, fluid is reabsorbed, reducing the need for intravenous fluid administration.

Inhalation Burn

Inhalation injury profoundly impacts the morbidity and mortality of burn injuries. Inhalation injuries may manifest as acute respiratory distress within the first 12 hours, adult respiratory distress within 1 to 5 days, or bronchial pneumonia later in the course of burn injury. It is seen in closed space fires and results from the chemical pneumonitis caused by inhalation of incompletely combusted materials. Significant inhalation may lead to carbon monoxide poisoning, which must be progressively treated with 100 per cent oxygen and monitoring of carboxyhemoglobin levels. Chest radiographic changes may not be apparent, and bronchoscopy is the most reliable diagnostic tool. Therapy depends on symptoms and ranges from oxygen supplement and bronchial toilet to mechanical ventilation.

MEDICAL TREATMENT

Anticipation and Treatment of Shock

Burns approaching or more than 20 per cent of BSA require intravenous fluids. Because the features of shock may be delayed, it is important to maintain a normal blood pressure by administration of intravenous fluids through a large-bore percutaneous catheter, ideally in a peripheral vein in a nonburned area. If such is not available, a jugular or subclavian catheter may be required. There is no need for corticosteroids.

Estimation of Fluid Requirements

The availability of the Brooke and Parkland formulas provides a working method for estimating the crystalline and colloid fluid needs of the burn patient within the first 48 hours by multiplying the formulated amount of fluid by the patient's weight in kilograms times the percentage of surface area burned (Table 4–3).

Fluid management is complemented by insertion of a Foley catheter and hourly measurement of urine output. Urine output should be maintained at 1 ml/kg in children and 0.5 to 1.0 ml/kg in adults.

TABLE 4–3. Fluid Resuscitation Formulas

Parkland formula	
First 24 hours	Lactated Ringer, 4 ml/kg/% BSA
	50% volume 1st 8 hours, 50% 2nd 8 hours
24–48 hours	Colloid increased and crystalloid decreased to maintain same output
Brooke formula	
First 24 hours	Lactated Ringer, 1.5 ml/kg/% BSA (up to 50% BSA)
	Colloid, 0.5 ml/kg/% BSA (up to 50% BSA)
	Free water, 1500 ml/m²/day
	50% volume 1st 8 hours, 25% 2nd 8 hours, 25% 3rd 8 hours
	50% volume given in 2nd 24 hours

BSA = Burn surface area

A nasogastric tube is inserted and gentle suction maintained for gastric decompression.

Systemic antibiotic therapy may be commenced and tetanus toxoid provided. If prophylactic antibiotics are used, penicillin to prevent early *Streptococcus* infection is the drug of choice.

Analgesics and sedatives are administered and the patient is kept warm to prevent hypothermia.

Prevention of Infection

Initial wound débridement is carried out and, if indicated, escharectomy is done. The high risk of deaths from respiratory and septic complications is highlighted by the fact that extensive thermal injury induces a significant degree of immuno-suppression. The reduced resistance to infection occurs at two levels: (1) Dermal level: The destruction of skin by a burn causes the loss of its barrier to infection. The development of an avascular eschar provides an ideal pabulum for microorganism growth. Thus early excision of an eschar is important. (2) The inflammatory reaction at the site of injury depends upon the cellular and humoral components of the immune system. Depression of both components is induced by thermal burns, predisposing the burn patient to respiratory infection, which may be aggravated by smoke inhalation. It may also predispose to systemic sepsis.

Among the important pathogens leading to wound and systemic sepsis are *Pseudomonas aeruginosa* and *Staphylococcus aureus*.

Although specific antibiotics are appropriate in the presence of positive blood cultures, there is no universal need for continuous systemic prophylactic antibiotic therapy except during periods of operative manipulations, if good local treatment and early escharectomy and skin grafting are carried out.

Penicillin and cephalosporins represent the most common antibiotics in appropriate cases, and the aminoglycosides may be added to the antibiotic regimen. *Candida* infections of significant degree may require amphotericin B for their control.

TOPICAL ANTIBIOTIC THERAPY

Because deep burn wounds become colonized by gram-positive cocci within 24 hours and within a week by gram-negative aerobes, it becomes important to keep the wound as bacterially uncontaminated as possible by appropriate topical therapy.

Silver sulfadiazine (Silvadene): This topical agent is available as a cream in a concentration of 1 per cent. It is widely used for moderate and major burns, being applied twice daily with dressings (closed) or without dressings (open). It does not cause pain. It provides chemotherapeutic control of the number of organisms in the wound. It does not cause any electrolyte abnormalities. It is effective against a variety of gram-positive and gram-negative organisms as well as *Candida albicans*. It may induce the development of resistant organisms, such as Enterobacteriaceae and *Pseudomonas aeruginosa*. Occasional hypersensitivity reactions may occur. It penetrates eschar poorly.

Silver nitrate (0.5 per cent solution in water): This is applied using multilayer compresses that are kept wet continuously. As a broad-spectrum agent that is minimally absorbed from the burn wound, it is chemoprophylactic, sterilizing the wound surface. Its application is a useful method of maintaining sterility prior to excision of whole-thickness wounds. It should not be used in infected wounds, in burn wound sepsis, or in the presence of an eschar. Apart from being messy, staining the skin and bedding, it may cause hyponatremia, hypokalemia, and, occasionally, methemoglobinemia.

Mafenide acetate (Sulfamylon): This carbonic anhydrase inhibitor may be used in infected, dirty wounds, in high-voltage electrical burns, and when other agents fail. It is applied twice daily to the wound, which is left open. Although it is effective in burn wound sepsis, superinfection by resistant organisms or fungi may develop after prolonged use. As it penetrates eschar and cartilage, it may be used in burns of the nose and ears. It is painful on application.

Nitrofurazone (Furacin): Applied twice daily under a burn dressing, it has a broad antibacterial spectrum, including staphylococci resistant to Silvadene. It does not penetrate eschar and may cause a metabolic acidosis.

Miscellaneous agents: Chlorhexidine gluconate, aminoglycosides such as gentamicin, bacitracin, and polymyxin B. Bacterial resistance occurs rapidly to these non–eschar-penetrating agents.

PREVENTION OF TETANUS

Tetanus toxoid, 0.5 ml, is given intramuscularly. Unimmunized individuals with a "tetanus-prone" wound should immediately be given antitoxin to bind any circulating toxin. Tetanus immune globulin (Laxoid) in a dose of 250 to 500 units is given, followed by a proper immunization schedule.

General Management

1. Hemoglobin estimation twice weekly for 3 weeks, with appropriate blood transfusions if necessary.

2. Nutrition: High protein intake orally, by nasogastric tube, or by parenteral nutrition should be provided, with vitamin supplement. A daily minimum intake of 3 g of protein per kilogram of body weight should be ensured.

3. Renal function is assessed in patients with burns greater than 30 per cent of BSA, with blood urea nitrogen estimated regularly so that renal failure can be recognized as early as possible.

4. Serum electrolyte levels should be regularly checked.

5. Urinalysis should be done for glycosuria, as the "pseudo-diabetes" of burns may cause nonketotic hyperglycemia and glycosuria, requiring the reduction of carbohydrate intake.

6. Sedatives should be given to allay apprehension and ensure sleep at night.

7. Narcotics in small doses are provided for pain relief.

8. Physiotherapy is provided to prevent respiratory infection. All joints are kept moving to prevent stiffness and contracture.

9. Maintenance of morale is an important factor.

Metabolic Requirements

Burn injuries cause a hypermetabolic state characterized by catabolism and depletion of energy stores. Inadequate nutritional support leads to progressive gluconeogenesis, protein depletion, and a state of starvation. Nutritional support should be instituted within the first day or two of injury with a caloric intake that provides protein sparing. Patients with large burns may require caloric intake of more than 5000 calories per day. The most commonly used formula is that described by Curreri.

Adult 24-hour caloric requirement = 25 kilocalories per kilogram
plus 40 kilocalories per per cent of surface area burned

Child 24-hour caloric requirement = 60–90 kilocalories per kilogram
plus 35 kilocalories per per cent surface area burned

Vitamin supplementation is beneficial.

Nutritional support is ideally provided by a feeding tube, although a feeding jejunostomy tube may be required in selected patients. Intravenous hyperalimentation may be necessary in selected situations, although risk of sepsis is significant. It also does not provide the salutory immunologic stimulus provided by enteral feeding.

OPERATIVE MANAGEMENT OF BURN WOUNDS

DÉBRIDEMENT

With the patient appropriately stabilized and adequately sedated or narcotized, the initial wound débridement is carried out. All blisters and loose skin are débrided, the wound is gently irrigated and washed, and the topical agent is applied. Subsequent wound débridement sessions can be conveniently carried out in the Hubbard tank if the patient is stable or in the bed if the patient is unstable.

ESCHAROTOMY

Eschar is the dry, leathery tissue seen in deep partial- and full-thickness burns. When circumferential, the eschar can compromise chest wall excursion and circulation in the extremities, requiring escharotomy (Fig. 4–4). An incision is made through the thickness of the eschar into underlying subcutaneous tissues. Electrocautery must be available to aid in hemostasis. If extremity escharotomy does not restore circulation, fasciotomy may be necessary.

EXCISION AND GRAFTING

Accurate early excision of all necrotic dermal and subcutaneous tissue followed by immediate grafting produces rapid primary healing with an optimal functional and cosmetic result. Early coverage of the burn wound also minimizes the immunosuppressive, infectious, and metabolic consequences of a large burn.

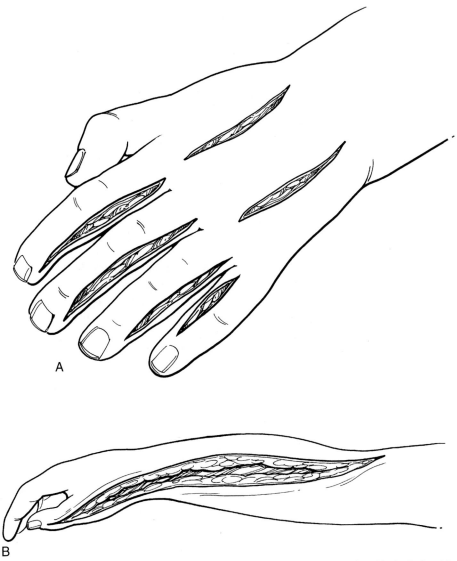

FIGURE 4–4. *A,* Preferred site for escharotomies to the digits. The ulnar side is preferred in the 2nd to 4th digits, avoiding subsequent scar on the radial side of the digit, which would compromise thumb-to-digit pinch. Escharotomy on the dorsum of the hand decompresses the dorsal interossei muscles. *B,* Radial escharotomy of the forearm is preferred to minimize risk of injury to peripheral nerves. Care must be taken to avoid injury to the superficial branch of the radial nerve.

Whether to use this approach in a given case depends on the size and depth of the wound, the amount of blood loss, and the total extent of the burn, as adequate skin graft donor sites may not be available.

If autograft sites are unavailable, sheets of cadaver allograft skin, split-thickness porcine skin, human amnion, or biologic or synthetic film may provide temporary wound cover. Cultured keratinocyte allografts may serve as a biologic dressing. Cultured keratinocyte autografts on a dermal substrate have also been used to cover large areas in patients with limited donor skin.

Autologous grafts are harvested with an electric dermatome at a thickness of 0.08 to 0.15 inches. Sheet grafts provide optimal cosmetic results and should always be used in the facial area. Meshed grafts at 1.5:1 give an acceptable cosmetic result and allow the escape of subgraft fluid. Mesh of 3:1 or even 6:1

may be necessary in large burns with a paucity of donor sites. In the face, sheet grafts are secured by 6–0 Vicryl sutures, whereas staples may be used elsewhere in the body. Sheet grafts may be left open and any subgraft fluid evacuated by rolling or by aspiration. Grafts of extremities or trunk are secured by wet dressings and fine mesh Kling roller gauze soaked in a dilute antibiotic-saline solution or by nonadherent Xeroform gauze (Sherwood Medical, St. Louis, MO) secured with dry gauze.

Management of Specific Areas

Face: Burns of the face are best treated by the "open" method. Most burns heal spontaneously. Failure to heal may require tangential excision and skin grafting.

Eyes: The eyelids often bear the brunt of injury. Maintenance of eye closure is best achieved by continual regrafting of the eyelid rather than tarsorrhaphy.

Ears: Sulfamylon is often used, as it penetrates cartilage and may prevent suppurative chondritis, which is destructive of the integrity of the ear. If cartilage becomes exposed, it requires conservative débridement until an adequate bed for split-thickness skin grafting is established.

Nose: Sulfamylon with its cartilage-penetrating quality is the preferred topical agent. Delayed nasal reconstruction may be necessary.

Hands: The critical factor in managing hand burns is adequate splinting within the first few days of injury and early and aggressive therapy. Early excision of burned tissue and immediate grafting preserve maximum function.

Trunk: Circumferential burns of the trunk carry a high mortality and create nursing difficulties. Early excision and grafting are ideal when possible.

ELECTRICAL BURNS

The burn may be due to the action of the heat or to the passage of the current. High-voltage injury causes more significant deep tissue injury. Alternating current, especially of low voltage, is more dangerous than direct current.

Pure heat burns occur by arcing of the current between two electrodes near the body. These "flash burns" behave like any thermal burn. The heat burn occurs when the victim is unable to release the active cable, with muscle spasm continuing until the current is switched off. Current burns may affect the heart, causing myocardial fibrillation, or the brain, causing coma. The burn results in a white central area surrounded by erythema. After 24 hours the local lesions become edematous, with development of a central slough. Because skin has a high resistance, greater burn effects are exerted on the deeper tissue. Damage to vascular intima and thrombosis lead to subsequent spread of tissue necrosis (Fig. 4–5). Escharotomy or formal fasciotomy may be needed.

The local treatment of current burn is determined by the degree of vascular involvement, with maximal effects delayed for some days. Management requires serial débridement. Once all dead tissue is definitively removed, early closure with skin grafts, flaps, or free tissue transfer is performed.

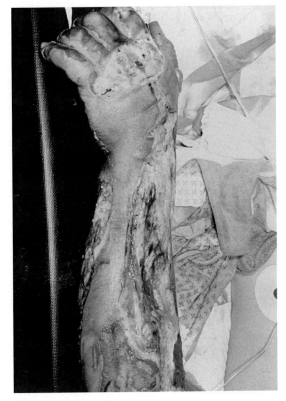

FIGURE 4–5. Electrical burn of the hand and forearm with extensive tissue necrosis.

CHEMICAL BURNS

Acid burns should be managed with copious irrigation with water. Sodium bicarbonate may be added to water to aid in neutralizing the acid. Hydrofluoric acid burns also require immediate application of 10 per cent calcium gluconate gel or direct injection of calcium gluconate. Alkali burns require prolonged irrigation with saline or 1 per cent acetic acid. Phosphorus burns are washed with a 1 per cent copper sulfate solution, which in turn must be removed with a second irrigation. Chemical burns are subsequently treated like thermal burns, with topical antimicrobials, early excision, and grafting of full-thickness injuries.

COLD INJURY

Frostbite occurs when tissue temperature is sufficiently low to cause ice crystallization of extracellular water. Water is drawn from the cells, with a cascading sequence of cellular death, tissue ischemia, and progression of injury. Frostbite may be superficial, involving skin only, or deep, with subcutaneous tissue involvement.

Frostbitten tissue is rapidly rewarmed by continuous immersion in water at 40 to 44°C. Wounds are managed by conservative débridement once tissue necrosis becomes clearly evident. Wounds are closed as necessary with grafts or flap transfer. Long-term sequelae including hypersensitivity, vasomotor instability, and sympathetic dystrophy are common following frostbite injuries.

BURN REHABILITATION

Attention is initially directed at preventing scar hypertrophy and contractures. Once deeper partial-thickness burns and grafted areas are healed, a compression garment is provided. Physical therapy, including range of motion and strengthening, is initiated or continued, and splints are used to avoid joint contractures. Despite aggressive management, however, burn patients may require multiple surgical procedures to maximize their functional and aesthetic outcome.

Scar Contractures

Scar contractures may require surgical release with Z-plasty, skin graft, flap transfer, and postexpansion tissue rearrangement. Long-standing joint contractures require attention to heterotopic bone, contracted or ossified joint ligaments and capsule, and shortened tendinous insertions. Growing children often require serial releases and grafting when burns involve flexor surfaces.

Unstable Wound

Burn scars may not withstand the rigors of life. Wounds that continually break down or ulcerate require excision and reclosure by appropriate means. Malignant transformation of an old burn wound may lead to the development of a squamous cell carcinoma (Marjolin ulcer).

Hand Reconstruction

Serious hand burns often require secondary procedures, including scar release with Z-plasty and split- or full-thickness grafts, tenolysis, and joint release.

Facial Reconstruction

Reconstruction ideally achieves a symmetric face with preburn facial contour. Skin should be homogeneous in terms of color and texture, and aesthetic units must be respected. Specific techniques depend on extent of injury, and each individual structure and feature must be evaluated. Serious facial burns require multiple reconstructive procedures, often over a period of years.

Suggested Readings

Arturson G, Hedlund A: Primary treatment of 50 patients with high-tension electrical injuries. Scand J Plast Reconstr Surg 18:111, 1984

Burke JF, Bondoc CC, Quinby WC Jr, et al: Primary surgical management of the deeply burned hand. J Trauma 16:593, 1976

Burke JF, Quinby WC, Bondoc CC: Primary excision and prompt grafting as routine therapy for the treatment of thermal burns in children. Surg Clin North Am 56:477, 1976

Cuono C, Langdon R, McGuire J: Use of cultured epidermal autografts and dermal allografts as skin replacement after burn injury. Lancet 2:1123, 1986

Curreri PW, Asch MJ, Pruitt BA Jr: The treatment of chemical burns: Specialized diagnostic, therapeutic and prognostic considerations. J Trauma 10:634, 1970

Curreri PW, Luterman A: Nutritional support of the burn patient. Surg Clin North Am 58:1151, 1978

Labandter H, Kaplan I, Shavitt C: Burns of the dorsum of the hand. Conservative treatment with intensive physiotherapy vs. tangential excision and grafting. Br J Plast Surg 29:352, 1976

Monaro WW, Ayvazian VH: Topical therapy. Surg Clin North Am 58:1157, 1978

Pruitt BA Jr, Levine NS: Characteristics and uses of biologic dressings and skin substitutes. Arch Surg 119:312–322, 1984

Reaves LE, Antonacci AC, Shires GT, et al: Fluid and electrolyte resuscitation of the thermally injured patient. World J Surg 7:566–572, 1983

CHAPTER 5

Grafts and Implants

SKIN GRAFTS

Skin may be transferred from one part of the body to another as a free graft. A segment of skin is detached from its donor area and placed on a raw surface elsewhere. The graft is allostatic, as it has no blood supply of its own. Skin grafts, like grafts of any other tissue or organ, may be (1) an autograft: The skin is transposed from donor to recipient site in the same individual; (2) an allograft or homograft: The transposition of tissue is between different members of the same genetic species, that is, human to human; (3) xenograft or heterograft: The transposition of tissue is between members of different and distinct genetic species, such as pig to human.

Types of Free Skin Grafts

Split-Thickness Skin Grafts. This is the most used graft in practice, and its size is limited only by the size of available donor area. The graft consists of epidermis and a variable amount of dermis (Fig. 5–1). The amount of dermis taken depends on the desired thickness of the graft. The greater the percentage of dermis in a graft, the less it contracts and the better the cosmetic result (Fig. 5–2). The thicker the graft, however, the greater the incidence of graft loss in poorly vascularized beds. Split-thickness grafts vary from 0.010 to 0.016 inch. Because dermis is left behind, the donor site heals by epithelialization.

Full-Thickness Grafts. This consists of epidermis and full thickness of dermis but no subcutaneous fat (Fig. 5–1). Because no epithelial cells remain, the donor area does not heal spontaneously and must be closed primarily.

Whereas a split-thickness graft tends to contract, the full-thickness graft does so to a much lesser extent. It also provides a graft of more normal color and

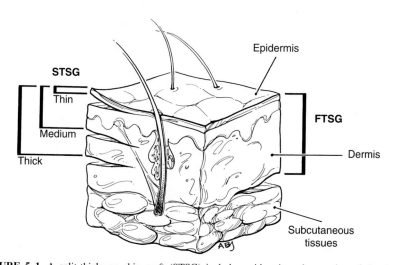

FIGURE 5–1. A split-thickness skin graft (STSG) includes epidermis and a portion of the dermis. Because dermis is left behind, the donor site heals by epithelialization. A full-thickness skin graft (FTSG) includes the epidermis and all layers of the dermis. Because no dermis is left behind, the donor wound must be closed primarily.

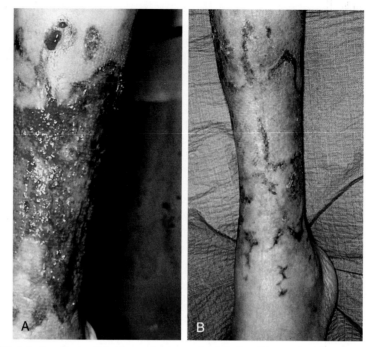

FIGURE 5–2. A well-vascularized superficial wound of the leg *(A)* treated with medium-thickness split-thickness skin graft *(B)*.

texture. It is the preferred graft in areas where graft contracture is to be avoided, such as the palm, or areas where cosmesis is important, such as the face (Fig. 5–3).

Composite Grafts. These grafts include skin and any underlying tissue such as subcutaneous fat or cartilage. A conchal composite graft is often used in nasal or eyelid reconstruction and includes postauricular skin attached to the underlying cartilage (Fig. 5–4). A composite graft from the helical rim includes anterior and

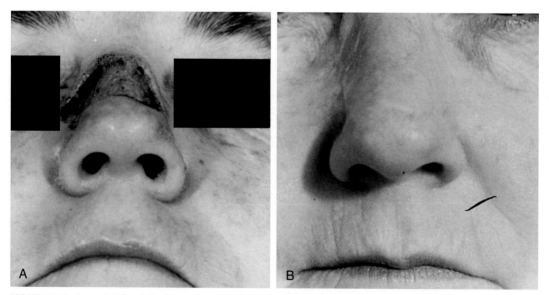

FIGURE 5–3. A nasal defect following excision of a basal cell carcinoma *(A)* treated with a preauricular full-thickness skin graft *(B)*. There is little graft contraction, and color and texture matches are satisfactory.

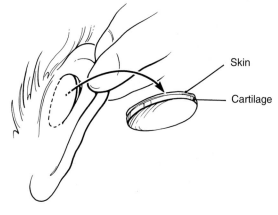

FIGURE 5–4. A composite conchal graft consisting of postauricular skin and underlying conchal cartilage.

posterior skin with an intervening layer of helical cartilage (Fig. 5–5). A composite graft of skin and subcutaneous tissue containing hair follicles is grafted from hair-bearing scalp to hairless scalp when doing hair transplants for baldness.

SURVIVAL OF FREE GRAFTS

Successful "take" of a free graft depends on a recipient site capable of producing capillary buds, accurate approximation of graft and recipient sites, prevention or evacuation of fluids under the graft, and prevention of shearing forces that might displace the graft.

Adherence of a free graft to its underlying bed occurs within a matter of minutes. The fibrinous adhesion consolidates within 0.5 hour, reflecting potential for a successful "take." After placement of a free graft, its nourishment is derived from tissue fluids. By the process of plasma imbibition, the fluid is derived from the recipient site bed and permeates between its cells. By the third day capillary loops derived from the bed grow into the graft to provide a permanent blood

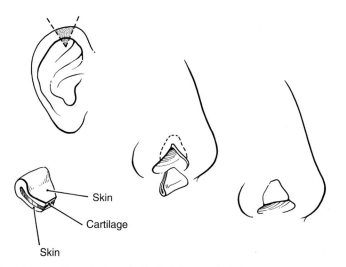

FIGURE 5–5. A composite graft from the helical rim may include a graft of cartilage sandwiched between two layers of skin. It provides an ideal graft for correction of notched deformities of the nasal ala.

supply, in addition to growth of capillaries across the marginal suture lines. This process is called inosculation.

Pressure dressings are not necessary for graft survival but do prevent accumulation of lymph or blood that might lift the graft off its bed.

CHANGES IN FREE GRAFTS

Contraction: The predilection for contraction of a free graft varies with the thickness of the graft and the rigidity of the donor site. The thinner the graft and the more mobile the soft tissue bed, the greater the degree of contraction. Across a flexor surface, the graft must be kept stretched for several months by splinting the joint. A graft under tension matures better than one that is slack.

Sensation: Return of sensation with temperature and pain perception usually occurs within 3 months.

Color change: The thicker the graft, the more likely it is to retain the color of the donor site. The best color results from full-thickness grafts kept under normal tension. Contraction causes a concentration of melanocytes, with a variable degree of early pigmentation that resolves slowly. In pigmented races, thick grafts may become darker than the surrounding skin.

Donor Sites

In elective skin-grafting procedures, the donor skin should resemble as closely as possible the skin around the recipient site. Because the thickness, texture, vascularity, hair-bearing feature, and appearance of skin vary according to the site of origin, proper selection of donor site becomes very important.

The donor site of small split-thickness grafts can usually be closed immediately by converting it into an elliptical wound and suturing it. If a large split-thickness graft has been taken, the area epithelializes from the residual hair follicles and sweat and sebaceous glands. Donor sites of split-thickness grafts may be protected by the application of bactericidal ointment covered with a fine mesh petrolatum-impregnated gauze. Epithelialization proceeds as long as blood and serum are allowed to drain from the donor site into the dressing, with prevention of local trauma and sepsis. Preferably the donor wound is dressed with an impermeable occlusive dressing such as Op-site (Smith & Nephew Ltd, Hull, England). This maintains a moist environment that is ideal for re-epithelialization and results in a significantly less painful donor site.

Because skin appendages are absent after taking a full-thickness graft, the residual wound must be closed primarily.

CUTTING GRAFTS

Cutting the graft varies with the thickness of the graft and the donor site selected. Three basic types of instrument are available:

Electrical or air-driven dermatome: A motor-driven dermatome permits the removal of long strips of skin 10 cm or less in width. The thickness of the skin graft can be altered by adjusting the calibrating knobs to alter the pitch of the blade, which moves back and forth like the blade of a hair cutter. The Brown dermatome knife blade is disposable. Other dermatomes include the Padgett, Stryker, and Castroviejo.

Sterile mineral oil is applied to the donor site to lubricate the movement of the dermatome. The dermatome is placed on the donor site with its flat undersurface at a slight downward angle, and as the instrument moves forward a constant pressure is applied to produce a well-cut graft.

Knives: The Humby knife was developed from the more primitive Blair and Ferris-Smith knives. It is manually powered and has adjustable rollers that control the thickness of the skin graft. It can produce long, narrow grafts of split-thickness skin from thigh, arm, or abdomen.

Drum dermatomes: Padgett and Reese drum dermatomes take uniform grafts but are cumbersome and difficult to use.

A full-thickness skin graft is taken when a whole skin graft has to fit the defect accurately. A pattern can be provided using aluminum foil, x-ray film, or a paper drape. In cutting the graft, no fat should be left on the graft. This can be accomplished either by accurate primary dissection or by removing any residual fat after the donor specimen has been excised.

FULL-THICKNESS DONOR SITES

Preauricular skin: Hairless preauricular skin in a female patient provides the best color and texture match for a facial graft. The donor incision lies in the preauricular creases, similar to a face-lift incision.

Postauricular skin: The posterior surface of the ear and the adjacent hairless mastoid area provide full-thickness skin that gives an excellent color and texture match when transplanted to the face, eyelids, or nose.

Upper eyelid: A small thin graft of upper eyelid can be taken from an adult, for repair of another eyelid, without deforming the donor site.

Supraclavicular skin: A large area of skin can be taken from the lower posterior triangle of the neck. It provides a good color and texture match for the face, but not as good as preauricular or postauricular skin. The donor area, however, may suffer the cosmetic effects of the skin removal.

Flexural skin: The antecubital flexure crease and the groin provide good donor sites for full-thickness skin for the face, hands, or fingers.

Preputial skin: This can be used for full-thickness grafting.

Expanded skin: Donor sites may be pre-expanded by tissue expansion techniques to provide a larger donor area that can then be closed primarily.

Biologic Skin Replacements

As with skin grafts, biologic skin replacement may include autogenic, allogenic, and xenogenic materials composed of fibrin products, collagen products, amnion, and cultured keratinocytes. Homograft and xenograft materials are used for limited periods, serving as a biologic dressing, whereas autograft materials may be used as a permanent substitute for skin in closing a wound.

Xenogenic Replacement. Frozen or lyophilized porcine skin is the most commonly used xenogenic material. It serves as a temporary skin substitute, reducing wound bacterial colonization and water loss.

Allogenic Replacement. Amnion is effective in reducing bacterial colonization, but it does little to minimize water vapor loss and requires an occlusive dressing. Because of its fragility, it has minimal practical use at this time.

Cultured Keratinocytes. Cultured allogenic keratinocytes are used as a temporary skin substitute and are effective in promoting the healing of chronic ulcers. Although the cultured cells do not survive for more than several days, they seem to stimulate proliferation and migration of host keratinocytes. The sheets of cells are extremely fragile, and clinical efficacy is improved if the cultured sheets are grown on a collagen substrate. This provides a stable material that can be trimmed and placed on a wound under an occlusive dressing. The wound is cleaned and fresh material placed every 5 days (Fig. 5–6).

Cultured autogenic keratinocytes have been used to re-epithelialize a multitude of wounds, including large full-thickness burns. The cells are cultured from small samples of skin taken from the patient. The main drawback in the use of autogenic skin culture is the weeks it takes to provide sufficient sheets for large wounds. They provide a protection against bacterial colonization and minimize loss of water vapor. Keratinocyte sheets are easily blistered or rubbed off and do not provide long-term stable coverage. The cells are best cultured on a dermal equivalent such as fibroblast collagen lattice, reconstituted collagen, and cross-linked bovine dermal collagen. This provides a much more stable skin substitute for permanent closure of a wound.

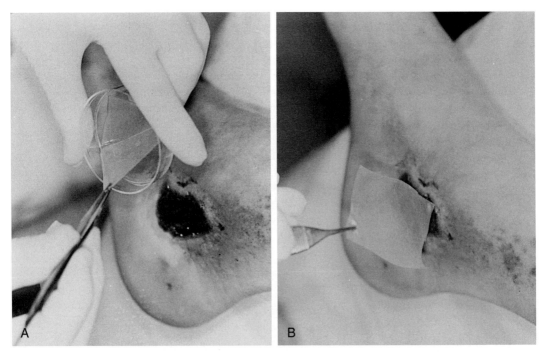

FIGURE 5–6. *A*, Keratinocytes have been cultured on a sheet of collagen substrate and stored in frozen state in a sterile Petri dish. *B*, The cultured keratinocytes and collagen substrate are placed on a wound under an occlusive dressing. The biologic dressing will be changed in 5 days.

CARTILAGE GRAFTS

The human body contains three types of cartilage: (1) *Hyaline cartilage* is compressible cartilage; it comprises joint cartilage, costal cartilage, nasal septum, and cartilage of the trachea and bronchi. (2) *Elastic cartilage* is rich in elastin. It is quite flexible and is the predominant cartilage in the external ear, nasal tip, and larynx. (3) *Fibrocartilage* has a dense fibrous matrix and is the primary cartilage of the intervertebral discs and tendinous insertions on bone.

Cartilage Autograft. Cartilage may be transplanted to a vascular recipient site where chondrocytes survive by diffusion of nutrients. Conchal cartilage grafts and nasal septal cartilage grafts are used for refinement of the nasal structures in aesthetic rhinoplasty as well as for major nasal and eyelid reconstructions. Sculpted costal cartilage grafts provide the scaffold for reconstruction of the external ear.

Cartilage Allograft. Clinical experience with irradiated cartilage allograft, preserved cartilage allograft, and lyophilized cartilage allograft has been satisfactory overall. The primary problems with cartilage allograft include the unpredictability of the degree of resorption and the potential for the grafts to warp with time. Cartilage allograft may provide time in children undergoing staged reconstructions and a reasonable source of cartilage if sufficient autologous cartilage is not available. When possible, the use of autologous cartilage is much more predictable and is preferred.

BONE GRAFTS

Bone consists of an outer cortex and a cancellous spongy inner layer (Fig. 5–7). Different bones have different composition of cortical and cancellous bone, and graft donor sites may be selected on the basis of this different structure. Bone may be either membranous or endochondral.

Membranous bone, which includes the bones of the face and skull, develops by intramembranous ossification, which is development by direct deposition of bone on a pre-existing vascularized mesenchymal layer. Endochondral bone, which includes the iliac crest ribs and long bones, develops by endochondral ossification, which is the development of bone from a cartilage precursor.

Nonvascularized Autologous Bone Graft

A bone graft must pass through an orderly repair process to become fully integrated. By the end of the process the bone graft has been fully resorbed and is replaced by deposition of new bone through "creeping substitution." The repair includes four stages: (1) Incorporation: The bone graft becomes adherent to surrounding tissues. (2) Osteoconduction: Capillary and cellular ingrowth takes place from the recipient bed along vascular channels of the bone graft. (3) Osteoinduction: New bone is formed as adjacent mesenchymal cells differentiate into osteocyte precursor cells. (4) Osteogenesis: Surviving osteocytes in the bone

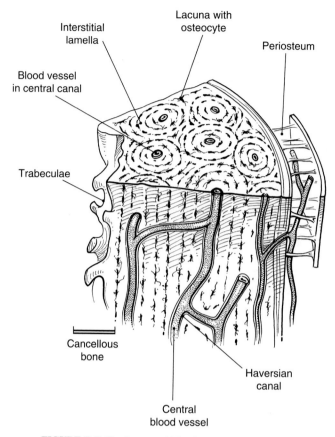

Interstitial
lamella

Lacuna with
osteocyte

Periosteum

Blood vessel
in central canal

Trabeculae

Cancellous
bone

Haversian
canal

Central
blood vessel

FIGURE 5–7. The layers and blood supply of a long bone.

graft contribute to the production of new bone. Osteogenesis plays a relatively small part in the repair of nonvascularized grafts.

Preferred sources for nonvascularized autologous bone grafts include the calvarium, ribs, and iliac crest.

Calvarial Graft. The calvarium is an ideal donor site for reconstruction of the facial skeleton due to its proximity and the acceptable donor incision. The outer table is used for small grafts. When a large graft is needed for significant craniofacial reconstructions, full-thickness calvarium is harvested, the inner and outer tables are separated, and one table is returned to reconstruct the donor defect while the second surface is transplanted to the recipient area (Fig. 5–8). Membranous bone is preferred in facial reconstruction, as these grafts demonstrate more rapid vascularization and significantly less resorption.

Iliac Bone Graft. The iliac crest and ilium are a rich source of both cortical and cancellous bone graft. Large blocks of endochondral bone may be harvested for appropriate reconstructions.

Rib Grafts. Rib grafts are bone that have the advantage of being soft and pliable. Two contiguous ribs may be harvested. If more graft material is required, every second rib is harvested to preserve chest wall contour. The rib grafts may be split, providing a rich source of cortical bone. Their curvature is ideal for reconstruction of mandibular defects and skull defects associated with cutis aplasia.

Vascularized Bone Grafts

Vascularized bone grafts may be harvested for transfer by microvascular techniques. The fibula with the peroneal vascular pedicle, the iliac crest with the deep circumflex iliac vascular pedicle, the rib with the posterior intercostal vascular pedicle, the lateral border of the scapula with the circumflex scapular vascular pedicle, and the radius with the radial artery pedicle may all be transferred in this fashion. Vascularized bone grafts heal like fractures, with survival of grafted osteocytes and repair by osteogenesis. Vascularized bone grafts are particularly important when bridging large defects and in areas with compromised recipient beds.

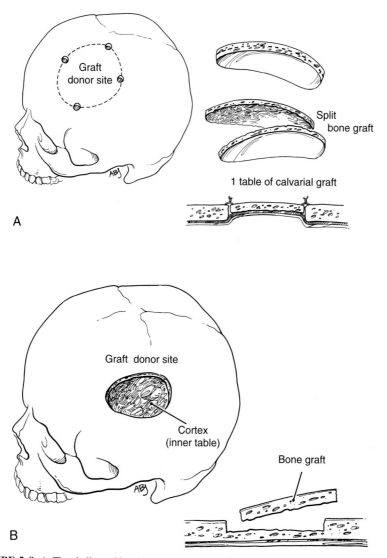

FIGURE 5–8. *A*, The skull provides a large source of membranous bone. Full-thickness calvarium is harvested and the inner and outer tables are separated. One table is returned to reconstruct the donor defect, and the second surface is transplanted to a recipient area. *B*, The outer table of calvarium may be harvested. The graft includes outer table and diploë layer, leaving the inner cortex undisturbed.

Bone Allograft

Allograft bone may be decalcified and freeze dried. Once reconstituted with saline, it provides a minimally immunogenic pasty scaffold for new bone formation. It is helpful in filling small gaps between autologous bone graft and adjacent bone or internally fixed osteotomy sites.

FAT

Fat may be transferred from a donor to a recipient site. Grafting of solid fat has proven disappointing because the fat generally resorbs. Fat may be aspirated and re-injected in small amounts into a recipient area. Fat injections are effective in correcting facial creases and wrinkles and may also be of benefit in correcting small contour deformities after liposuction. Evidence to date suggests that the fat resorbs within 6 to 12 months.

COLLAGEN

Injection of bovine collagen has been used for the correction of facial wrinkles and creases and of small contour deformities. Injectable collagen is available in two forms, either as processed bovine collagen (Zyoderm) or as a glutaraldehyde cross-linked derivative of Zyoderm (Zyplast). Zyoderm is best injected into the superficial dermis, whereas Zyplast is injected into deeper layers of the dermis. Zyoderm is resorbed within 3 to 4 months and Zyplast within 6 months, requiring repeat injections to maintain the clinical results. Patients must be skin tested on two occasions 8 weeks apart prior to initiating treatment because of the risk of local hypersensitivity reactions.

ALLOPLASTIC MATERIAL

Methyl Methacrylate. Methyl methacrylate is an ester of acrylic acid and an excellent material for reconstruction of cranial defects. Methyl methacrylate polymer in a powdered state is mixed with a liquid monomer. As it slowly hardens it can be introduced and shaped to recontour a defect. The material hardens within 6 to 8 minutes. Once hardened, a final contouring is accomplished with high-speed electrical bone burrs.

Hydroxyapatite. Hydroxyapatite may be used for both onlay and inlay grafts. It is a calcium phosphate, which is an important mineral component of both bone and coral. When placed in contact with bone, it stimulates formation of new bone and becomes tightly bonded to adjacent bone. It has proven clinically beneficial in orthognathic procedures, avoiding the need for autogenous bone grafting.

Proplast. Proplast is a porous material that allows ingrowth of fibrous and vascular tissues. Proplast I is composed of polytetrafluoroethylene (PTFE) and black carbon fibers, whereas proplast II is a combination of PTFE and white aluminum oxide fibers. Both materials have been used for augmentation of the facial skeletal components.

Silicone. Silicone includes a multitude of polymers composed of the element silicon, oxygen, and a variety of organic materials. The silicones used for medical implantation are a dimethylsiloxane polymer containing silicone, oxygen, and methane. The degree of polymerization of dimethylsiloxane determines its liquid, gel, or solid state. Numerous implants of varying consistency have been used in reconstructive procedures. The most common implants include breast prosthesis, testicular prosthesis, and solid silicone implants for chest wall deformities. Dimethylsiloxane polymers are also used to coat injection needles and disposable syringes.

Suggested Readings

Birch J, Branemark PI: The vascularization of a free full-thickness skin graft. I. A vital microscopic study. Scand J Plast Reconstr Surg 3:1, 1969

Clemmesen T: The early circulation in split-skin grafts: Restoration of blood supply to split-skin autografts. Acta Chir Scand 127:1, 1964

Edgerton MT, Hansen FC: Matching facial color with split thickness skin grafts from adjacent areas. Plast Reconstr Surg 25:455, 1960

Gallico GG: Permanent coverage of large burn wounds with autologous cultured human epithelium. N Engl J Med 381:448, 1984

Hanker JS, Giammura BC: Biomaterials and biomedical devices. Science 242:885, 1988

Morykwas M: Synthetic and biologic skin replacements. Probl Gen Surg 2:192, 1994

Robson MC, Krizek TJ: Predicting skin graft survival. J Trauma 13:213, 1973

CHAPTER **6**

Flaps

DEFINITION

A flap, in contrast to a free skin graft, consists of tissues transferred from their bed to an adjacent or distal area while retaining a functioning vascular attachment. The vascular attachment supplies arterial inflow and provides venous outflow at the base or pedicle of the flap.

The arterial and venous vessels remain in their native bed in a "pedicled flap" or are anastomosed by microvascular techniques to recipient vessels in a "free flap." A flap with two separate vascular attachments to its donor area is called a bipedicled flap.

Types of Flaps

Skin flap: skin and subcutaneous tissue
Muscle flap: muscle alone, which may be covered with a split-thickness skin graft
Myocutaneous flap (musculocutaneous flap): muscle with overlying subcutaneous tissue and skin
Fascial and fasciocutaneous flaps: fascia alone or fascia with overlying subcutaneous tissue and skin
Osteocutaneous flap: flap with multiple tissues, usually including bone, a cuff of muscle, fascia, and skin. Alternatively, bone can be carried alone on a vascular pedicle as an osseous flap.

SKIN FLAPS

VASCULAR DETERMINATION

Depending on the vascular characteristics, a flap may be one of the following:

Random pattern flap: These flaps lack specific vessels but are based on a "random" blood supply from the intradermal and subdermal plexus. The circulation through the capillary network becomes less reliable distally, limiting the length of these flaps (Fig. 6–1).
Axial pattern flap: This is a single-pedicled flap with a defined arteriovenous system running along its long axis. The axial vascular system permits the flap to be comparatively long because the flap can be raised along the entire

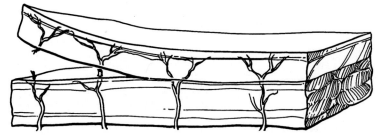

FIGURE 6–1. The blood supply to a random pattern flap is based on blood vessels in the intradermal and subdermal plexus. There is no defined vessel entering the flap, and circulation becomes less reliable distally.

length of the vessels (Fig. 6–2). The flap may also include a random portion distal to the axial vessels, allowing an even longer flap.

Island flap: The soft tissue around the vascular pedicle is dissected away so that the flap is attached only to the axial vessels. The mobility of the flap is greatly increased, permitting its rotation through an arc of 180 degrees or greater. A neurovascular island flap can be designed by including a nerve within an axial vascular pedicle, thereby permitting the skin to retain sensation.

Specific Axial Vascular Flaps

Deltopectoral Flap. Situated transversely on the anterior chest wall with its medial base along the sternal border, the flap has the perforating branches of the internal mammary artery as its axial vascular source. The flap is raised deep to the fascia, baring the underlying pectoralis major muscle up to the anterior surface of the deltoid.

In resurfacing defects in the vicinity, it can be moved to the lower face and neck, cheek, and parotid and mastoid regions.

Groin Flap. Based medially, it lies along the line of the groin. It uses as its arteriovenous axial system the superficial circumflex iliac vessels, which are incorporated into the flap as it is raised at the level of the deep fascia (Fig. 6–3). It is used for resurfacing the hand and as a local flap.

Hypogastric Flap. This is an inferiorly based flap on the lower abdomen. The superficial epigastric vessels provide its axial vascular system. The flap is raised at the level of the Scarpa fascia. It is used locally to replace suprapubic defects and distantly for resurfacing the hand.

Forehead Flap. Based on the supratrochlear or supraorbital vessels, the forehead flap can be used to repair large facial defects around the nose and lower eyelid.

Indications for skin flaps are full-thickness wounds with minimal dead space and one of the following conditions: (1) An avascular recipient site prohibiting skin grafting—bare bone, cartilage, or tendon—or following irradiation. (2) Cosmesis better provided by a flap than a skin graft. (3) Restoration of sensation by a neurovascular island flap. (4) Need to provide padding over bony prominences.

Flap survival can be augmented by a "delay procedure." Arterial blood supply and venous drainage provide the necessary nourishment to the flap via its pedicle, but it is the subdermal plexus in the areolar tissue on which final survival

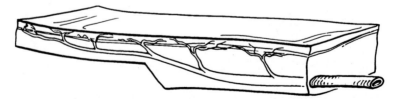

FIGURE 6–2. An axial pattern flap has a defined arteriovenous system running along its axis. The flap can be elevated along the entire length of these vessels and may also carry a random portion distal to the axial portion of the flap.

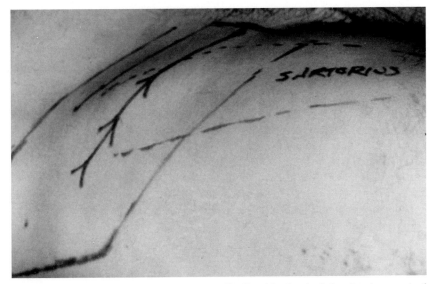

FIGURE 6–3. The groin flap is an axial pattern skin flap. The flap is designed to incorporate the superficial circumflex iliac artery and vein.

depends. The subdermal plexus can undergo hypertrophy and re-orientation of its vessels if a delay procedure is done and enough time is allowed to elapse. By making two parallel incisions and undermining the designated flap, the blood supply from each side is cut off and survival of the flap depends on the two end attachments. Over the ensuing 2 weeks the blood vessels become rearranged to run along the long axis of the flap. Once this axial blood supply becomes established, survival of the flap is possible with the division of one end (Fig. 6–4).

Principles of Flap Repair

1. Planning: A decision must be made regarding the type of flap and the method of its transfer. In general, planning should be done in reverse by back-planning the order of the operative steps.

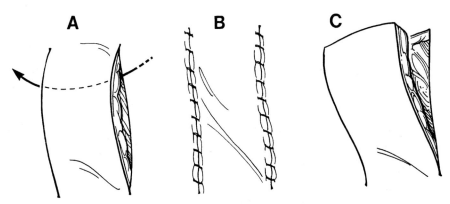

FIGURE 6–4. The delay procedure: *A,* An incision is made along the two parallel edges of the flap, and the flap is undermined. *B,* The incisions are closed, leaving blood flow to the tissues through either end. *C,* The flap is elevated in 10 to 14 days, by which time flow is well established along the long axis of the flap. The delay procedure greatly increases safety in elevation of a random pattern flap.

A. Choice of best donor area: Color match, availability of enough tissue, the patient's age and general status, the disfigurement of the donor area, and the need for immobilization are all considered.

B. A pattern of the defect is made to represent the amount of skin required for coverage.

C. The pattern of the flap is placed on the defect and moved back to the donor area, ensuring that once the patient is anesthetized there will be no problems with the prograde movement of the flap.

2. Size of the flap: A margin of reserve should be allowed for. It is possible to trim a flap that is a little too large, but one that is too small cannot be made bigger.

3. Closure of donor area: This may be done by direct suture after undermining the area or by application of a free graft.

4. Prevention of flap failure

A. Tension on the flap compromises arterial inflow and flap viability.

B. Venous congestion may occur because the flap is too long for adequate venous drainage, or the flap may be kinked. Suture removal or repositioning before vessels thrombose may salvage the flap.

C. Hematoma under the flap with subsequent infection must be avoided by early examination and evacuation of any fluid or blood collection. Prevention by suction drainage is a wise precaution.

Types of Skin Flaps

LOCAL SKIN FLAPS

Rotation, Transposition, and Interpolation. These have in common a pivot point and an arc through which the flap is rotated. (1) Rotation flap: A semicircular flap of skin and subcutaneous tissue that rotates about a pivot point into the defect that is to be closed (Fig. 6–5). (2) Transposition flap: A rectangular or square flap

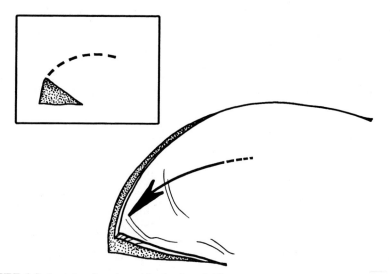

FIGURE 6–5. A rotation flap: A semicircular flap of skin and subcutaneous tissue is rotated about a pivot point into the defect.

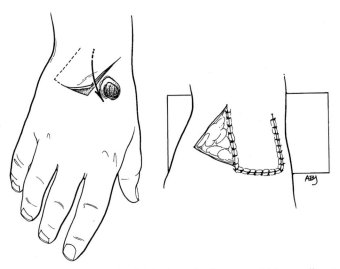

FIGURE 6–6. A transposition flap: The flap is elevated and transposed into an adjacent defect. The donor defect is either closed primarily or skin grafted.

of skin and subcutaneous tissue that transposes around a pivot point into an adjacent wound (Fig. 6–6). Variants include the bilobed flap, Z-plasty, and the rhomboid flap. The rhomboid flap can be made only in an area of loose skin and is designed for closure of a rhomboid defect with angles of 60 and 120 degrees (Fig. 6–7). (3) Interpolation flap: A flap of skin and subcutaneous tissue rotated in an arc around a pivot point into a nearby but distinct defect with intervening normal tissue between the two. A necessarily long pedicle must pass over the intervening tissue.

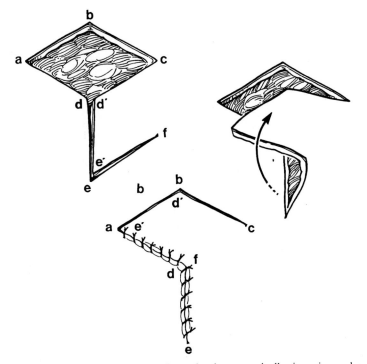

FIGURE 6–7. A rhomboid flap: The flap is advanced and transposed, allowing primary closure of the donor wound.

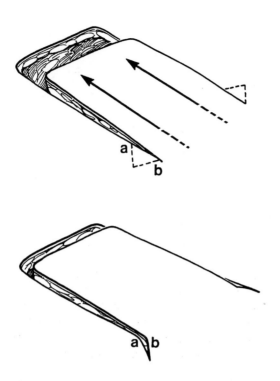

FIGURE 6–8. An advancement skin flap may be facilitated by excision of Burow's triangles at its base.

Advancement Flap. An advancement flap depends on a certain amount of stretching of the skin in moving it in a straight line to fill the defect. There are certain modifications: (1) The single-pedicled advancement flap is a rectangular or square skin flap that is simply stretched forward. Burow's triangles may be removed at the base to facilitate advancement (Fig. 6–8). (2) V-Y advancement is created by a V-shaped incision made in the skin. The skin on each side of the V is advanced, and the incision is then closed by suture as a Y (Fig. 6–9). The lengthening that results from this method can be used to lengthen the columella of the nose, eliminate lip notches, and close small defects. (3) The double-pedicled flap in its simplest form is a relaxing incision. The flap is undermined and advanced, maintaining pedicles at either end.

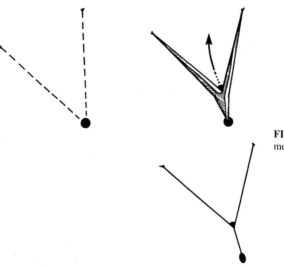

FIGURE 6–9. A V to Y advancement flap.

DISTANT SKIN FLAPS

These flaps are constructed some distance from the defect and may be transferred to it in one of two ways.

Direct Transfer. The donor flap is designed after measuring the defect. The flap is raised and its vascularity assured. The donor area is closed. The recipient area is prepared, and the flap is used to cover the entire defect. The pedicle and proximal flap carrying the blood supply bridge normal tissues. Vessels grow into the inset distal flap over 2 to 3 weeks. The flap no longer depends on its original pedicle, which may be divided and unneeded tissue discarded. The flap is inset at the proximal recipient site, and the original donor site is tidied up. A groin flap is a skin flap from groin to a defect on the hand, which is positioned under the flap (Fig. 6–10). A trunk flap may be transferred to any part of the arm or hand. Cross-arm flaps, although impractical, can be created when a contralateral flexor or extensor surface of the upper arm or forearm is used as a donor flap for defects on hand and fingers as well as the face. The Tagliacozzi flap is transferred in two stages from the medial arm to the face. Cross-leg flaps are possible when the knee joint is sufficiently supple for the two limbs to be appropriately positioned so that the flap can be used to provide stable coverage of exposed tendon or bone on the foot, ankle, lower leg, or knee. A forehead flap is shown in Figure 6–11.

Indirect Transfer. In this technique, currently rarely used, a carrier such as the wrist is used as an intermediary in bringing the flap from a distance to the defect in a staged manner. Reconstruction of face, lips, or ears can be done using indirect transfer from the neck as a bipedicled tubed flap with its long axis in the direction of the flexion creases. After 6 weeks' maturation, the flap can be transferred directly or waltzed in several stages at 3-week intervals. With the Crane principle, 2 to 3 weeks after transposing a flap, subcutaneous tissue is left on the recipient site over bone, tendon, or cartilage for coverage by a split-thickness graft and the main flap is returned to the donor site.

Postoperative Characteristics of Successful Skin Flaps

1. Color and texture are maintained.
2. Hair growth and sebaceous secretion characteristic of the donor site are retained.
3. Sensation is lost after flap transfer but may return within 6 to 18 months.
4. The flap provides a durable cover over bony prominences.
5. The flap continues to grow at the same rate as body growth.
6. The excess bulkiness of the flap may be reduced by removing subcutaneous tissue with preservation of the subdermal plexus, either by suction lipectomy or direct surgical thinning.

COMPOSITE FLAPS

A composite flap is created when underlying fascia, muscle, bone, or cartilage is incorporated into the skin flap. These flaps include musculocutaneous, fasciocuta-

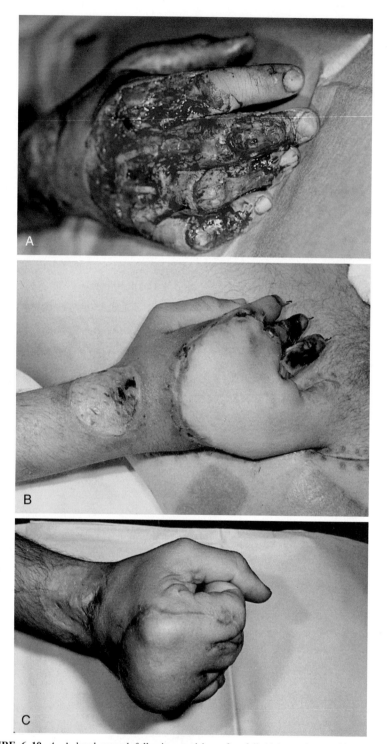

FIGURE 6–10. *A,* A hand wound following excision of a full-thickness burn with exposure of underlying tendons and joints. *B,* A groin flap has been elevated and sutured to the hand wound. Over the course of 3 weeks, sufficient vascularity will grow from the hand to the overlying flap that it is no longer dependent on its pedicle. *C,* At a second procedure, the pedicle to the groin flap is divided, the flap is inset into the hand, and the groin donor wounds are closed.

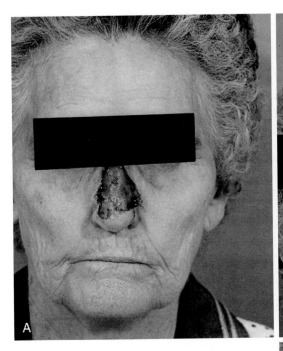

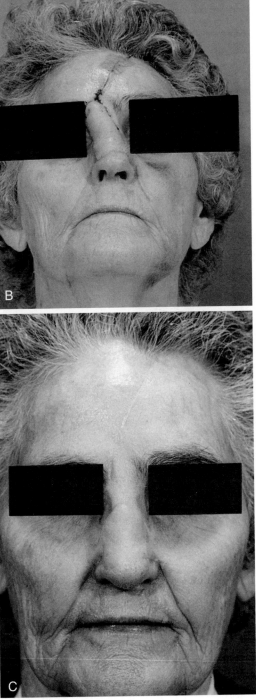

FIGURE 6–11. *A,* A full-thickness defect of the nose with exposure of underlying bone and cartilage. *B,* An island flap of forehead skin is transferred onto the nasal defect. The flap is supplied by the supratrochlear vessels. *C,* After 2.5 weeks, sufficient vascularity grows from the nose into the distal flap. The flap pedicle is resected and the forehead flap inset into the nose. The inferior aspect of the donor wound is closed.

neous, and osteocutaneous flaps (Fig. 6–12). Each component element can also be raised on a vascular pedicle as muscle, fascia, or osseous flaps.

MUSCLE AND MUSCULOCUTANEOUS FLAPS

A muscle may be detached from its normal origin and insertion and transposed on its vascular pedicle to an adjacent area. Alternatively, the vascular pedicle may be dissected and detached at its origin and the muscle unit transferred by microvascular techniques as a free flap. Muscle flaps provide a permanent additional blood supply to the recipient area. Muscle obliterates rigid cavities and wounds with dead space and aids in combatting low-grade infections once all devitalized tissue is débrided. The exposed surface of muscle provides an excellent recipient area for split-thickness skin graft if skin is not transposed with the muscle unit.

Muscles are supplied by arteriovenous systems branching from major segmental vessels. Arteries enter the muscle and ramify before giving off multiple perforators, which pass through the muscle into overlying subcutaneous tissue and skin. These perforators join with the subdermal and dermal plexus, enabling large paddles of skin to be taken with the underlying muscle (Fig. 6–13). Most muscles have a dominant vascular pedicle that provides the pivotal point for the flap's rotational mobility. This vascular pedicle provides the flap's "axis of rotation." When transposing a muscle flap, the "arc of rotation"—that is, its reach—is determined by the mobility of the flap on its vascular pedicle, and this arc determines the area that may be covered by the flap (Fig. 6–14). Muscle flaps may also be advanced as a V-Y advancement, as in the case of the hamstring muscles for ischial defects, or turned over on its perforating vessels, as in the case of the pectoralis major muscle turnover flap for sternal wounds. Clearly the muscle to be

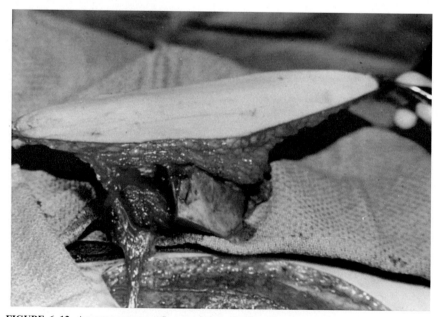

FIGURE 6–12. An osteocutaneous flap consisting of skin, subcutaneous tissue, and iliac bone has been raised from the iliac crest. The vascular pedicle, composed of the deep circumflex iliac artery and vein, is seen entering the flap.

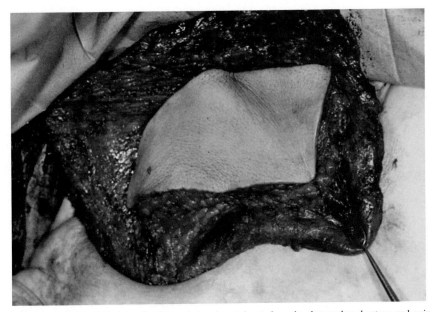

FIGURE 6–13. The latissimus dorsi muscle has been elevated on the thoracodorsal artery and vein. Perforating vessels from the muscle into the overlying subcutaneous tissue and skin enable a paddle of skin to be harvested and transferred with the muscle.

transferred must be expendable, as its functional loss should not detrimentally affect the donor area.

When transposing a muscle flap for the purposes of wound coverage, the innervation to the flap is usually divided to hasten atrophy of what could otherwise be a bulky soft tissue cover. If, however, muscle is being transferred for functional

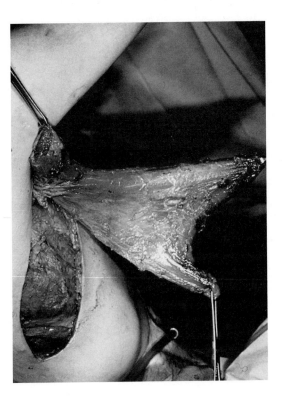

FIGURE 6–14. The arc of rotation of a flap is determined by its vascular pedicle. The latissimus dorsi flap pedicle may be transferred anteriorly to the chest wall, superiorly to the neck, or posteriorly to the midline of the back. The limit of transfer is that point beyond which excessive tension would be placed on the vascular pedicle.

purposes, innervation to the flap is carefully preserved. This is true in the case of muscle-tendon transfers in the extremities, transfer of innervated muscles for facial re-animation after seventh nerve injury, and transfer of innervated gluteus or gracilis muscle for replacement of rectal sphincters.

It is also possible to use only a portion of the muscle, leaving the bulk of the muscle with its innervation, origin, and insertion intact and functioning. This is possible in muscles with a large surface area such as the latissimus dorsi, pectoralis major, gluteus maximus, serratus anterior, and trapezius muscles. This technique is critical, for example, when using a portion of the gluteus maximus muscle in ambulatory patients. A segment of the muscle is used to cover a wound while sufficient muscle is left undisturbed with intact innervation.

Classification of Musculocutaneous Flaps

This is based on certain anatomic variables:

1. Anatomic source of muscle's arterial pedicles
2. Number of pedicles
3. Size of pedicles
4. Angiographic pattern of muscle vasculature
5. Location of pedicles in relation to the muscle's origin and insertion

Commonly Used Muscle and Musculocutaneous Flaps

RECONSTRUCTION OF HEAD AND NECK DEFECTS

Temporalis Muscle. The temporalis muscle, after arising from the floor of the temporal fossa of the skull, converges to a tendon that is inserted into the borders and inner surface of the coronoid process of the mandible. One of the masticatory muscles, it is expendable because the masseter and pterygoid muscles continue to permit mastication. In the infratemporal fossa, immediately below the foramen ovale, the mandibular nerve divides into its motor and sensory branches. The temporal muscle is innervated by the temporal branch of the mandibular nerve, which arborizes to the segments of the muscle.

The maxillary artery, one of the terminal branches of the external carotid artery, is directed forward to the ramus of the mandible and gives off two deep temporal branches that reach the pterygoid surface of the muscle above its insertion and course longitudinally toward the upper portion of the muscle, giving branches to the various muscular segments. Venous drainage occurs along companion tributaries to the pterygoid plexus.

The temporal muscle is used for (1) muscle transfer in facial palsy with segments routed to activate the eye, upper and lower lips, and corners of the mouth; (2) coverage of defects around the coronoid process; (3) coverage of intraoral defects in the cheek, pharynx, and palate; and (4) obliteration of defects in the orbit.

The temporalis fascia with its vascular supply from the superficial temporal artery is available as a free fascial flap for coverage of defects.

Trapezius Muscle. This triangular muscle is situated in the upper back with its base toward the vertebral column. Each muscle has an extensive origin from the spines of all the thoracic and seventh cervical vertebrae, the supraspinous ligaments, the ligamentum nuchae, and the medial third of the superior nuchal line of the occipital bone.

Converging laterally to the shoulder, the muscle is inserted into the lateral third of the clavicle on its posterior aspect as well as into the medial border of the acromion and upper margin of the scapular spine. It receives its nerve supply from the spinal accessory (11th cranial nerve) and from the cervical plexus (C3-C4). The transverse cervical artery provides the main blood supply to the muscle. As a branch of the thyrocervical trunk, it enters the deep surface of the trapezius muscle and divides into ascending and descending branches. The occipital artery also provides branches to the cervical part of the muscle.

The best flap design is a paddle made parallel to the dorsal vertebrae, pivoting the flap at the root of the neck. The secondary defect can usually be closed primarily.

The trapezius muscle is used for (1) coverage of dural defects; (2) coverage of defects in the cervical and thoracic spine; (3) postradiation coverage of parietal or temporal areas; and (4) coverage after removal of head and neck tumors.

RECONSTRUCTION OF THE TRUNK

Pectoralis Major Muscle. This triangular muscle has its base at the sternum and its apex at the arm. It has a broad origin from the medial half of the front of the clavicle, the anterior surface of the sternum and cartilages of the upper six ribs, and the aponeurosis of the external oblique muscle.

The muscle fibers converge to form a bilaminate tendon, which is inserted into the lateral lip of the bicipital groove of the humerus. It is innervated by the medial and lateral pectoral nerves derived from the brachial plexus.

Its major blood supply is derived from the thoracoacromial artery, which is a branch of the subclavian artery. Equally important are the perforating branches of the lateral thoracic and superior intercostal arteries. The thoracoacromial artery lies on the medial border of the pectoralis minor, then pierces the clavipectoral fascia and divides into four branches—pectoral, clavicular, acromial, and deltoid. The multiple segmented blood supply with its rich source of collateral anastomoses provides scope for segmentation of the muscle.

The pectoralis major muscle is used to (1) cover defects over the shoulder; (2) by transposition unilaterally or bilaterally, cover defects after excision of the sternum in post-sternotomy infections; (3) plug intrathoracic pleurocutaneous fistulas; and (4) reconstruct head and neck defects.

Latissimus Dorsi Muscle. This is the widest muscle of the back. It is thin and aponeurotic in its attachment to the vertebral column. It arises along the middle line from the spinous processes of the six lower thoracic vertebrae, from the lumbar fascia, and from the posterior part of the outer lip of the iliac crest as well as from the lowest three ribs and the inferior angle of the scapula. Its fibers are directed laterally and upward and converge to be inserted, after turning around the lower border of the teres major, by a tendon into the bottom of the bicipital groove in front of the teres major. It receives its nerve supply from the thoracodorsal branch of the brachial plexus. The muscle is primarily an extensor and medial rotator of the arm.

Its dominant blood supply is derived from the thoracodorsal artery, a branch of the subscapular artery. Paravertebral posterior perforating arteries provide the main blood supply to the distal part of the muscle.

The latissimus dorsi flap is usually elevated on its thoracodorsal pedicle so that the flap can be swung as a pendulum and cover many areas within its reach. It can also be based distally by preserving the paravertebral perforators with division of the muscle insertion and its proximal pedicle to cover defects of the abdomen, flank, and lower thoracolumbar area.

The latissimus dorsi muscle is used to (1) reconstruct breast using the upper two thirds of the muscle; (2) repair defects of chest wall, back, abdomen, and upper limb; and (3) repair defects of the head and neck.

Rectus Abdominis Muscle. This muscle arises from the pubic crest and symphysis and ascends to be inserted into the xiphoid cartilage and into the fifth, sixth, and seventh costal cartilages. The muscle is divided transversely by three and occasionally four tendinous intersections, known as lineae transversae, through which it is firmly attached to the anterior wall of the rectus sheath. Its nerve supply is derived from the 5th through 12th intercostal nerves.

The epigastric arcade is formed by the superior and inferior epigastric arteries anastomosing to form an arcade that gives off two rows of perforating vessels that are situated paramedially and perforate the anterior rectus sheath to supply the overlying skin. The accompanying venae comitantes have valves permitting one-way flow toward the liver. The communications between deep and superficial vascular arcades give the overlying skin a dual blood supply, permitting transfer of the transverse island abdominal flap for breast reconstruction.

The rectus abdominis receives an additional segmental blood supply through the segmental intercostal vessels, which enter the muscle posteriorly for free anastomosis with the epigastric arcade.

The inferior epigastric artery is the larger of the two main vessels, but the entire muscle can survive on either of these two pedicles. Muscle segments are also capable of surviving on intercostal branches only.

The rectus abdominis muscle is used in the following ways: (1) As a transverse island abdominal flap for breast reconstruction (TRAM flap). It provides a breast mound consisting of autogenous tissue without the need for a prosthesis. The flap is based on the superior epigastric artery, with a skin island situated at the umbilical level. (2) As coverage for mediastinal wound infection, complementary to the use of the pectoralis major, after aortocoronary bypass. The entire muscle is based on the superior epigastric artery (Fig. 6–15). (3) As coverage for defects of the upper thigh and perineum area if the flap is based on the inferior epigastric artery. The muscle may also be transposed intra-abdominally to fill pelvic defects following pelvic exenteration.

Gluteus Maximus Muscle. The most superficial muscle of the buttocks, the gluteus maximus has a fleshy origin from the posterior fifth of the iliac crest, the posterior layer of the lumbar fascia, and the back of the lower part of sacrum, coccyx, and sacrotuberous ligament. Its fibers are directed downward and laterally to be inserted into the strong iliotibial tract of the thigh and into the rough gluteal tuberosity above the linea aspera of the femur. It is innervated by the inferior gluteal nerve.

The superior and inferior gluteal arteries, derived from the hypogastric (internal iliac) artery, provide its blood supply. The two vascular pedicles enter the

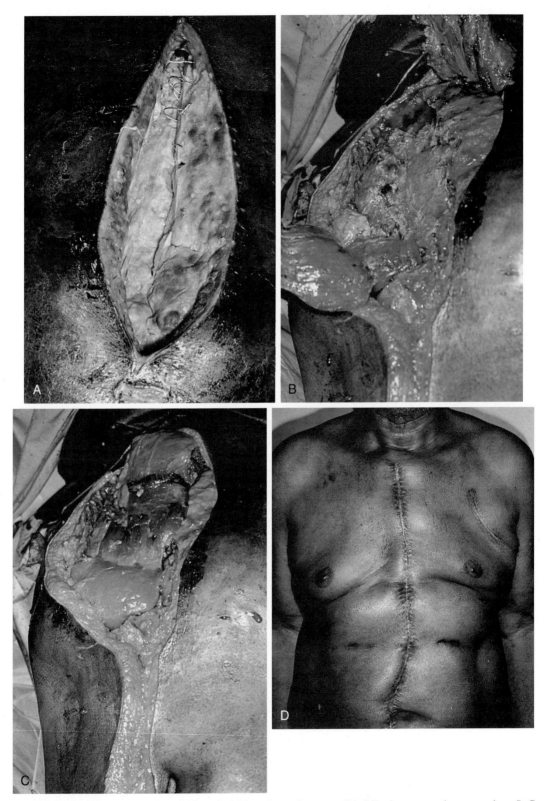

FIGURE 6–15. *A,* A patient has developed mediastinitis and sternal osteomyelitis following an open heart procedure. *B, C,* The wound, including infected bone and cartilage, must be excised, leaving significant dead space and exposed heart. *D,* The wound has been closed with a rectus abdominis muscle and single pectoralis muscle and the skin closed over the muscle flaps.

posterior medial muscle belly from beneath the sacrum to supply the superior and inferior components of the muscle.

Released from its insertion in the femur, the musculocutaneous flap provides coverage of defects in the ischium and sacrum, as the unit can be rotated upward or downward. Its use in paraplegics reduces the impact of the muscle's loss of function. When used in ambulatory patients, only segmental transfer is practical.

RECONSTRUCTION OF LOWER EXTREMITY

Tensor Fascia Lata Muscle. Situated in the upper third of the thigh, this muscle arises from the anterior superior iliac spine, and its fleshy belly descends to be inserted into the iliotibial tract of the fascia lata within 6 inches of its origin. Situated between the sartorius and gluteus medius muscles at its origin, its nerve supply is derived from the superior gluteal nerve.

Its vascular pedicle is the transverse branch of the lateral circumflex artery, which comes off the profunda femoris artery to enter the muscle about 3 inches below the muscle's origin. The vascular pedicle permits the flap to have a wide arc of rotation anteriorly and posteriorly, especially if designed as an island. The inclusion of the lateral cutaneous nerve of the thigh in the flap permits retention of sensation in the flap.

The tensor fascia lata is used for (1) coverage of defects over the pubis, and (2) reconstruction of the lower abdomen.

Gracilis Muscle. This superficial, long, thin, flat muscle extends from its origin at the medial margin of the pubis and adjacent inferior pubic ramus to its insertion by its flat tendon into the medial surface of the tibia under cover of the sartorius insertion. Its nerve supply comes from branches of the obturator nerve.

Its vascular supply consists of four pedicles along the deep aspect of the muscle. The predominant pedicle is the first and largest one from the medial femoral circumflex artery. It enters the muscle about 4 inches from the pubic tubercle. The entire muscle can survive off this pedicle, with viability of overlying skin over the proximal half of the muscle. The pedicle determines the arc of rotation. The distal blood supply of the muscle derives from a branch of the superficial femoral artery.

The gracilis muscle is used for (1) vaginal reconstruction after pelvic exenteration, (2) perineal and penile reconstruction, and (3) as a free microvascular flap for resurfacing of lower extremity defects.

Rectus Femoris Muscle. This fleshy prominence in front of the thigh arises from the pelvis by a straight head attached to the anterior inferior iliac spine and a reflected head from the rough groove on the outer surface of the ilium just above the acetabulum. The two fuse to form a single tendon that spreads out to the fleshy fibers, terminating in a tendon that joins the quadriceps femoris aponeurosis to form a common tendon for insertion to the upper edge and sides of the patella. The femoral nerve provides its motor innervation.

Its vascular supply comes directly from the lateral circumflex artery, which enters the muscle about 4 inches below its origin and provides the pedicle that determines its arc of rotation. Just before penetrating the muscle, the artery divides into superior and inferior branches. The upper branch can, however, sustain the entire muscle if the inferior branch is divided.

The rectus femoris is used for (1) reconstruction of lower abdominal defects,

(2) reconstruction of perineum or groin, and (3) intra-abdominal coverage and support of the pelvic floor.

Gastrocnemius Muscle. This uppermost superficial calf muscle has two heads of origin—a medial head arising from the upper aspect of the medial femoral condyle, just below and behind the insertion of the adductor longus, and a lateral head with a tendon of origin in a pit on the outer surface of the lateral femoral condyle, just above the attachment of the popliteus muscle. The fleshy fibers of the two heads unite along the midline by an aponeurosis, which terminates with the soleus in a common tendon, the tendo Achilles, into the calcaneus. Its nerve supply is from the medial popliteal nerve.

Its vascular supply is from the sural branches of the popliteal artery. Each muscle has an independent blood supply, which permits use of each as a separate unit. Each pedicle enters its head close to its origin, where it divides and runs down the muscle parallel to its fibers. The medial gastrocnemius is the larger of the two heads and can be transposed or rotated around the medial or lateral side to cover defects of the knee or upper half of the lower leg.

Soleus Muscle. This large, flat muscle arises from the head and upper third of the posterior surface of the fibular shaft, as well as the soleal line of the tibia, and from a thick fibrous arch over the large blood vessels of the back of the leg, and merges with the tendon of insertion. Its nerve supply is from the medial popliteal nerve.

Its vascular supply is predominantly from the popliteal vessels, but distally it receives blood via perforating branches of the posterior tibial artery.

The soleus muscle is used in two ways: (1) Based on its proximal pedicles and detached from its tendon of insertion, the soleus can be used to cover midtibial defects. (2) Based on its distal segmented vascular supply, the muscle can be turned down for coverage of small ankle defects.

It is becoming increasingly apparent that many muscle units can be used to reconstruct or provide coverage for pathologic lesions. The functional deficit that may occur from the use of such units varies at different sites and in different patients. Awareness of such anticipated functional deficits and disclosure of the potential resulting defect should be shared with the patient in planning and carrying out such reconstructive musculocutaneous flaps.

Other muscles that have been used as flaps with or without associated skin territory for reconstruction of local deficiencies or defects include the internal oblique, serratus anterior, pectoralis minor, biceps femoris, vastus medialis and lateralis, and intrinsic foot muscles.

FASCIOCUTANEOUS FLAPS

These flaps include fascia, subcutaneous tissue, and skin. They are relatively easy and quick to raise and are well vascularized. They are an excellent source of tissue because they provide a relatively thin flap, avoid the need for sacrifice of a muscle, and are readily available in all regions of the body. A rich system of vessels passes through intermuscular septa, giving off branches that perforate the fascia and divide to join with the rich subdermal plexus of vessels. Three distinct anatomic types of fasciocutaneous flap may be elevated on this system of septocutaneous vessels.

Random Fasciocutaneous Flap

The pedicle is supplied by multiple fasciocutaneous perforators at the base of the designed flap. These perforators arise from the septocutaneous vessels and, after perforating the fascia, divide into multiple branches that anastomose with similar branches from adjacent septocutaneous vessels. This radial pattern, formed by the terminal branches of the septocutaneous system, provides a rich network of vessels. These flaps are available only as pedicle-based flaps (Fig. 6–16A).

Axial Fasciocutaneous Flaps

The flap is based on an axial artery with its venae comitantes running just beneath or just above the fascia. This artery is a branch from another septocutaneous artery or major artery. The flap is oriented axially along the vessel (Fig. 6–16B). Examples of this flap include the following:

Posterior calf fasciocutaneous flap, based on a descending branch of the popliteal artery
Scapular and parascapular flaps based on the circumflex scapular artery
Lateral arm flap based on the posterior radial collateral artery
Deltoid flap based on the posterior circumflex humeral artery
Temporoparietal flap based on the temporal vessels

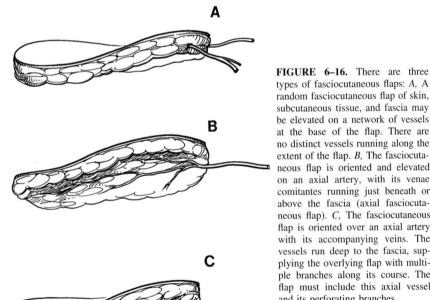

FIGURE 6–16. There are three types of fasciocutaneous flaps: *A,* A random fasciocutaneous flap of skin, subcutaneous tissue, and fascia may be elevated on a network of vessels at the base of the flap. There are no distinct vessels running along the extent of the flap. *B,* The fasciocutaneous flap is oriented and elevated on an axial artery, with its venae comitantes running just beneath or above the fascia (axial fasciocutaneous flap). *C,* The fasciocutaneous flap is oriented over an axial artery with its accompanying veins. The vessels run deep to the fascia, supplying the overlying flap with multiple branches along its course. The flap must include this axial vessel and its perforating branches.

A second type of axial fasciocutaneous flap is based on multiple small branches passing through the intermuscular septum from a major deep vessel (Fig. 6–16C). Examples of this flap include the following:

Peroneal island flap based on the peroneal vessels
Radial forearm flap based on the radial artery

Axial fasciocutaneous flaps, whether based on a major artery or a branch of a major artery, may be used as pedicled flaps or transferred as free fasciocutaneous flaps. Branches from these axial vessels may directly supply adjacent bone, allowing transfer of vascularized bone. Common examples of these osteocutaneous flaps include the following:

Radial forearm osteocutaneous flap with a segment of radius
Scapular flap with a segment of the lateral border of the scapula
Fibular free flap based on the peroneal artery
Deep circumflex iliac flap carrying a segment of iliac crest

Suggested Readings

Carriquiry C, Costa MA, Vasconez LO: An anatomic study of the septocutaneous vessels of the leg. Plast Reconstr Surg 76:354, 1985
Cormack GC, Lamberty BGH: A classification of fasciocutaneous flaps according to their patterns of vascularization. Br J Plast Surg 37:80, 1984
McCraw JB, Vasconez LO: Musculocutaneous flaps: Principles. Clin Plast Surg 7:9, 1980
McGregor IA, Jackson IT: The groin flap. Br J Plast Surg 25:3, 1972
McGregor IA, Morgan C: Axial and random pattern flaps. Br J Plast Surg 26:202, 1973
Orticochea M: History of the discovery of the musculocutaneous flap method as a substitute for the delay method. Ann Plast Surg 11:63, 1983.
Ponten S: The fasciocutaneous flap: Its use in soft tissue defects of the lower leg. Br J Plast Surg 34:215, 1983
Reinisch JF: The pathophysiology of skin flap circulation. The delay phenomenon. Plast Surg 15:436, 1985

CHAPTER **7**

Tissue Expansion

Tissue expansion has added a new dimension to the techniques available for reconstructive surgery. It has helped overcome the limitations imposed by lack of available local tissue so that large defects can now be handled expeditiously, using expansion techniques to facilitate the use of well-tested reconstructive procedures.

As a living organ, skin responds dynamically to mechanical stress. The skin envelope responds to incorporate accumulated subcutaneous fat in the development of obesity. It responds in similar fashion to the rapidly expanding abdomen during pregnancy. Primitive tribes in Africa and Central America have long appreciated that the labial soft tissues and ear lobes could be stretched to immense proportions by slow mechanical stress. These observations led to the clinical application of mechanical skin expansion as an initial step in some reconstructive procedures. First used in postmastectomy breast reconstruction, the procedure has been extended to augmentation of soft tissue to facilitate the advancement of wound edges for direct closure as well as for the rotation and transposition of skin and fasciocutaneous and musculocutaneous flaps.

Tissue expansion stretches available local tissue, generating increased tissue for reconstruction of defects without unduly compromising the donor area. It also avoids the need for transfer of distant, dissimilar skin and soft tissue. Infection, prosthesis extrusion, and necrosis of overlying skin are all potential complications that can be minimized by diligent attention to proper performance of the procedure, careful follow-up of patients, and adherence to the principles of skin and soft tissue expansion.

Expander Prosthesis

The prosthesis consists of a silicone bag connected to a self-sealing injection port. This port is connected to the prosthesis by a length of tubing, or the implant may have a self-contained port (Fig. 7–1). The port is distinct from the main expander, and a needle is easily inserted for saline injection. As saline is injected into the port, it passes into the expander, which is progressively inflated. As the expander inflates, it stretches the overlying tissues.

Prostheses may be round, rectangular, or tubular in shape, ranging in volume from 10 to 1000 cc, although any size or shape can be custom fabricated.

Technique of Expansion

Choice of donor site is determined by the desire to transfer tissue from an area of close proximity to the defect, because this tissue is most similar to the tissue being replaced.

The incision for placement of the prosthesis is made in an area that will be either well hidden or incorporated into the incision for the subsequent reconstructive procedure (Fig. 7–2). The pocket is dissected for comfortable placement of the expander, and meticulous hemostasis is ensured. The valve is placed about 5 cm away in a separate pocket if a distant valve is used. The valve is positioned so as not to be over a bony prominence or in a location subject to prolonged pressure.

After wound closure, saline is introduced into the prosthesis in a volume sufficient to obliterate the dead space in the pocket. Subsequent inflations are

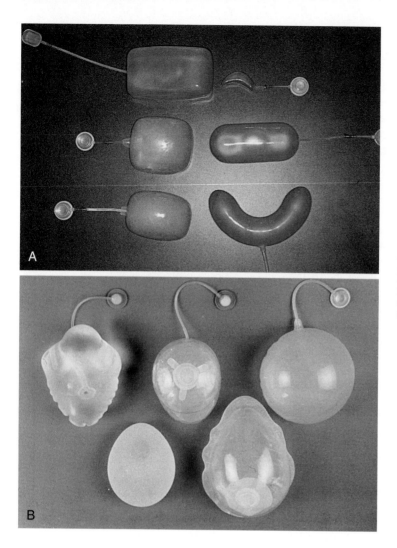

FIGURE 7–1. *A*, Expander prostheses with distant injection ports. *B*, Expander prostheses used for breast reconstruction. Both integrated and distant injection port prostheses are available.

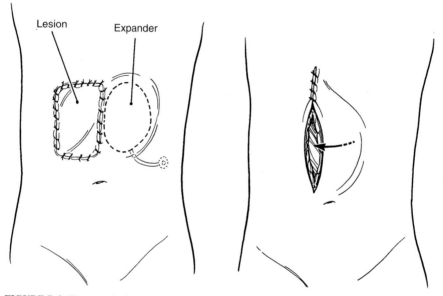

FIGURE 7–2. The expander is usually placed through an incision adjacent to the lesion. Once adequate expansion has been achieved, the prosthesis is removed and the loose tissue is advanced or transposed into the defect.

commenced about 2 weeks later when the wound has developed sufficient tensile strength.

The prosthesis is inflated by introducing a needle into the valve with injection of saline until the skin feels tense or discomfort is engendered. Capillary refill is used as a test of capillary perfusion, and inflation is discontinued before capillary perfusion is compromised. On the average, the interval between injections is 7 days but may vary from 4 to 14 days, the objective being to develop tissue for optimal cosmetic reconstruction and not to develop tissue as rapidly as possible. As the expander fills, overlying tissues are stretched. These tissues relax during the interval between inflations, allowing serial stretching or expansion at each inflation. The inflations are continued until sufficient tissue has been generated or clinical experience suggests undue compromise of tissues if expansions are continued. Definitive reconstruction is then accomplished using the expanded soft tissues.

TISSUE RESPONSE TO EXPANSION

The major changes occur in the dermis with fibroplasia, increased collagen deposition, and realignment of collagen fiber. A marked increase in vasculature occurs, especially at the junction of the developing periprosthetic capsule and the adjacent dermal tissue. The skeletal muscle becomes thin and compacted, and adipose tissue undergoes atrophy.

Complications

Complications of expansion include hematoma, seroma, infection, extrusion, leakage, and deflation. Hematoma is avoided by meticulous hemostasis, and seroma is minimized by obliteration of dead space with conservative inflation of the prosthesis at placement. Infection is unusual in clean wounds, although placement of expanders adjacent to open or infected wounds does carry a significant rate of periprosthetic infection. Mechanical problems, including leaking and deflation, can be minimized by careful handling of the prosthesis and injection ports. If they do occur, the implant can be readily replaced in the previously dissected pocket.

Extrusion of the implant is a potentially serious complication because it can compromise the tissue needed for reconstruction. Care must be taken to dissect an adequate pocket for the prosthesis, avoiding pressure on the wound edge. The implant must be well seated to prevent displacement under adjacent skin graft or unstable tissue, and folds in the silicone wall are adjusted to prevent pressure areas. Injection ports are placed away from positional pressure points. Should a partial extrusion or exposure occur late in expansion, topical antimicrobials are used to coat the implant. Expansion is continued for a short period, and definitive reconstruction is accomplished once prolonging expansion is no longer expedient.

REGIONAL EXPANSION

The Breast

Tissue expansion was initially used to facilitate breast reconstruction in postmastectomy patients with insufficient chest wall tissue for simple placement of a permanent implant. Current mastectomy procedures leave the pectoralis major intact so that the prosthesis can be placed beneath the pectoralis major as well as the serratus anterior and origin of the rectus abdominis. Expansion is initiated 2 weeks after placement of the implant and the implant is inflated at weekly intervals until inflation is 50 to 70 per cent greater than the final desired volume. The longer the fully inflated expander is left, the greater the likelihood of simulating an inframammary crease, and one might wait several months before replacing the inflated expander with a permanent implant (Fig. 7–3).

Placement of an expander prosthesis is an ideal technique in immediate breast reconstruction following mastectomy. After the mastectomy is accomplished, the expander prosthesis is placed in a subpectoral and subserratus pocket, taking care to separate the implant from the subcutaneous mastectomy space with a myofascial layer. Enough saline is introduced into the expander to obliterate dead space. Once the wound is healed, expansion and reconstruction are completed.

Expansion and reconstruction of the breast can be used in a similar manner for breast deformities due to burns, trauma, or congenital aplasia, as in Poland syndrome. Poland syndrome patients have skin and subcutaneous tissue that are contracted or deficient and require expansion through a transaxillary or inframammary incision before a reconstructive implant can be placed. If the contralateral breast is still growing, the expander is an effective temporizer. It is placed under the hypoplastic breast in adolescent patients and serially inflated to maintain symmetry with the normal breast. This provides an ongoing dynamic reconstruction of the aplastic chest with great psychological benefit.

Trunk and Extremities

Expansion of the trunk, the upper extremity above the elbow, and the lower extremity above the knee are readily accomplished because they all tolerate expansion quite well. Expanders are placed around the defect (Fig. 7–4) and, once surrounding tissues are fully expanded, they can be advanced or transposed as full-thickness flaps into the adjacent defect. This is very effective after excision of large lesions or unsightly skin grafts.

In the extremities the expansion technique may be used after excision of tattoos, large nevi, congenital lesions, large scars, or skin grafts.

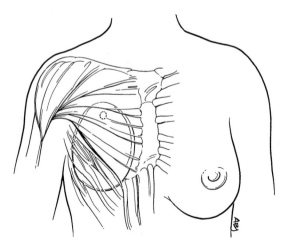

FIGURE 7–3. The tissue expander is ideally placed beneath the pectoralis major, the origin of the serratus anterior, and the origin of the rectus abdominis muscles when expanding chest wall soft tissue for breast reconstruction.

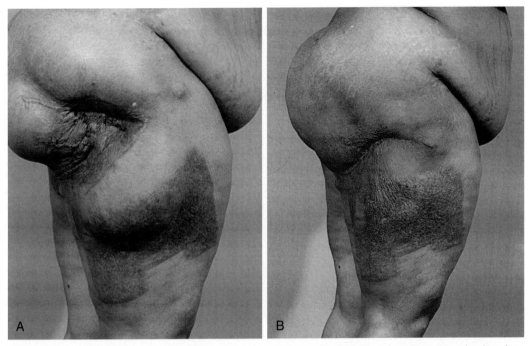

FIGURE 7–4. A patient with a soft tissue tumor initially treated with excision and skin graft. *A*, Three expanders have been placed circumferentially around the defect. *B*, Following 6 weeks of inflations, sufficient tissue has been generated that the depressed graft site may be excised and a primary closure achieved.

Expansion below the elbow and knee should be done very carefully, as the risks of infection and extrusion are high. Care must be used in crush-injured tissues, with compromise of venous and lymphatic drainage, because they do not tolerate expansion well.

Scalp

Repair of scalp abnormality due to congenital defect, trauma, burn injury, tumor extirpation, or alopecia is facilitated by tissue expansion (Fig. 7–5). The expander is placed deep to the galea immediately over the periosteum. After 6 to 8 weeks of serial inflations, the expanded tissue is advanced, rotated, or transposed into the defect. Placement of expanders must be carefully planned so that ultimate tissue mobilization can use the temporal and occipital vessels. Hair growth in rearranged tissues must be oriented relative to normal direction, hairlines, and cowlicks.

Forehead

Forehead expansion aids in the reconstruction of defects due to removal of congenital lesions or tumors, and traumatic tissue loss. The prosthesis is placed beneath the frontalis muscle overlying the periosteum using an incision above the hairline or in an area that must be incised in the definitive reconstruction.

Pre-expansion of forehead flaps has facilitated the use of the forehead in reconstructing nasal defects. Expansion over a 6-week period generates enough

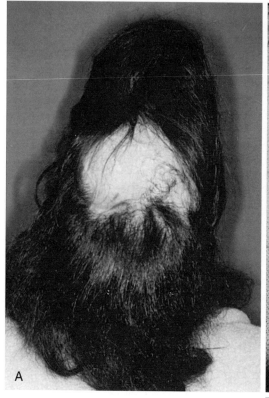

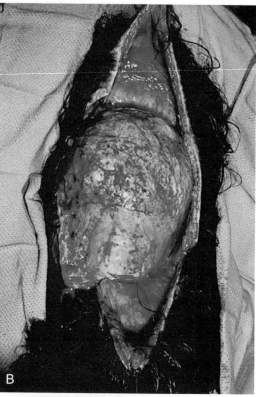

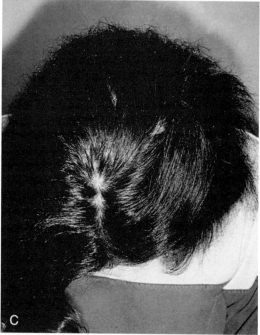

FIGURE 7–5. The scalp responds well to tissue expansion. *A*, An area of alopecia following a burn injury. Expanders have been placed in the anterior and posterior hair-bearing scalp and inflated over a 6-week period. *B*, Following removal of expander prostheses, the remaining scalp has been significantly stretched for tension-free transfer into the defect. *C*, Postoperative view following closure of the defect with minimal rewidening of the scar.

tissue for reconstruction of the skin surface and, by folding the flap on itself, for the nasal lining as well. The capsule that forms around the prosthesis is best removed to avoid a thick, amorphous nasal reconstruction.

Face and Neck

Reconstruction of the face requires attention to function, symmetry, color, and texture of the facial skin. In planning placement of the prosthesis, attention must be paid to where scars will lie when the expanded flaps are advanced and to hair pattern or, in the case of children, expected hair pattern.

When expanded flaps are rotated or advanced to periorbital and perioral regions, the flaps must be secured to underlying fascia and periosteum to minimize subsequent contracture and distortion of the eyes and mouth.

The central face is ideally covered with a large cheek rotation flap, so that the suture lines lie in the infraorbital area, along the border of the nasal aesthetic unit, and into the nasolabial fold. In placing the prosthesis, the dissection is carried out between the subcutaneous tissue and the superficial fascial layer over the parotid capsule without injuring the facial nerve branches.

Lower face reconstruction is best served by tissue expansion of the neck. Over 800 cc of expansion can be provided via two expanders without compromising the many anatomic structures in the neck. The implant is best placed external to the platysma (Fig. 7–6).

For reconstruction of the lateral face, the maximal amount of tissue should be generated in the preauricular area and in the posterior neck below the hairline. The flap, based inferiorly and laterally, can then be rotated medially to reconstruct a lateral facial defect.

Ear

Ear reconstruction requires a sufficiency of non–hair-bearing skin, and this can be provided by expansion of the skin overlying the mastoid area. Once adjacent soft tissue is available for comfortable placement of a costal cartilage framework, the definitive reconstruction is carried out. Usually, the capsule that forms around the ear must be removed to get sufficient tissue thinness for adequate definition of the underlying framework.

Expansion of Myocutaneous and Fasciocutaneous Flaps

The latissimus dorsi, pectoralis major, and trapezius are important myocutaneous flaps used in the reconstruction of large head and neck defects after tumor excision or traumatic injuries.

These flaps can be significantly expanded in situ, facilitating difficult reconstructions. The expander is placed deep to the muscle and inflated weekly for up to 8 weeks, attaining a volume of 600 to 800 cc. The expanded muscle becomes

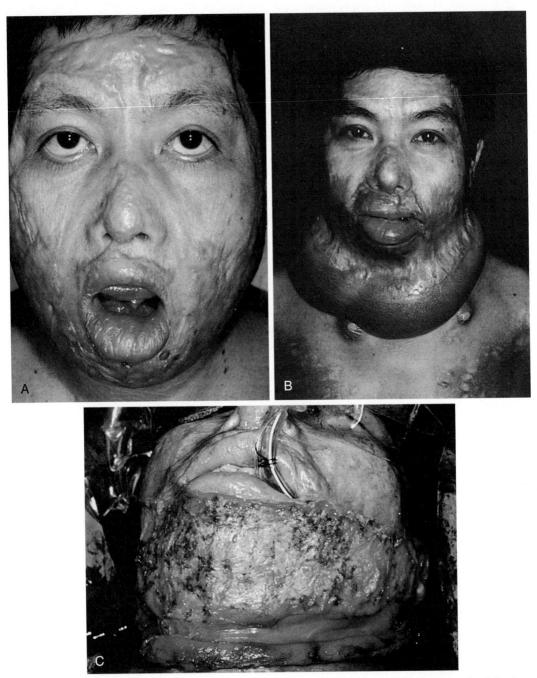

FIGURE 7–6. The elasticity of skin allows safe expansion in all areas of the body. *A,* Hypertrophic scarring following a deep partial-thickness burn. *B,* Tissue expanders have been placed in the neck and each has been inflated to a volume of 400 cc over an 8-week period. *C,* Burn scar from the lower lip margin to the level of the thyroid cartilage has been removed and sufficient skin stretching has been achieved to advance the unburned neck skin to close the defect *(D).* (From Marks MW, Argenta LC, Thornton JW: Burn management: The role of tissue expansion. Clin Plast Surg 14:543, 1987.)

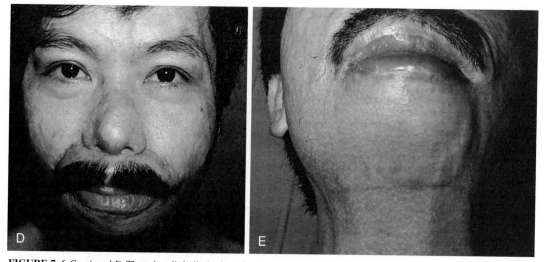

FIGURE 7–6 *Continued E,* There is a little limitation of neck extension. (From Marks MW, Argenta LC, Thornton JW: Burn management: The role of tissue expansion. Clin Plast Surg 14:543, 1987.)

significantly thinner, which is advantageous because of the reduced bulk. Expansion causes sufficient stretching of the overlying skin and soft tissue that very large flaps can be harvested with primary closure of the donor site. This is also true following expansion of fasciocutaneous flaps such as the lateral arm, radial forearm, and scapular free flaps.

Full-Thickness Grafts

Full-thickness skin graft donor sites must be closed primarily, often limiting the amount of skin that is available. This is especially true for facial grafts, best obtained from donor sites above the clavicle. Pre-expansion of donor skin generates more skin for grafting and facilitates primary closure of the donor site.

Suggested Readings

Argenta LC, Marks MW, Pasyk KA: Advances in tissue expansion. Clin Plast Surg 12:159, 1985

Argenta LC, Watanabe MJ, Grabb WC: The use of tissue expansion in head and neck reconstruction. Ann Plast Surg 11:31, 1983

Austad ED, Thomas SB, Pasyk K: Tissue expansion: Dividend or loan. Plast Reconstr Surg 78:63, 1986

Becker H: The permanent tissue expander. Clin Plast Surg 14:519, 1987

Manders EK, Graham WP, Schenden JM, et al: Skin expansion to eliminate large scalp defects. Ann Plast Surg 12:305, 1984

Manders EK, Schenden MJ, Furrey JA, et al: Soft-tissue expansion: Concepts and complications. Plast Reconstr Surg 74:493, 1984

Neumann CG: The expansion of an area of skin by progressive distention of a subcutaneous balloon. Plast Reconstr Surg 19:124, 1957

Pasyk KA, Argenta LC, Austad ED: Histopathology of human expanded tissue. Clin Plast Surg 14:435, 1987

Radovan C: Breast reconstruction after mastectomy using the temporary expander. Plast Reconstr Surg 69:195, 1982

Radovan C: Tissue expansion in soft-tissue reconstruction. Plast Reconstr Surg 74:842, 1984

CHAPTER **8**

Microvascular Surgery

The development of the operating microscope in 1921 set the stage for small vessel anastomosis. Jacobson and Suarez in 1960 successfully anastomosed blood vessels with an external diameter of 1.0 mm. By 1964 not only were partially amputated, nonviable fingers being revascularized, but the successful replantation of a completely amputated upper extremity was accomplished. Vessels with diameters of 0.5 mm are now routinely anastomosed in microvascular procedures.

The modern microscope has a fiberoptic light source and magnification that ranges from 6 × to 40 ×. Focal length can be changed through interchangeable lenses, but 200 mm is most popular.

Microinstruments and microclamps have been designed and perfected to satisfy clinical demand. Microsutures are monofilamentous of fine caliber between 18 and 24 μm swaged to atraumatic needles with diameters of 75 to 140 μm. Prolene suture or 9-0, 10-0, and 11-0 nylon suture is most commonly used for microvascular anastomoses, depending on vessel caliber.

MICROSURGICAL TECHNIQUE

1. Proper vessel preparation: Flap artery and vein should be débrided under high-power microscopic examination. Only adventitia should be handled and properly trimmed.
2. Preparation for anastomosis: After adequate exposure of the recipient site, the artery is visualized microscopically. Topical application of vasodilatory agents such as papaverine is provided if vascular spasm is present. The artery is divided or arteriotomy performed and good pulsatile flow ensured. The vein is similarly prepared and vessel ends are irrigated with heparinized saline.
3. Anastomosis performed: Whether to create an end-to-end or end-to-side anastomosis depends on the degree of luminal discrepancy and the expandability of the recipient vessel. The vessels are approximated and clamps adjusted to hold them in position without tension. Anastomosis is accomplished by one of three end-to-end techniques or an end-to-side technique (Fig. 8–1).
   a. 180° stay sutures: Two stay sutures of prolene or nylon on hand-honed, swaged microneedles are placed 180 degrees apart. This separates the front and back walls. After the front wall interrupted sutures are in place, the clamp is rotated through 180 degrees and the posterior wall is sutured. The fewest sutures are placed at right angles to the vessel wall to minimize the incidence of anastomotic clotting.
   b. Triangulated anastomosis: Three stay sutures are placed 120 degrees apart from each other. Light tension is placed on two stay sutures, and intervening sutures are placed. This is repeated with each set of two stay sutures.
   c. Back wall anastomosis: Sutures are placed in the back wall first, and the anterior wall is then approximated. This avoids the need to rotate the clamped vessels.
   d. End-to-side anastomosis: After arteriotomy is performed in the recipient vessel, an end-to-side anastomosis is accomplished.
4. Demonstrate patency of the anastomosis:
   a. Flicker test: The vessel distal to the anastomosis is gently partially occluded by lifting it with closed forceps. Blood is seen to pulsate or "flicker" through the narrowed segment.
   b. Double-occlusion "milking" test: The vessel distal to the anastomosis is

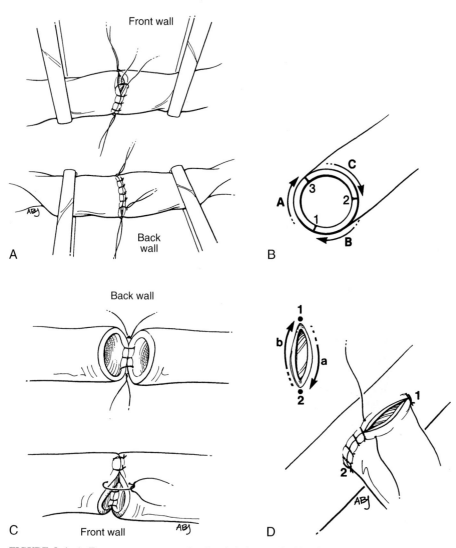

FIGURE 8–1. *A*, Two stay sutures are placed and tied on each side of the anastomosis 180 degrees apart. The anterior wall is then closed with simple interrupted sutures. The vessel is turned over between the two clamps and the back wall closed with simple interrupted sutures. *B*, The anastomosis may be triangulated by placing the first three sutures 120 degrees apart. Simple interrupted sutures are then used to close each segment between the stay sutures. *C*, If there is insufficient space to flip the vessel and its clamps back and forth, the anastomosis may be accomplished by the back-wall-first technique. After the back wall is approximated, closure is continued anteriorly across the front wall. *D*, Illustration of an end-to-side anastomosis.

doubly occluded and milked. As the proximal forceps is released, rapid filling of the milked segment is noted (Fig. 8–2).

5. Whether artery or vein should be anastomosed first depends on relative access for the second anastomosis and whether flow is to be restored only after both anastomoses are completed. If there is a question of which vein in a flap or replanted part is to be used, flow is restored in the artery after completion of the anastomosis. Backflow through the vein or veins is then evaluated and appropriate venous anastomosis accomplished. Arterial flow may also be re-established prior to vein anastomosis if transplanted or replanted tissues have had a prolonged ischemia time.

6. If there is doubt about the patency of an anastomosis, it should be revised.

7. Vein grafts are necessary if there is a sufficient gap between the donor and recipient sites, preventing a primary tension-free closure.

8. A bolus of 5000 U of heparin may be administered intravenously. Alternatively, a 100-ml bolus of low molecular weight dextran is given and continued at 20 ml postoperatively. Some prefer avoiding anticoagulation to minimize risk of postoperative hematoma.

Postoperative Management of Replanted Tissue

Apart from monitoring the patient's general status, it is imperative that signs of flap distress be noted at the earliest time and any necessary re-exploratory revision of vascular anastomosis be carried out.

Whether compromise is due to arterial or venous problems can be gauged by five basic parameters: (1) *Color*: With arterial occlusion, skin becomes pale and white. A cyanotic purple hue represents venous occlusion. (2) *Capillary refill* is decreased in poor arterial flow but is rapid if the problem is venous. (3) *Tissue turgor* is decreased with impaired arterial inflow but increased from the engorgement of venous impedance. (4) *Bleeding* on pin-prick is notably absent with arterial occlusion. With venous occlusion, a continuous purple ooze occurs. (5) *Temperature* of the flap drops quickly with arterial occlusion but very slowly with venous occlusion. Blood flow checks may use digital pulse oximetry, Doppler ultrasonography, and temperature thermocouples.

Pathogenesis of Microsurgical Failure

Early or late failure of a revascularization procedure may occur because of failure to attend to general systemic factors or to local intraoperative or postoperative detail. Proper preventive measures reduce the incidence of this catastrophe,

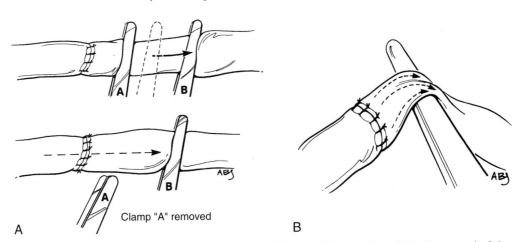

FIGURE 8–2. *A*, Patency of the anastomosis may be tested by the milking technique. Following removal of the proximal clamp, adequacy of flow is determined by speed of flow toward the distal clamp. *B*, Adequacy of flow may be determined by gentle narrowing of the posterior wall. Rapid flow should be noted over the partially occluding clamp.

whereas early diagnosis permits early ameliorative action with re-exploration of the vascular anastomoses.

1. Systemic factors
   a. Hypovolemia with failure to restore circulating blood volume
   b. Hypercoagulable states such as polycythemia, thrombocythemia, and vascular spasm due to smoking or local infiltration of epinephrine
2. Local factors
   a. Anastomotic errors leading to thrombosis
      1. Major vessel size discrepancy
      2. Intimal flap
      3. Partial suture occlusion of lumen
      4. Anastomosis completed under tension
   b. Occlusion of pedicle
      1. Intrinsic: vessels kinked, twisted, or injured
      2. Extrinsic: compression of vessels by edema, hematoma, skin closure, or tight dressing leading to impaired arterial inflow or venous drainage

REPLANTATION

The development of microneurovascular surgery has enabled replantation of amputated digits and limbs and assurance of the part's survival. It needs to be stressed, however, that survival of a replanted part lacking adequate function may represent a liability rather than a benefit. Careful patient selection, with emphasis on technical factors that result in an optimal range of motion and sensory perception of the replanted part, becomes very important.

Contraindications to Elective Replantation of Digits

1. Absolute contraindications
   a. Serious associated injuries that have priority
   b. Extensive injury or multiple areas of injury of the affected part which preclude a good functional result
   c. Significant systemic disorder creating danger of operation, including advanced age
2. Relative contraindications
   a. Single-digit amputation: Replantation requires a lengthy procedure and 4 to 5 days in the hospital and often ends with significant work loss and a stiff finger. Alternatives must be carefully discussed. Replantations distal to the insertion of the flexor superficialis generally result in excellent function and may be worthwhile in single-digit replants.
   b. Avulsion injuries: The extensive laceration of vessels and nerves proximal to the apparent amputation site may compromise a successful outcome.
   c. Warm ischemia time greater than 6 hours leads to irreversible muscle damage. If the part is kept cooled, replantation may be delayed for up to 12 hours. Fingers that have no muscle may be replanted after prolonged ischemia.
   d. Contamination of the part should not prevent its replantation unless the

tissues are so impregnated with foreign material as to make débridement impossible.

Salvage Replantation

Despite the above prohibitions, attempts at salvage replantation are justified in (1) children: Results are usually good with time for rehabilitation and planning future vocation; (2) multiple digit loss: Reconstruction is based on the greatest potential for restoration of function; and (3) thumb replacement, which is essential whenever possible (Fig. 8–3).

Technical Considerations

1. Upon arrival at the hospital, a thorough clinical examination is done, and any necessary investigations and resuscitative procedures are completed.
   a. Prophylactic antibiotics are commenced.
   b. Tetanus prophylaxis is administered.
   c. Radiographic studies of the affected extremity and of the amputated part are carried out.
   d. The patient is transferred to the operating room.
2. A double team of surgeons is generally advisable.
   a. Anesthesia: Axillary block with 0.5 per cent bupivacaine (Marcaine) and epinephrine provides upper limb anesthesia for 8 hours. Complementary sedation with diazepam and narcotics provides for a totally relaxed patient.

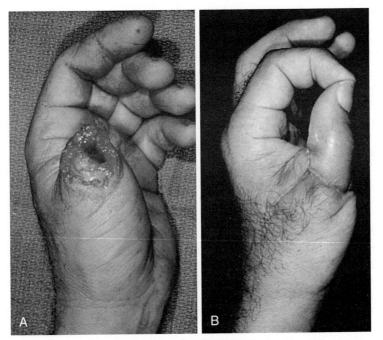

FIGURE 8–3. Preoperative *(A)* and postoperative *(B)* views of a replanted thumb.

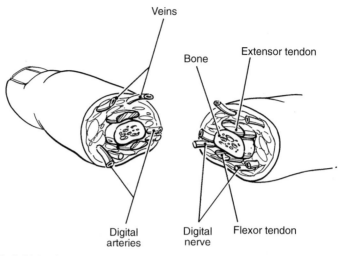

FIGURE 8–4. Digit reimplantation requires meticulous reapproximation of multiple structures. The bone is fixed first, followed by flexor tendon and at least one digital artery. The digital nerves are repaired, and the extremity is turned over and the extensor tendon is repaired. Ideally at least two veins should be repaired and the skin loosely reapproximated.

General anesthesia, however, minimizes patient movement and facilitates harvesting of vein or skin grafts.

b. Preparation of the components: The primary team, after application of a tourniquet, dissects out the neurovascular structures, tendons, and bone of the proximal limb while the secondary team carries out the same maneuvers on the distal amputated part (Fig. 8–4). Once the corresponding structures have been dissected out, identified, and labeled, the proximal tourniquet is removed, having obtained clamp control of the vascular structures.

c. Skeletal management: Using the previously performed radiographs for guidance, the fractured bone ends are débrided and shortened without compromising function. Solid fixation of the bone ends is accomplished, using compression plates for metacarpals, radius, ulna, and humerus. Intraosseous wiring, pin fixation, or plate fixation may be used for the phalanges.

d. Tendon repair of the flexor tendon is accomplished with loupe magnification using 4-0 synthetic nonabsorbable suture. The extensor tendon may be repaired at this time or following repair of the volar arteries and nerves.
Stabilization of bone and tendons reduces risk of disruption of the subsequent neurovascular procedures. At this juncture the operating microscope is introduced into the field.

e. Vascular anastomoses: The least traumatized artery is repaired first. Once flow is re-established, bleeding through transected veins is identified and vein repair is accomplished. Ideally, two veins are repaired. If time permits, a second artery may be repaired, although this is not practical in multiple digit replacements.

f. Neural anastomoses are performed following arterial repair or at a final stage prior to skin closure.

g. Loose skin closure concludes the operation, either by loose approximation of the skin edges or by application of a split-thickness graft or a flap, depending on local circumstances.

3. Postoperative management: Careful monitoring of the circulation is carried out. Active motion is commenced as soon as practical to prevent contracture, joint stiffness, or adhesion of tendons to the surrounding tissues.

FREE TISSUE TRANSFER

A free flap represents a composite mass of tissue with a vascular pedicle that is removed operatively from one part of the body and immediately transferred to a distant recipient site where vascular integrity is restored by microvascular anastomosis (Fig. 8–5). The groin flap was first transferred as a free flap in 1972, and since then the vascular anatomy of numerous muscle, musculocutaneous, fascial, fasciocutaneous, bone and osteocutaneous flaps has been described. Numerous flaps are available for free tissue transfer; several of the more common flaps are described below:

Muscle and Musculocutaneous Flaps

Latissimus Dorsi. A large flat muscle, it arises from the spinous processes below T5, the lower four ribs, and the posterior iliac crest. The fibers converge to insert in the intertubercular groove of the humerus. The muscle is supplied by the thoracodorsal artery, which arises from the subscapular artery, which is the third branch of the axillary artery. The muscle may be expended with little to no disability, as its functions are compensated for by the actions of adjacent synergistic muscles.

Rectus Abdominis. The rectus abdominis free flap is based on the muscle's inferior pedicle. The inferior epigastric artery originates from the external iliac artery just above the inguinal ligament and provides an arterial pedicle 3 to 3.5 mm in diameter. The vein, which is about 4 mm in diameter, drains into the external iliac vein. This large-caliber pedicle provides a technically easy free tissue transfer (Fig. 8–6). A large transverse skin paddle up to 40 cm in length can be taken with the muscle, which originates from the pubic crest and inserts on the fifth through seventh ribs.

Serratus Anterior. This flat muscle is supplied by a branch of the thoracodor-

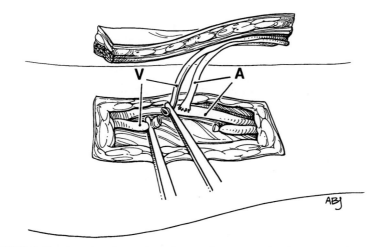

FIGURE 8–5. Free tissue transfer requires microvascular anastomosis of an artery and vein. The flap is then inset, avoiding any kinking of the donor or recipient vessels.

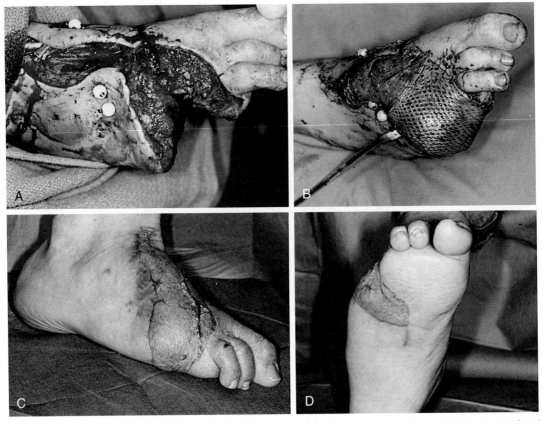

FIGURE 8–6. *A,* Preoperative review of a lawn mower injury to a foot. *B,* The rectus abdominis muscle has been transferred to the foot, and its vessels have been anastomosed to the anterior tibial artery and its vena comitans. *C, D,* Three months postoperatively the wound is well healed, and the soft tissue contour is adequate for ambulation and the wearing of shoes.

sal artery. It arises from the first through eighth ribs and inserts on the medial border of the scapula. It is innervated by the long thoracic nerve, and the lower slips of the muscle may be used as a free muscle transfer for facial reanimation. Sacrifice of the entire muscle leads to a winged scapula and weakness on raising the arm above horizontal.

Pectoralis Minor. A small flat muscle, it may be transferred on the thoracoacromial vessels. It is innervated by the lateral pectoral nerve and may be used for facial reanimation.

Gracilis. The gracilis is an ideal muscle for small wounds and has also been used in facial reanimation procedures. The muscle arises from the symphysis pubis and pubic arch and inserts below the medial condyle of the tibia. It is an adductor of the thigh and a leg flexor, but adjacent synergistic muscles compensate for its loss. The muscle has several pedicles, but free tissue transfer is based on the medial femoral circumflex artery branching from the profunda femoris artery. The vessel caliber is about 1.5 mm in diameter with two adjacent venae comitantes.

Gluteus Maximus. A robust flap, it carries significant subcutaneous tissue and skin and may be used for postmastectomy breast reconstruction. It is usually transferred on the superior gluteal artery and is technically difficult because of the short vascular pedicle. The muscle is an important hip extender and lateral rotator of the thigh, and the inferior portion of the muscle must be spared in ambulatory patients.

Fascial and Fasciocutaneous Flaps

Temporoparietal Flap. The temporoparietal fascia lies between the subcutaneous tissue hair follicles above and the superficial temporal fascia below. The superficial temporal artery and vein lie quite superficial in the fascia. On occasion the vein is absent or inadequate for microvascular anastomosis, and the posterior auricular vein may be used. The flap is thin and ideal for covering hand and foot defects. The flap must be covered with a skin graft. It may also be used to contour facial deformities resulting from atrophy of subcutaneous tissues.

Scapular Flap. The scapular free flap provides a large paddle of skin and subcutaneous tissue up to 30 cm in length. The flap is based on the circumflex scapular vessels, which exit the triangular space between the teres major, teres minor, and triceps. The flap may be designed either transversely or obliquely along the lateral border of the scapula on the descending branch of the circumflex scapular vessels (Fig. 8–7).

Radial Forearm Flap. The forearm provides an ideal donor site for a flap composed of thin skin with minimal subcutaneous tissue. The flap is designed along the length of the radial artery, which averages 2.5 mm in caliber, providing an easy technical anastomosis. A sensate flap is provided by including the superficial radial nerve and antebrachial cutaneous nerve. The thin tissues of the forearm provide an ideal flap for reconstruction of the penis.

Lateral Arm Flap. This flap also provides a thin flap of skin and subcutaneous tissue. The flap is based on the profunda brachii artery, which has a caliber of 1.5 to 2 mm. This artery arises from the brachial artery inferior to the teres major muscle and runs in the spiral groove of the humerus with the radial nerve. The vessel has a caliber of 1.5 to 2 mm. The posterior cutaneous nerve of the arm and forearm provides a sensate flap.

Groin Flap. The first flap used in free tissue transfer, it is based on the superficial circumflex iliac artery. This vessel originates from the femoral artery 2 to 4 cm below the inguinal ligament. Vessel caliber is about 2.5 mm in diameter. The advantage of this flap is its well hidden donor scar, although in many cases the amount of subcutaneous tissue in the area does not lend itself to an ideal skin flap.

Bone and Osteocutaneous Flaps

Fibula. The fibula is expendable as a bone flap, provided that the distal fourth of the fibula is left undisturbed to provide ankle stability. The fibular free flap is an ideal vascularized bone graft for repair of segmental long bone defects. It can also be osteotomized to reconstruct large mandibular defects. The flap supports

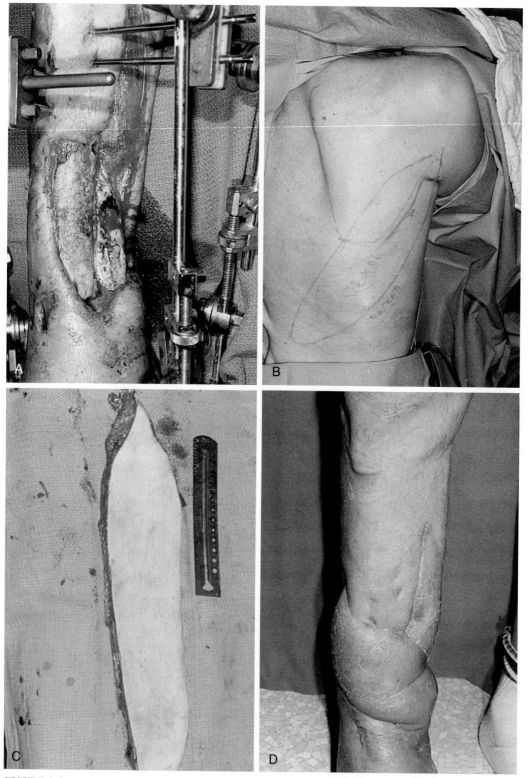

FIGURE 8–7. *A*, Large soft tissue defect over a comminuted tibial fracture. *B*, A 10 × 30 cm parascapular flap has been designed to include the descending branch of the circumflex scapular vessels. *C*, The flap has been harvested with an adequate arterial and venous pedicle. *D*, One year postoperatively the patient's bone is well healed and he has stable soft tissue coverage.

overlying skin if an osteocutaneous flap is desired. The fibular free flap is supplied by the peroneal artery, which has a caliber of 2 to 2.5 mm (Fig. 8–8).

Iliac Crest–Deep Circumflex Iliac Artery Flap. The iliac crest can be harvested with overlying soft tissue and skin based on the deep circumflex iliac artery. This vessel has a diameter of 1.5 to 2.5 mm and arises either from the external iliac artery above the inguinal ligament or from the femoral artery below the inguinal ligament. This flap provides a large segment of bone effective in reconstruction of significant mandibular defects.

Scapular Flap. The lateral border of the scapula may be harvested with a scapular free flap. Branches from the circumflex scapular artery to the periosteum over the lateral border of the scapula must be carefully preserved.

Radial Forearm. A segment of radius may be incorporated into a radial forearm flap. Approximately 40 per cent of the circumference of the radius may be safely harvested. The flap has the advantage of providing a bone graft with very thin overlying soft tissue and skin but is compromised by potential donor site morbidity.

Specialized Tissue Transfer

Toe Transfer. Toe transfers have proven effective in reconstruction of significant traumatic and congenital hand deformities. Either the great toe or a subtotal great toe transfer may be used for functional aesthetic thumb reconstructions. The second toe may be used for thumb reconstruction but is better reserved for digit reconstructions. Generally patients undergoing digit reconstruction have had amputation of four digits. A combined second and third toe transplant provides sensate digits against which a thumb can be opposed for functional hand reconstruction. The blood supply to the great toe is from the first dorsal metatarsal

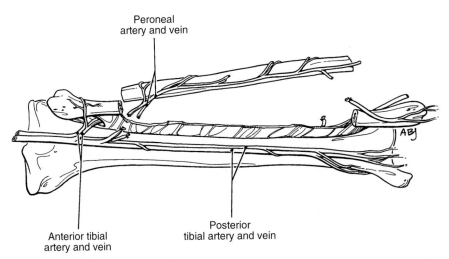

FIGURE 8–8. Bone may be transferred by microvascular technique. The fibula is transferred on the peroneal artery and its vena comitans, which runs along the axis of the bone and provides segmental perforating vessels.

artery, which is the terminal portion of the dorsalis pedis artery. The dorsalis pedis artery has a diameter of about 2.5 mm, which fits well in an anastomosis with the radial artery. The saphenous vein is used for venous drainage and matches the 3.5 mm diameter of the cephalic vein at the wrist. The second toe is generally transferred on the first dorsal metatarsal artery, although the plantar arteries may at times be preferable donor vessels.

Jejunum. The jejunum may be used as a free tissue transfer for the reconstruction of esophageal and pharyngeal defects. A segment of jejunum distal to the ligament of Treitz is harvested, and pedicle vessels are identified in the segment's mesentery.

Omentum. Omentum may be transferred on the right gastroepiploic vessels. It has been used to recontour facial defects in which overlying skin is adequate and transfer of skin is not required.

MICRONEURAL REPAIR

Structure of Nerve Trunk

The nerve fibers represent the basic anatomic unit of a peripheral nerve. Motor, sensory, and sympathetic fibers gather together to form a fascicle, which, with its tubular perineurium and its contained endoneurium, represents the macroscopic nerve unit. Fascicles are grouped together to form a nerve trunk.

Fibers may be myelinated, being covered with myelin, then Schwann cells, basement membrane, and endoneurium. Unmyelinated fibers lack the myelin coat.

Fascicles are enclosed in a sheath of interfascicular epineurium. The complete trunk is enclosed in a connective tissue layer of epifascicular epineurium (Fig. 8–9). Blood vessels, lymphatics, and nervi nervorum pass through the epifascicular epineurium into the nerve trunks.

The fascicular patterns of a nerve trunk may vary along its length:

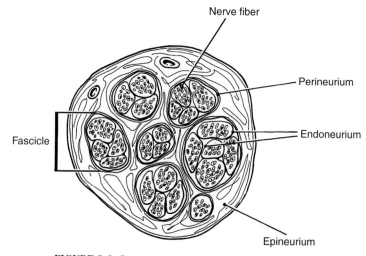

FIGURE 8–9. Cross-sectional anatomy of a myelinated nerve.

1. Monofascicular pattern: The nerve trunk consists of a single fascicle without any interfascicular epineurium.
2. Oligofascicular segment
    a. Minimal interfascicular epineurium is found between the two to four fascicles combined in the nerve segment.
    b. Five to 10 fascicles are located in the nerve segment, with significantly more interfascicular epineurium between the fascicles. This creates difficulty in the coaptation of the fascicles, requiring interfascicular dissection and individual coaptation in nerve repair.
3. Polyfascicular nerve segment: The nerve trunk consists of many fascicles.
    a. Without group arrangement: The fascicles vary in size, with a great deal of interfascicular tissue.
    b. With group arrangement: The fascicles of different sizes are arranged in groups, each with more than 10 fascicles.

Nerve Tissue Damage

Trauma to nerve tissue causes damage and fibrosis of the connective tissue components, progressing to fascicular constriction. The clinical effects can be categorized by whether the fibrosis affects (1) the epifascicular epineurium around the nerve trunk, (2) the interfascicular epineurium, or (3) the endoneurium involving the endoneural space.

After nerve section, structural changes occur above, at the site of, and below the level of transection, and wallerian degeneration occurs distal to the axonal division, leaving demyelinated empty endoneurial sheaths. The terminal motor and sensory endings also degenerate.

Proximal to the level of division, the nerve cell swells and Nissle granules appear, indicating active protein synthesis that is maximal at 4 to 14 days as axonal regeneration occurs. The axons must grow and cross the site of division for re-innervation of the appropriate motor or sensory nerve endings. Pure sensory and pure motor nerves regenerate better than mixed nerves.

The correlation between peripheral nerve injury and loss of function can be defined according to Sunderland's five grades:

I. Axon intact; no wallerian degeneration; no conduction at site of lesion; conduction distal to lesion
II. Axons interrupted; wallerian degeneration
III. Endoneurium interrupted but fascicular pattern intact
IV. Fascicles interrupted; continuity preserved by connective tissue
V. Continuity interrupted

Seddon's classification defines three types of nerve injury and is probably a more widely used classification:

1. Neurapraxia: A well-localized injury to the nerve blocks conduction at this point. Axonal continuity with normal conduction is preserved both distal and proximal to the lesion. Spontaneous and complete recovery occurs within several weeks.
2. Axonotmesis: In this injury there is disruption of axonal continuity. This results in an interruption of conduction and is followed by axonal degeneration distal to the injury. The connective tissues of the epineurium and endoneurium

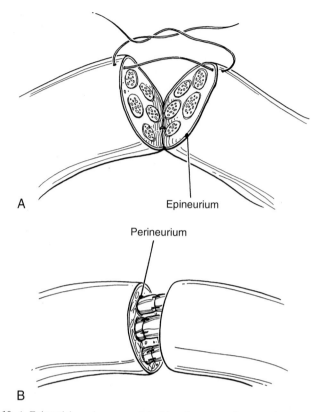

A

Epineurium

Perineurium

B

FIGURE 8–10. *A,* Epineurial repairs accomplished by placement of sutures through epineurium only. *B,* Perineurial repair is accomplished by approximation of groups of fascicles.

are uninvolved, allowing spontaneous regeneration in many of these injuries. If regeneration is delayed, the nerve may require decompression in the zone of injury.

3. Neurotmesis: The entire nerve, including axons and connective tissues, are interrupted. Axons distal to the injury degenerate. Degeneration also occurs proximal to the injury but to a much lesser degree. These injuries must be surgically repaired.

Nerve Repair

Magnification has facilitated the performance of fascicular repair and grafting. Epineurial and perineurial nerve repair are equally successful by microsurgical methods owing to accuracy of suture placement and avoidance of collateral injury (Fig. 8–10). Either technique requires proper fascicular orientation and suturing under magnification, avoiding tension. The minimal number of fine sutures (10-0 nylon) is used to maintain accurate alignment and apposition. Fasciculi with distinct topographic characteristics can readily be matched and apposed with a few sutures per group.

Epineurial Repair. This is the easiest method of repair. Sutures are placed through epineurium only. Intraneural components of the nerve are not dissected but are coupled as the sutures are tied around the nerve's circumference.

Perineurial Repair. Epineurium is dissected off underlying fascicles. Groups of fascicles may be coupled with sutures through the perineurium or individual fascicles dissected and coupled. Perineurial repair must be meticulously accomplished under high-power magnification to avoid injury and fibrosis of endoneurial tissues.

Factors Determining Functional Recovery

1. Age: Swifter functional recovery occurs in children because of cortical adaption, not because of swifter regeneration.

2. Associated injury: Devascularization, infection, or neuronal disruption leads to fibrosis and scarring, with impedance to axonal penetration at the site of division.

3. Primary nerve repair at the time of injury has the advantages of working in an unscarred area, minimal tension on the repair, and minimal degeneration of the end organ. Motor fascicles can be stimulated directly. Secondary repair is preferred for wounds with extensive soft tissue damage. As maximal axonal regeneration occurs by the 10th day, a case may be made for delayed primary repair, but potential difficulties with dissection, hemostasis, and tissue identification outweigh the physiologic factor.

NERVE GRAFTING

Nerve grafting is necessary to bridge nerve defects due to loss of nerve substance or secondary retraction. Grafts are also indicated for nerve transfer procedures, as in cross-facial nerve graft or the neurotization of the brachial plexus by intercostal nerves. Grafts should be reversed when inserted to prevent fascicular growth into nerve branches.

Donor Nerves

Sural nerve: This nerve is the most popular donor graft. Sacrifice results in minor loss of sensation on the lateral foot. Grafts longer than 30 cm can be harvested. The nerve has minimal branches and a dense fascicular pattern (Fig. 8–11).

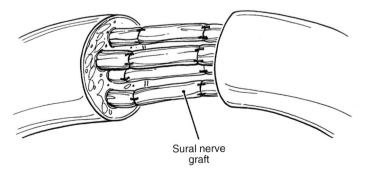

Sural nerve
graft

FIGURE 8–11. Tension on the nerve repair must be avoided. Cable grafts are used to bridge a wide nerve defect.

Medial and lateral antebrachial cutaneous nerves: These are an excellent source of graft for digital nerve repair, although segmental loss of forearm sensation is uncomfortable in some patients.

Superficial radial nerve: Anatomically this is a good donor nerve, but sacrifice may result in painful donor site neuromas.

Terminal branches of the posterior interosseous nerve: These are excellent donor sources for distal digital nerve injuries.

Suggested Readings

Millesi H: Nerve grafting. Clin Plast Surg 11:105, 1984

Nunley JA: Microscopes and microinstruments. Hand Clin 1:197, 1985

O'Brien BMcC: Reconstructive microsurgery of the upper extremity. J Hand Surg 15:316, 1990

Seddon HJ: War injuries of peripheral nerves in wounds of the extremities. Br J Surg (War Surg Suppl.) 2:325, 1948

Sunderland S, Bradley KC: The cross-sectional area of peripheral nerve trunks devoted to nerve fiber. Brain 72:428, 1981

Terzis JK: Clinical microsurgery of the peripheral nerve: The state of the art. Clin Plast Surg 6:247, 1979

CHAPTER 9

Craniofacial Surgery

THE SKULL

Anatomy

The Vault. The vault is rounded, strong, and elastic in consistency so that a blow may injure the underlying brain without necessarily fracturing the bone.

The Base. The many fissures and foramina of the base weaken and make it more susceptible to fracture. It consists of three fossae: (1) the anterior fossa, which contains the frontal brain lobes; (2) the middle cranial fossa, which contains the temporosphenoidal lobes; and (3) the posterior cranial fossa, which contains the occipital lobes, cerebellum, and medulla.

Structure. The skull is composed of an outer and inner table of compact bone, separated by a loose layer of cancellous bone known as the diploë. The smooth, thicker, and stronger outer table derives its blood supply from the pericranium and diploë, whereas the thinner, more fragile, and grooved inner table receives its blood supply from the diploë only. There are sutures between the various vault bones and, radiologically, these, as well as the vascular markings of the meningeal and diploë vessels, may resemble fracture lines.

Sutures (Fig. 9–1). (1) The coronal suture divides the frontal from the parietal bones. (2) The sagittal suture separates the parietal bones in the midline. (3) The lambdoid suture marks off the occipital from the parietal and temporal bones. (4) The squamosal suture separates the squamous temporal bone from the parietal bone and great wing of the sphenoid. (5) The metopic suture persists in the midline in about 8 per cent of cases and is situated between the two frontal bones. Normally, this suture fuses at about the fifth year.

Development of the Skull

The normal skull develops from a membranous capsule that encloses a growing brain. The base very soon become cartilaginous. Ossification centers appear in each of the bones of the vertex and extend toward each other. As these bones fuse, any residual portions of membrane gradually disappear, leaving only the membrane that forms the fontanelles. This process of development is normally complete by the end of the second year.

The mastoid antrum is well developed at birth, but the mastoid process and air cells begin to develop at the end of the second year, and during this time the facial nerve is very superficial and hence vulnerable to an ill-planned incision.

The frontal sinus does not exist at birth either, developing as an outgrowth from the nose during the first year of life, becoming evident at 8 years of age, and attaining complete development at 17 years of age.

The maxillary antrum is present in rudimentary form at birth, completing its development during adolescence. Small separate areas of ossification occasionally develop between the parietal and occipital bones, and these are termed *wormian bones.*

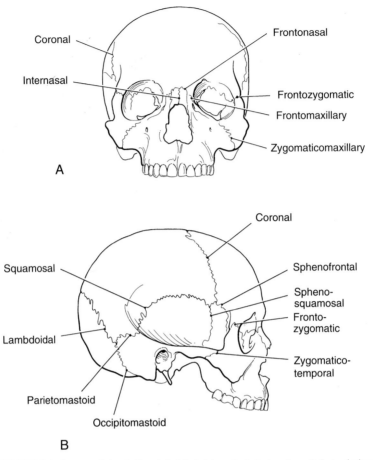

FIGURE 9–1. Sutures of the skull and facial skeleton. *A*, Anterior view. *B*, Lateral view.

Development of the Face

The face develops from five processes that surround an opening situated at the front end of the embryo, known as the stomodeum (Fig. 9–2).

The six primitive visceral arches are composed of mesoderm and covered with ectoderm and entoderm. The first or mandibular arch differentiates into two parts—the maxillary and mandibular processes. Its cartilage disappears ventrally but persists dorsally as the incus and malleus of the middle ear.

The cartilage in the second or hyoid arch forms the lesser cornu and part of the body of the hyoid bone, the stylohyoid ligament, and the styloid process of the temporal bone.

The third arch cartilage develops into the remainder of the hyoid bone and its greater cornu.

The fourth and fifth arch cartilages form the thyroid cartilage. The stomodeum, which appears at the end of the second week of intrauterine life below the expanded forebrain, is the first expression of the oral cavity.

The mandibular processes of the first arch join in the floor of the stomodeum to form the lower jaw and the structures connected with the floor of the mouth.

The five processes that surround the stomodeum are (1) *the frontonasal process*: Growing down from the roof of the stomodeum, it differentiates into a median and two lateral nasal processes. The appearance of olfactory pits divides

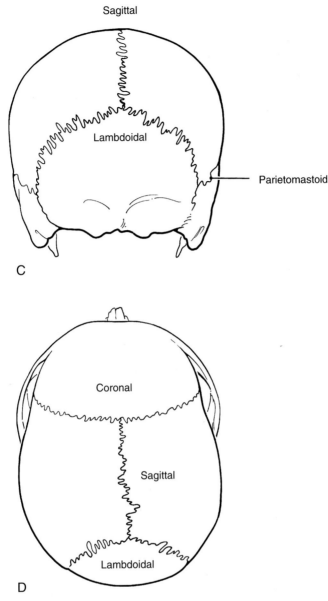

FIGURE 9–1 *Continued. C,* Posterior view. *D,* Superior view.

the frontonasal processes into three. (a) A median process known as the medial nasal process. (b) Two lateral nasal processes: the medial nasal process develops a bulge on each side known as the globular process. (c) The median, nasal, and globular processes form the premaxilla. The lateral nasal process forms the side of the nose only. (2) *The maxillary processes*: One on each side forms the cheek and the whole of the upper lip except the philtrum, as well as most of the upper lip and the palate. (3) *The mandibular process* on each side, referred to previously.

ANOMALIES OF CRANIOFACIAL DEVELOPMENT

Anomalies of craniofacial development may be due to residual clefts at sites of normal fusion of the embryologic components, or developmental skull abnormalities.

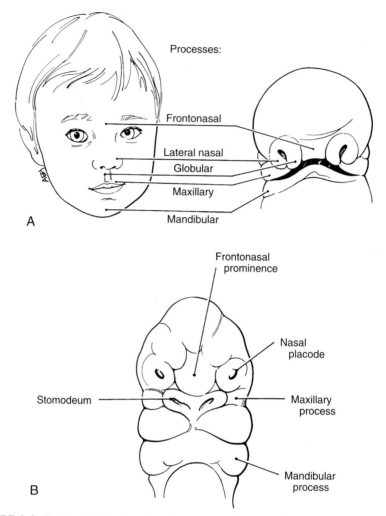

FIGURE 9–2. The face *(A)* develops from five processes that surround an opening in the embryo known as the stomodeum *(B).*

Residual Clefts

Maxillary hypoplasia and deficiency are often associated with the development of facial clefts. Exorbitism and nasomaxillary recession are frequently present, with malocclusion between the maxillary and mandibular dentition. The work of Tessier provided correlation between the pattern of facial clefts and their potential cranial extensions. The presence of a facial cleft should lead to awareness and search for complementary cranial defects. The Tessier classification is as follows (Fig. 9–3):

No. 0 cleft: Hypoplasia or absence of nasal columella, philtrum of lip, nasal septum, and premaxilla. Conversely, excess of the median nasal tissue causes a bifid nose with broadening of the nasal septum and a tilted premaxilla. It may extend into the cranium as a No. 14 cleft.

No. 1 cleft: The conventional cleft lip, with cleft between globular process and maxillary process accordingly extending through the dome of the nostril. The skeletal defect passes through the alveolar process between the central and lateral incisor teeth. It may extend into the cranium as a No. 13 cleft.

No. 2 cleft: The cleft as above is compounded by hypoplasia and distortion of the alar rim, with the alveolar defect extending as a widened notch between the nasal bone and the frontal process of the maxilla. It may extend into the cranium as a No. 12 cleft.

No. 3 cleft: The oro-naso-ocular cleft extends into the lower eyelid medial to its punctum and represents total failure of fusion between the frontonasal and maxillary processes. It may extend into the upper lid and orbital rim as a No. 11 cleft.

No. 4 cleft: An oro-ocular defect, this cleft commences lateral to the philtrum, skirting the nose and ending in the lower eyelid. The implication embryologically is that the cleft begins lateral to the nasal process rather than the globular process. It may extend into the cranium as a No. 10 cleft.

No. 5 cleft: Commencing at the oral commissure of the upper lip, the cleft penetrates the cheek to end near the middle of the lower eyelid into the lateral third of orbit, drawing lip and eyelid toward each other. The skeletal pathway from the premolar alveolus to lateral to the infraorbital foramen may lead to prolapse of the orbital contents into the maxillary sinus.

No. 6 cleft: A small coloboma of the outer lower eyelid and a descending cleft through the zygomaticomaxillary suture with involvement of inferior orbital rim. Hypoplasia of zygomatic soft tissues and an antimongoloid slant to the eyelid are seen.

No. 7 cleft: Oto-mandibular dysostosis; hemifacial microsomia; first and second branchial arch syndrome: This varies in degree from a pre-auricular skin tag to the complete form with macrostomia at the oral commissure, a furrow across the cheek toward a microtic auricle, hypoplasia of the muscles of mastication, tongue, and soft palate, and absence of the parotid gland and duct. Skeletal abnormalities include hypoplasia or absence of the mandibular ramus or condyle with flattening of the ramus. The zygomatic arch may be absent. Deafness may be present owing to absence of the middle ear ossicles. It is more common in males and may be bilateral. Facial (seventh) nerve paralysis may be due to agenesis of the facial muscles, aberrant nerve pathway in the temporal bone, or hypoplasia of its intracerebral components. The

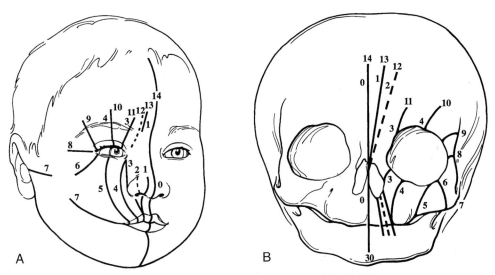

FIGURE 9–3. Tessier's classification of craniofacial clefts.

associated presence of ocular dermoid and vertebral abnormalities represents the Goldenhar syndrome.

No. 8 cleft: The cleft runs from the lateral canthus of the eye, with obliteration of the fornix, to the temporal area. A dermoid may be found at the lateral canthal coloboma. The skeletal defect is present at the zygomaticofrontal suture.

No. 9 cleft: A defect in the lateral third of the superior orbital rim results in a deep soft tissue groove that divides the upper eyelid.

No. 10 cleft: An underlying defect of the middle third of the superior orbital roof causes a fronto-orbital encephalocele to fill the gap and displace the orbit downward and outward, causing an asymmetric orbital hypertelorism. It may coexist with a No. 4 cleft.

No. 11 cleft: A cleft in the medial third of the superior orbital rim causes a small coloboma, with extension of the furrow through the eyebrow over the defect to the frontal hairline. It may coexist with a No. 3 cleft.

No. 12 cleft: An extension of cleft No. 2 into the cranium with the bony defect directed between maxilla and frontal bone causes the cleft to be lateral to the olfactory groove with involvement of the ethmoid.

No. 13 cleft: There is an extension of cleft No. 1 as a cranial prolongation, medial to the eyebrow as the cleft passes through the nasal bone, ethmoid, and olfactory groove, with widening of the cribriform plate. Orbital hypertelorism is always present.

No. 14 cleft: Affecting the midline as in cleft No. 0, there are two forms: (a) hypoplasia: There is poor forebrain differentiation with orbital hypotelorism, cyclopia, midline cleft, and false median cleft lip; (b) frontonasal dysplasia: Excess tissue results in a frontonasal encephalocele or a corrugated bifid nose and orbital hypertelorism. There is an increased distance between the medial cantha. Intellect is usually normal.

Treacher Collins Syndrome. This malformation, also known as mandibulofacial dysostosis or Franceschetti-Klein syndrome, is considered by Tessier to represent a combination of clefts 6, 7, and 8. Inherited as an autosomal dominant trait, the condition is characterized by bilateral symmetric hypoplasia of the zygomas. No. 6 cleft is represented by the coloboma of the lateral third and absence of eyelashes of the medial two thirds of the lower eyelid. The microtia, mandibular deformity, absence of the zygomatic arch, and deafness characterize No. 7 cleft with the absence of malar prominences.

Developmental Skull Abnormalities

FAILURE OF SKULL OSSIFICATION

Congenital cranial aplasia: The skull bones remain soft or membranous so that minor skull injuries become very serious. Reconstruction requires multiple rib grafts.

Encephalocele: There is persistence of a congenitally abnormal opening in the skull, permitting intracranial contents to protrude through it. The usual sites for such a defect are in the occipital, parietal, frontal, nasal, and nasopharyngeal regions. The protruding dura and associated contents represent a cephalocele and may be of three varieties: (1) Meningocele: A protrusion of the meningeal membranes with cerebrospinal fluid content only. (2) Meningoencephalocele: Brain substance as well as meninges is present in the protruding membranes. (3) Meningoencephalocystocele: A portion of one of the lateral ventricles is contained within the cerebral protrusion.

Frontoethmoidal encephalocele: Also called a nasal encephalocele, the defect lies anteriorly between the frontal bone and ethmoid. The failure of this midline closure of bone and subsequent abnormal facial skeletal development result in hypertelorism and orbital dystopia. Correction requires application of craniofacial techniques.

Congenital dermal sinus: A midline sinus communicates through a small defect in the skull with an intradural or extradural dermoid.

PREMATURE CLOSURE OF CRANIAL SUTURES

A firm fibrous union normally occurs between the bones of the skull vault by the time a child is 6 months old. If one or more of the cranial sutures becomes prematurely obliterated by ossification, deformity of the vault results. Virchow correctly postulated that with premature closure of a cranial suture, inhibition of growth at right angles to the involved suture and compensatory overexpansion at the open sutures to accommodate the normal brain development both occur.

CRANIOSYNOSTOSIS

This may be primary, owing to premature obliteration of the sutures with cerebral compression, or it may be secondary to underlying microcephaly.

The general effects of primary craniosynostosis are (1) cranial deformity: The pattern of deformity depends on which sutures are involved (Fig. 9–4); (2) ocular abnormalities: Proptosis with disturbance of extraocular movements may proceed to papilledema, optic atrophy, and blindness; (3) potential for progressive mental deficiency, sometimes with an associated seizure disorder; (4) associated congenital abnormalities such as syndactyly, facial clefts, or cleft palate; (5) restriction of facial growth with faciosynostosis which further distorts the facial appearance.

Patterns in Craniosynostosis (Table 9–1)

Premature Closure of the Coronal Suture

Unilateral Synostosis. A palpable ridge is present at the site of fusion, with increased vertical dimension and elevation of the orbit on the ipsilateral side. The facial midline and chin are deviated to the contralateral side. Viewed from above, the calvarium has an oblique orientation defined as plagiocephaly.

Bilateral Synostosis. Simple bilateral coronal synostosis causes recession of the forehead without any facial abnormalities. A palpable ridge across the crown is present at the sites of the synostoses. General physical examination demonstrates no other abnormalities and specifically normal digits. Bilateral coronal synostosis

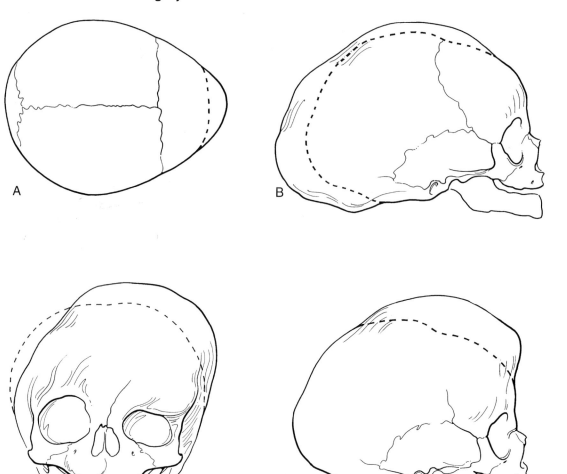

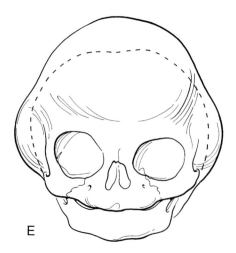

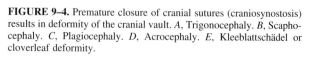

FIGURE 9–4. Premature closure of cranial sutures (craniosynostosis) results in deformity of the cranial vault. *A*, Trigonocephaly. *B*, Scaphocephaly. *C*, Plagiocephaly. *D*, Acrocephaly. *E*, Kleeblattschädel or cloverleaf deformity.

TABLE 9–1. Patterns of Craniosynostosis

Type	Suture	Description
Trigonocephaly	Metopic	Keel-shaped anterior cranium with pointed forehead
Scaphocephaly	Sagittal	Long narrow cranium
Plagiocephaly	Unilateral coronal	Ipsilateral frontal flattening, contralateral frontal bossing, and occipital bulging
Posterior plagiocephaly	Unilateral lambdoid	Ipsilateral occipital flattening with contralateral bulging
Brachycephaly	Bilateral coronal	Short anteroposterior dimension and wide transverse dimension
Acrocephaly/turricephaly	Bilateral coronal (untreated)	"Tower skull" with increased height of the cranium
Oxycephaly	Multiple	Pointed head with a posteriorly tilted forehead
Kleeblattschädel	Multiple	Trilobed "cloverleaf" cranium

in conjunction with other synostosis is seen in a multitude of craniofacial syndromes.

CROUZON SYNDROME. In this genetically autosomal dominant condition with craniofacial dysostosis, bilateral coronal synostoses result in a calvarium with a shortened anteroposterior dimension and an increased bitemporal dimension (brachycephaly). Other sutures may be involved, leading to acrocephaly or oxycephaly. The forehead is recessed and the skull's inner table has a copper-beaten appearance. The shallow orbits cause exorbitism with mild orbital hypertelorism and divergent strabismus. The hypoplastic retruded midface is associated with crowding of the maxillary dentition on the constricted arch. Although the mandible is smaller than normal, relative mandibular prognathism with retrusion of the chin is present. The diminished size of the oronasopharynx leads to inspiratory impedance with episodes of obstructive sleep apnea.

Although the digits are normal, ankylosis of the elbow joints and subluxation of the head of the radius are occasionally present.

APERT SYNDROME. A flattened high forehead with digital markings of the inner table of the skull is associated with exorbitism, mild orbital hypertelorism, and divergent strabismus. The skull deformity is characterized by brachycephaly or acrocephaly. Faciosynostosis results in midface recession and collapsed maxilla with a high arched palate. Pseudoprognathism is present, causing anterior dental malocclusion with an open bite. Upper airway obstruction may occur.

The feature specific to the syndrome is a symmetric osseous and soft tissue syndactyly of hands and feet, often with fusion of the three central digits. Radial deviation of the distal phalanx of the thumb is present. The syndrome is designated acrocephalosyndactyly. Some degree of mental retardation may occur, and the development of acne vulgaris during adolescence is often seen to affect the face and forearms.

PFEIFFER SYNDROME. The craniofacial parameters are similar to, although milder than those in Apert syndrome. The specifically characteristic features are the broadened thumbs and big toes. If syndactyly is present, it is mild and confined to web integuments only. The syndrome is autosomal, and no intellectual impairment is present.

CARPENTER SYNDROME. Acrocephalopolysyndactyly is defined by the associated presence of polydactyly as the unique characteristic of this syndrome, in addition to the syndactyly of fingers and toes. In addition to coronal synostosis, premature fusion of other sutures may occur. Mental retardation is usually present in this autosomally recessive condition.

SAETHRO-CHOTZEN SYNDROME. There is a low frontal hairline on a backward-sloping forehead with characteristic bilateral eyelid ptosis. The midface and intellect are normal. Soft tissue syndactyly is often present between the second and third fingers and toes in this autosomally dominant condition.

Metopic Synostosis. If the midline suture between the frontal bone fuses prematurely, the palpable ridge on the forehead causes the V-shaped contour (trigonocephaly) with recession of the lateral part of the orbits and mild orbital hypotelorism. Neither intellectual nor any other physical impairments are present.

Sagittal Synostosis. One of the most common forms of synostosis, this has no associated intellectual effects. A palpable ridge is present along the suture with prominence of the frontal and occipital regions, causing an upside-down boat-shaped deformity (scaphocephaly).

Multiple Synostosis. Frequently accompanied by hydrocephalus, premature closure of the coronal, lambdoid, and temporoparietal sutures as well as the metopic suture, this may occur alone or in patients with Crouzon, Apert, or Carpenter syndrome. The cranial vault has a trilobular deformation with the brain bulging through the open sagittal suture. This cloverleaf or kleeblattschädel anomaly is easily recognizable clinically.

Orbital Hypertelorism. Hypertelorism results from failure of the orbits to attain their normal medial position. The intercanthal and interpupillary distances are increased, and enlarged ethmoids fill the space between the orbits. It often occurs as part of other syndromes, including craniofacial clefts and encephaloceles.

Mild cases of hypertelorism may be corrected by a subcranial approach, but more severe cases with intercanthal distances of 35 mm and greater require a transcranial approach. The transcranial approach is also indicated when the cribriform plate is positioned inferior to the front nasal suture or a coexisting encephalocele is present.

MANAGEMENT OF CRANIOFACIAL MALFORMATIONS

The integration of the multiple specialties involved in the diagnosis, treatment, and rehabilitation of patients with craniofacial malformation depends upon the leadership of the reconstructive surgeon. The operative collaborators include neurosurgeons, oral and orthodontic specialists, otolaryngologists, and anesthesiologists versed in the details of the problems. Audiologists, neuroradiologists, and speech pathologists provide the diagnostic and rehabilitation parameters so vital in functional rehabilitation and so necessary to complement the structural improvements provided to the patient with craniofacial deformity.

Clinical Evaluation

The pattern of the craniofacial malformations needs proper definition:

1. The nature of the soft tissue abnormalities and the need for augmentation of any deficiencies
2. The degree of dental malocclusion
3. The nature and degree of bony abnormality
4. The degree of symmetry or asymmetry of the osseous structures
5. The degree of orbital involvement and its effect on visual acuity
6. The relative position of the maxilla
7. The degree of mandibular development.

Radiologic examinations should include cephalometric films. Computed tomographic (CT) studies and MR imaging provide information about intracranial pathology.

Analysis of the skeletal deformities and of the relationship between osseous and soft tissue structures is best provided by cephalometry, whereas photocephalometry can provide guidance in planning treatment. The necessary osteotomies can be planned on transparencies, and lateral cephalograms outline the soft tissue profiles in relation to the mandibular, maxillary, and cranial base structures.

Because the state of the teeth determine the success of operations on the maxilla and mandible, proper hygiene and dental restoration are important.

Principles of Surgical Intervention

Correction of craniofacial deformity should be carried out as early as possible in children, taking advantage of the rapid expansion of the brain in the first year of life. Control of exorbitism and the psychological benefits of early repair also provide dividends in the child's and parents' pursuit of normalcy.

PRINCIPLES OF EARLY INTERVENTION

In children less than 1 year of age, the presence of associated hydrocephalus requires neurosurgical remedy. Hydrocephalus can be determined in the neonate by ultrasonography, but in older children CT scanning is necessary. Positive contrast studies, via either the lumbar route, subarachnoid space, or ventricular system, may be necessary to identify the anatomic site of obstruction before a ventriculoperitoneal shunt is performed. Alternative shunts include the ventriculoatrial and ventriculopleural shunts.

Techniques limited to strip or linear craniotomy do nothing for the facial deformity, requiring major craniofacial repair later if the synostosis at the cranial base is not remedied. This causes persistence of the flattened forehead, the shallow anterior cranial fossa, and the orbital exorbitism.

PRINCIPLES OF DEFINITIVE CRANIOFACIAL CORRECTION

The contributions of Tessier, Munro, Le Fort, and Converse have resulted in the procedures of frontal bone advancement, intracranial and subcranial Le Fort advancement, and monoblock or craniofacial advancement, as well as maxillary and mandibular osteotomies. These procedures can now be performed within the first year of life without interference with subsequent facial growth and development.

Craniofacial Dysostosis

Tessier first mobilized the frontal bone in 1971, and Marchac devised the "floating forehead." In 1978, Marchac introduced the concept of fronto-orbital remodeling for craniosynostosis by a rocking advancement of the supraorbital bar and the upper forehead (Fig. 9–5). Refinements of frontocranial remodeling have led to improved results in management of craniofacial dysostosis.

Optimal treatment requires advancement of the frontal bone in the early months of life. Craniotomy is performed through a transcoronal approach. The anterior skull is removed, reshaped, or rotated 180 degrees and advanced. Additionally, release of the sutures of the anterior cranial base and of the frontosphenoidal, frontoethmoidal, and frontozygomatic sutures is essential. The natural expansion of the brain then directs the facial skeleton in a forward direction.

The supraorbital block may also be advanced by an osteotomy through the anterior cranial base extending into the lateral orbital walls. Cranial defects are allowed to fill in naturally in younger patients, but in children over 4 to 5 years of age the advancement is filled in surgically with bone dust and split cranial grafts.

Orbital Advancement

Osteotomy and mobilization of the orbits may be required for the correction of hypertelorism, encephalocele, orbital dystopia, exophthalmos, and enophthalmos. The orbital wall can be mobilized by either a subcranial or an intracranial approach. The intracranial approach is preferred for moderate to severe hypertelorism, with intercanthal distance of greater than 35 mm, associated encephalocele, and a low-lying cribriform plate.

A frontal bone flap is elevated through a transcoronal approach. The frontal lobe is elevated and retracted, and orbital osteotomies are fashioned. In the case

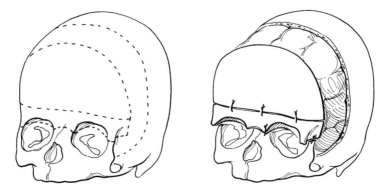

FIGURE 9–5. Frontal orbital remodeling by advancement of the supraorbital bar and frontal bone.

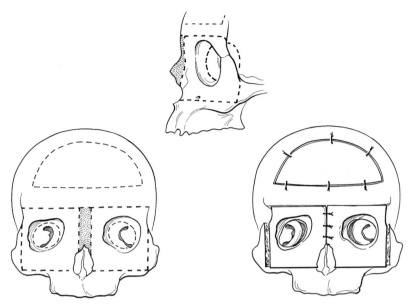

FIGURE 9–6. Orbital osteotomies to correct hypertelorism.

of hypertelorism, the interorbital ethmoid bone is resected and the orbits are repositioned (Fig. 9–6).

The medial canthal tendons are reinserted and a lateral canthoplasty is performed if necessary. Nasal reconstruction is difficult in these cases and requires a variety of techniques, including bone graft, remodeling of nasal cartilages, and soft tissue techniques to lengthen or shorten the nose.

Monoblock Frontofacial Advancement. A circumorbital osteotomy combined with Le Fort III osteotomies allows fronto-orbital and facial advancement as one unit. It is reserved for brachycephalic children and cannot be done safely in adults because of risk of resorption of the frontal bone advancement flap (Fig. 9–7).

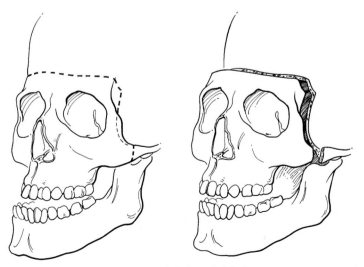

FIGURE 9–7. Monoblock frontofacial advancement.

Facial Bipartition. This craniofacial approach to the orbits as well as vestibular exposure of the maxilla allows for correction of hypertelorism combined with maxillary expansion (Fig. 9–8).

Maxillary Reconstruction

The dentoalveolar and skeletal abnormalities associated with facial deformities may result in maxillary protrusion or midface retrusion due to maxillary hypoplasia.

Cephalometrics. This refers to measurements describing the relationship of facial skeletal components to each other and to the cranium. The critical measurements relate to the cranial base, maxilla, mandible, maxillary teeth, and mandibular teeth. A variety of cephalometric analyses have been advocated, including horizontal, vertical, and angular analysis, each providing numerical norms for skeletal relationships (Fig. 9–9). The maxilla and mandible may each be protruding (prognathic), retruded (retrognathic), or normally positioned (orthognathic). Each component may also be too long or too short, hypoplastic or hyperplastic.

Dental Occlusion. Occlusion is determined by physical examination and dental impressions. Models may be fabricated and cut to determine appropriate mobilization of the jaws to improve occlusion. Evaluation determines occlusal plane, maxillary and mandibular midline relationship, relationship of maxillary and mandibular incisors, and relationship of cuspids and first molars. The relationship of the molars is best defined by the Angle classification, which describes three main types of occlusion. It is based on the relative position of the mesiobuccal

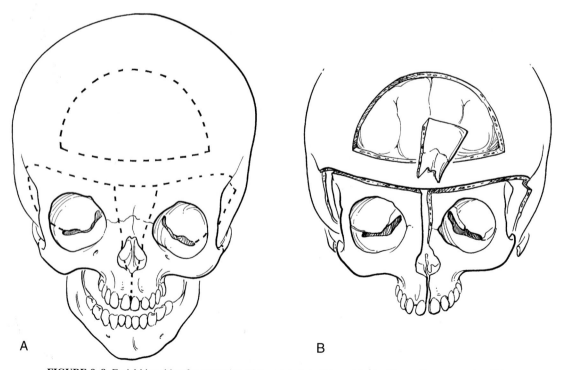

A   B

FIGURE 9–8. Facial bipartition for correction of hypertelorism *(A)* combined with maxillary expansion *(B)*.

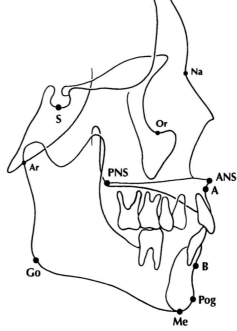

FIGURE 9–9. The relationship of facial skeletal components to each other and to the cranium is measured by cephalometric analysis. Important cephalometric landmarks include the nasion (Na), orbitale (Or), sella (S), articulare (Ar), posterior nasal spine (PNS), anterior nasal spine (ANS), point A on the maxilla (A), point B on the mandible (B), menton (Me), gonion (Go) and pogonion (Pog). Vertical and horizontal dimensions may be determined by the relationship of these critical landmarks to each other. (From Zide B, Grayson B, McCarthy JG: Cephalometric analysis. Parts I–III. Plast Reconstr Surg 68:816, 1981. Copyright © Williams & Wilkins.)

cusp of the maxillary first molar to the mesiobuccal groove of the mandibular first molar (Fig. 9–10).

Neutrocclusion (Class I). In normal occlusion the mesiobuccal cusp of the first maxillary molar occludes against the mesiobuccal groove of the mandibular first molar.

Distocclusion (Class II). The buccal cusp of the maxillary first molar is anterior to the mesiobuccal groove of the mandibular first molar. This may be seen with a retruded mandible or a protruding maxilla.

Mesiocclusion (Class III). The buccal cusp of the maxillary first molar is posterior to the mesiobuccal groove of the mandibular first molar. This may be seen with a protruding mandible or a retruded maxilla.

Occlusion may be further defined by the relationship of the arches to each other. Premature occlusion of the molars results in an anterior open bite (Fig. 9–11), and premature occlusion of the incisors causes a posterior open bite. Discrepancy in a lateral direction results in a cross-bite (Fig. 9–12).

Facial Osteotomies. The facial skeleton can be approached via three incisions: (1) bicoronal scalp incision, (2) conjunctival or subciliary cutaneous incision, and (3) buccal vestibular incision.

Le Fort III Osteotomy. Appropriate osteotomies may be combined with orbital advancement by an osteotomy at the nasofrontal junction, which continues backward across the medial wall of the orbit to the orbital floor. Another osteotomy is fashioned at the frontozygomatic suture line. An osteotomy through the lateral orbital wall continues inferiorly and posteriorly across the maxilla and through the

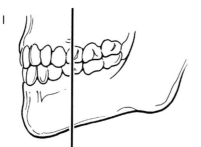

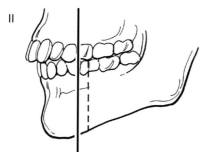

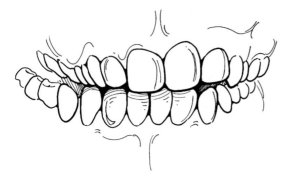

FIGURE 9–10. Angle's classification of occlusion is determined by the relationship of the first permanent maxillary and mandibular molars. Class I (neutrocclusion): The maxillary first molar mesiobuccal cusp is aligned with the mandibular first molar mesiobuccal groove. Class II (distocclusion): This may occur as a result of a protrusion of the maxilla or retrognathia of the mandible. The maxillary first molar mesiobuccal cusp sits anterior to the mesiobuccal groove of the mandibular first molar. Class III (mesiocclusion): This is seen with retrusion of the maxilla or prognathia of the mandible. The mesiobuccal cusp of the maxillary first molar lies posterior to the mesiobuccal groove of the mandibular first molar.

FIGURE 9–11. Anterior open bite due to premature occlusion of the molars.

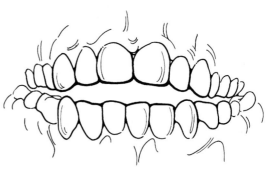

FIGURE 9–12. Cross-bite is seen with lingual malposition of the maxillary teeth relative to the adjacent mandibular teeth.

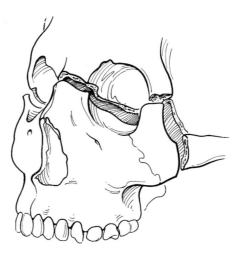

FIGURE 9–13. Le Fort III osteotomy for maxillary advancement.

pterygomaxillary fissure. Pterygomaxillary disjunction is then carried out, and the facial skeleton is loosened and advanced with special disimpaction forceps. The Le Fort III advancement (Fig. 9–13) is then consolidated with miniplate fixation at the nasofrontal junction, lateral orbital wall, and pterygomaxillary fissure.

Le Fort II Osteotomy. Marked retrusion of the nasomaxillary area can be remedied by the Le Forte II osteotomy. The osteotomy begins at the nasofrontal junction, extends into the medial orbital wall, and then passes below the zygoma to the pterygomaxillary junction (Fig. 9–14).

Le Fort I Osteotomy. Dental malocclusion due to an abnormality of the lower maxilla or dentoalveolar deformity may be corrected with a low transverse osteotomy of the maxilla. The osteotomy is continued into the pterygomaxillary fissure, and the maxillary segment is repositioned with plates and screws (Fig. 9–15).

Mandibular Correction

The interrelationship between concurrent anomalies of the mandible and maxilla on the one hand and the effect of maxillary asymmetry on mandibular growth on

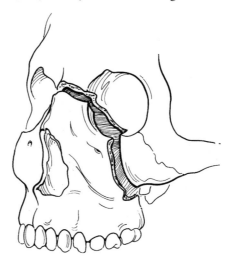

FIGURE 9–14. Le Fort II osteotomy for maxillary advancement.

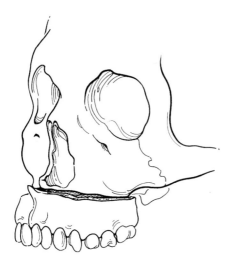

FIGURE 9–15. Le Fort I osteotomy for maxillary advancement.

the other hand requires a cogent surgical strategy for correction of mandibular malformation.

1. Symmetric defects: Early reconstruction of the mandible may be considered in patients with the Treacher Collins syndrome because the defects are symmetric and replacement of the missing bulk of bones aids in restoration of functional matrix.

2. Asymmetric defects: One school of thought advocates that all mandibular surgery be postponed until facial skeletal growth has been completed. Thus, in hemifacial microsomia (No. 7 cleft), reconstructive mandibular surgery should be delayed, as it should be in anterior open-bite situations and in the treatment of prognathism.

Exposure of the mandible may be via an intraoral or an extraoral approach. The intraoral approach provides good access without leaving observable scars. The extraoral approach has advantages in providing access to the ramus. For exposure of the body and ramus, a combined intraoral and extraoral approach has merit.

Procedures are of two types: osteotomies and distraction osteogenesis.

Osteotomies include vertical osteotomy of the ramus, sagittal split osteotomy of the ramus, step osteotomy of the mandibular body for increase in length, and horizontal osteotomy for correction of microgenia or underdevelopment of the chin. Although all the above osteotomies have a place, the sagittal split osteotomy is the preferred option because it permits rapid bone consolidation (Fig. 9–16). It can be done through an intraoral incision, and the wide surface contact permits greater discretion in the positional change of the fragments. Plate fixation avoids the need for prolonged intermaxillary fixation.

Osteotomy for advancement or lengthening of the mandible may require bone grafts at the osteotomy site coupled with plate fixation to provide a rigid skeletal mobilization with minimal risk of relapse. This mandates precise mobilization, repositioning, and fixation of skeletal components.

Distraction osteogenesis allows a slowly progressive mobilization that can be continued until optimal positioning has been accomplished. A corticotomy is performed along traditional osteotomy sites. Pins are fixed in and behind the segment to be moved, gradually distracting the segment from the rigid craniofacial skeleton. The progressing gap (usually 1 mm/day) fills in with new bone, avoiding the need for bone grafts and rigid fixation (Fig. 9–17).

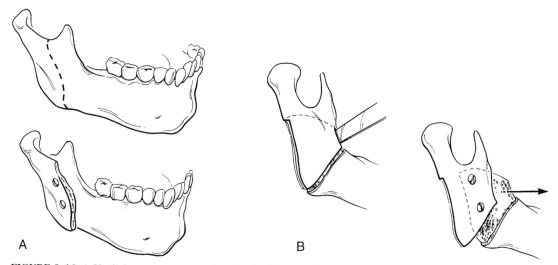

FIGURE 9–16. *A*, Vertical ramus osteotomy with setback of the mandible and lag screw fixation. *B*, Sagittal split osteotomy for mandibular advancement with lag screw fixation.

CORRECTION OF FACIAL SKELETAL DEFORMITIES

Hemifacial Microsomia

Also known as "the first and second branchial arch syndrome," the condition is usually unilateral but occasionally bilateral. Mandibular pathology is the characteristic deformity noted and is due to hypoplasia of the temporomandibular and pterygomandibular complexes. Associated deformities of the ear, orbit, and maxilla must also be addressed. In a mild deformity, bone and cartilage grafts correct the contour deformities. More severe deformities require mandibular and maxillary osteotomies to correct a malaligned occlusal plane. Aplasia of the glenoid fossa or mandibular ramus is corrected with costal cartilage grafts. Although uncommon, there can be hypoplasia of the entire zygomatic complex, requiring rib or cranial bone graft reconstruction. Inferior displacement of the orbit is corrected by a craniofacial approach and osteotomy repositioning. Once the craniofacial skeletal

Area for
new bone growth

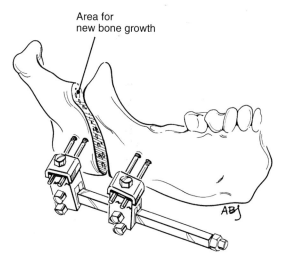

FIGURE 9–17. Distraction osteogenesis. A corticotomy is performed and pins are fixed to each segment. The pins are attached to a device that enables distraction of the two segments by the turn of a screw. The screw is turned daily, distracting segments by 1 mm per day. The progressing defect fills in with new bone. Solid union is accomplished once distraction is completed.

architecture has been restored, appropriate soft tissue repair of the cheek and reconstruction of the ear may be carried out. Correction of facial nerve paralysis is also planned.

Treacher Collins Syndrome

This deformity is generally bilateral, with symmetric involvement of each side of the face. Soft tissue reconstruction is directed at the palpebral coloboma, macrostomia, and external ear deformities. The hypoplastic or aplastic malar bones and mandible are corrected with bone grafts or segmental osteotomies, depending on severity.

Fibrous Dysplasia

Fibrous dysplasia is characterized by an enlarging facial mass composed of fibrous and osseous tissue. It may be monostotic, involving a single bone, or polyostotic. If polyostotic, it may be associated with the Albright syndrome (hyperparathyroidism, skin pigmentation, and precocious sexual development). Fibrous dysplasia typically involves the frontal and sphenoid bones, the maxilla, and the mandible. Treatment should be directed at excision of involved bones if possible and reconstruction with bone grafts.

With the development of craniofacial operative techniques in the management of craniofacial deformities, these methods have now become applicable to the management of craniofacial traumatic deformities as well as repair of defects due to surgical ablation of extensive malignancies.

Suggested Readings

Converse JM, Wood-Smith D, McCarthy JG: Report on a series of 50 craniofacial operations. Plast Reconstr Surg 55:283, 1975

Le Fort R: The classic reprint: Experimental study of fractures of the upper jaw. I and II. (Translated from French by Paul Tessier). Plast Reconstr Surg 50:497, 1972

Le Fort R: The classic reprint: Experimental study of fractures of the upper jaw. III [Translated from French by Paul Tessier]. Plast Reconstr Surg 50:600, 1972

Marchac D: Radical forehead remodeling for craniostenosis. Plast Reconstr Surg 61:823, 1978

Marchac D, Renier D: Treatment of craniosynostosis in infancy. Clin Plast Surg 14:61, 1987

Munro IR: Treatment of craniofacial microsomia. Clin Plast Surg 14:177, 1987

Munro IR, Sabatier RE: An analysis of 12 years of craniomaxillofacial surgery in Toronto. Plast Reconstr Surg 76:29, 1985

Tessier P: Anatomical classification of facial, craniofacial and latero-facial clefts. J Maxillofac Surg 4:69, 1976

Tessier P: The definitive plastic surgical treatment of the severe facial deformities of craniofacial dysostosis. Crouzon's and Apert's disease. Plast Reconstr Surg 48:419, 1971

Van der Meulen JC, Mazzola R, Vermey-Keers C, et al: A morphogenetic classification of craniofacial malformations. Plast Reconstr Surg 71:560, 1983

CHAPTER 10

Cleft Lip and Palate

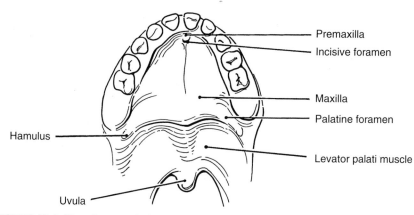

FIGURE 10–1. The palate extends from the incisive foramen to the uvula, includes the hard and soft palates, and is referred to as the secondary palate. The structures anterior to the incisive foramen are the premaxilla, alveolus, and upper lip and are referred to as the primary palate.

THE CLEFT DEFORMITY

The congenital anomaly known as cleft lip represents an abnormality of fusion between the medial nasal component of the frontonasal process and the maxillary process. It predominantly affects the upper lip and is placed laterally, the cleft running between the philtrum and the lateral part of the upper lip. Clefts of the lip and palate are separate components of a common embryologic problem. The "primary" palate refers to the lip, premaxilla, and alveolus, whereas the secondary palate includes the soft and hard palate posterior to the incisive foramen (Fig. 10–1).

Clefts of the lip and palate are classified according to the anatomic structures involved.

1. Cleft of primary palate (cleft lip)
   a. Unilateral (Fig. 10–2)
      (1) Incomplete: involves the lip only
      (2) Complete: involves the structures of the primary palate, including lip, nasal floor, and alveolus
   b. Bilateral (Fig. 10–3)
      (1) Incomplete: involves the lip only

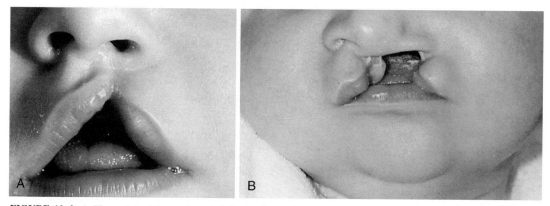

FIGURE 10–2. *A*, The unilateral incomplete cleft lip involves only one side of the lip. *B*, The complete unilateral cleft lip involves the structures of the primary palate on one side, including the lip, nasal floor, and alveolus.

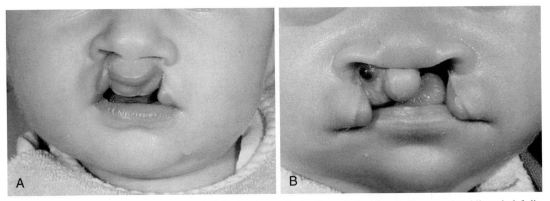

FIGURE 10–3. *A*, The bilateral incomplete cleft lip involves only the lip on both sides. *B*, The complete bilateral cleft lip deformity involves the lip, nasal floor, and alveolus on both sides. The deformity may be incomplete on one side and complete on the other side.

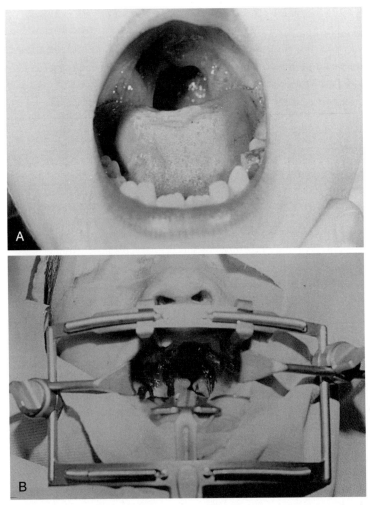

FIGURE 10–4. A cleft of the secondary palate may be incomplete, involving the soft palate or the soft palate and a portion of the hard palate *(A)*, or complete, involving the entire palate to the incisive foramen *(B)*.

(2) Complete: involves lip, nasal floor, and alveolus
2. Cleft of secondary palate (Fig. 10–4)
   a. Incomplete: involves the soft palate or the soft palate and part of the hard palate
   b. Complete: involves the soft palate and hard palate to the incisive foramen
3. Combination of clefts involving primary and secondary palate (Fig. 10–5)

Principles of Cleft Lip Repairs

A variety of operative procedures are available using local tissue in order to increase the length of the lip on the cleft side. Equally important is the need to redirect the fibers of the orbicularis oris muscle with their proper approximation.

In a complete unilateral cleft lip, the orbicularis muscle fibers proceed horizontally from the corner of the mouth toward the midline. At the margins of the cleft the muscle fibers turn upward to insert into the base of the nose.

In a bilateral cleft the muscle fibers exhibit the same architecture, but the prolabium has no muscle fibers having been replaced by connective tissue.

The objectives of repair are (1) to restore lip symmetry; (2) to create a normal philtrum with a Cupid's bow with preservation of the mucocutaneous white line, a full vermilion, and a normal-appearing tubercle; (3) to restore nostril floor symmetry with lengthening of the columella and to reshape the nasal tip when necessary; and (4) to create an inconspicuous scar.

Timing of Surgical Repair

Despite controversy about whether repair should be carried out during the first week of life or later, conventional wisdom tends to follow the "rule of tens": (1) Delay until the child is 10 weeks of age, permitting the lip tissues to develop. (2)

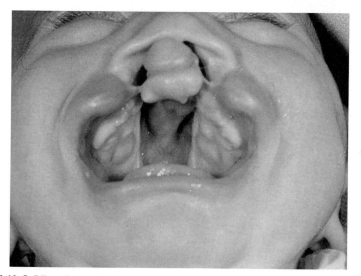

FIGURE 10–5. Bilateral complete cleft lip and palate. The vomer is evident in the midline posterior to the protruding premaxilla.

The child should weigh 10 pounds. (3) Hemoglobin should be 10 g/dl. (4) The white cell count should be below 10,000/cm^3.

Etiology

Although no causative factors are known in this condition that affects about one child per 1000 births, some known associations increase the incidence of lip clefts:

1. Chromosomal abnormalities
    a. Trisomy 13–15: 75 per cent incidence
    b. Trisomy 18
    c. Trisomy 21 (Down syndrome)
2. Pierre Robin syndrome (micrognathia)
3. Genetic factors
    a. Familial incidence
    b. Exogenous effects: irradiation
4. Rubella

Prerepair Management

The presence of a cleft lip does not, on its own, cause difficulty with feeding, either by breast or by bottle.

Guides to Operative Management

Three categories of unilateral cleft lip can conveniently be used in planning operative repair: microform cleft lip, incomplete cleft lip, and complete cleft lip.

The associated nasal deformity can be classified as mild or moderate. In the mild form, despite a widened alar base, the alar contour is normal with a normal dome projection. In the moderate form, the widened alar base is associated with hypoplasia of the alar cartilage with marked deepening of the alar crease as well as underprojection of the alar dome.

The Microform Cleft. A furrow or scar along the lip with a vermilion notch and an imperfect white roll is associated with vertical shortness of the lip. Nasal deformity is often present. During general anesthesia for repair of the cleft, the palate should be examined for the presence of a submucous cleft. The lip cleft can be repaired in a straight line fashion by an elliptical excision of the scar and vermilion if there is no vertical tip shortening on the affected side. The lip is then closed in two layers. The muscles and mucosa are approximated by three mattress sutures tied on the mucosal side. The skin is closed by fine interrupted nylon sutures. If the vertical shortening is greater than 1 to 2 mm, a rotation advancement repair is used.

The presence of a mild nasal deformity can be dealt with during late adolescence, when a rhinoplasty may be done. Alternatively, if the nasal deformity progresses with growth, then alar mobilization and correction can be accomplished at about 4 years of age.

Unilateral Incomplete Cleft Lip. It is essential that the soft tissues of the lip be rearranged so that the vertical scar line is broken and a central fullness is produced. This prerequisite is satisfied by fashioning muscle flaps by the various techniques described by Blair and Brown, Le Mesurier, Tennison, Randall, and Millard. The techniques described by Millard are most frequently used.

The incomplete cleft is identified by a varying degree of vertical separation of the lip, but the nasal sill is intact, providing a Simonart band. The Millard rotation advancement flap is the most commonly used technique for the incomplete cleft, as it is easily planned with a minimal amount of tissue sacrifice. The scar is inconspicuous as it skirts the philtral ridge, and the nostril is restored without notching. Repair of the incomplete unilateral cleft lip is similar to that described for repair of a complete cleft.

Unilateral Complete Cleft Lip. This cleft is characterized by separation of the lip, nostril sill, and alveolus. The secondary palate may remain intact, but often the entire palate may be cleft.

The maxillary alveolar components may vary in their relationship to each other: (1) A narrow separation, but the two segments are on the same horizontal plane; that is, there is no "collapse." (2) A narrow separation but the lateral maxillary segment is positioned lingually in relation to the arch configuration of the medial dental ridge; that is, there is collapse. (3) A wide separation with no collapse. (4) A wide separation with collapse.

The strategy of surgical management depends on the configuration of the cleft:

1. The narrow, noncollapsed cleft can be readily repaired by the rotation-advancement technique with concurrent correction of the nasal deformity.

2. The narrow, collapsed cleft may be handled by preoperative palatal orthopedic expansion, commenced at 2 weeks of age and continued until lip repair is performed. Many proponents, however, proceed with definitive repair at 3 months of age and delay palatal expansion until mixed dentition at 6 to 9 years of age.

3. The wide, noncollapsed cleft can be improved by preliminary lip adhesion, although most surgeons reserve lip adhesion for only the widest of clefts with a diminutive lateral element.

4. The wide, collapsed cleft may be treated by palatal expansion to correct the collapse, with subsequent lip adhesion and an appliance to control the segments as the cleft narrows.

Lip Adhesion. This procedure may have a place in highly selected unilateral and bilateral wide clefts. It is achieved by temporarily bringing together the lip margins so as to line up the maxillary arch in proper position for a secondary definitive procedure under less tension. For bilateral clefts the procedure may be performed bilaterally or each side may be done separately with a 2- to 3-month interval between the procedures.

Millard Repair. The peaks of the Cupid's bow are determined and labeled on the medial side of the cleft at p and p'. The same point is located on the lateral side of the cleft. The incision on the lateral lip follows the mucocutaneous line into the nostril and is joined by another incision along the alar base. On the medial aspect of the cleft, a line of incision from point p' follows the mucocutaneous line

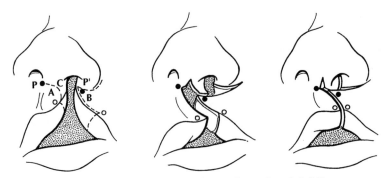

FIGURE 10–6. Millard repair of a complete unilateral cleft lip.

into the nostril, and a second incision is carried from the base of the columella to the opposite philtral ridge. The rotation-advancement procedure produces three flaps: Flap A rotates interiorly, flap B is advanced into the space vacated by flap A, and the proximal flap C at the alar base creates the new nasal sill. The mucosal, muscular, and skin layers are approximated and sutured (Fig. 10–6).

Randall Repair. The unilateral cleft lip repair described by Randall remains an effective and popular means of repair (Fig. 10–7).

Bilateral Cleft Lip. The clefts on each side may be complete or incomplete. The most important clinical consideration in these cases is the state of the prolabium and the premaxilla. Repair in these cases is complicated by scarcity of tissue in the prolabium and columella and by premaxillary displacement.

With the forward displacement of the premaxilla, the two maxillary segments tend to collapse medially. Cleft lip repair in these patients is complicated by

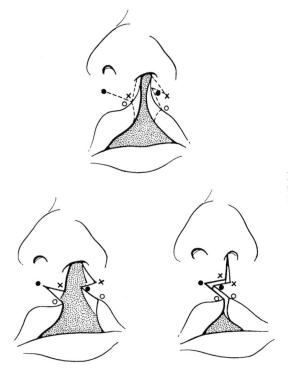

FIGURE 10–7. Randall's modification of the Tennison unilateral cleft lip repair.

tension on the repair line, which displaces the prolabium. It may also cause wound disruption and result in an unsightly scar.

Reduction of prolabial tension can be achieved by the application of an orthodontic device that moves the prolabium backward and the two lateral maxillary segments outward (Georgiade-Latham device).

Once arch relationships have been established, the cleft repair is performed at about 10 weeks of age, at which time associated soft palate repair may be done.

Some proponents recommend repair of the bilateral cleft without specific attention to the protruding premaxilla. The repaired lip remodels the premaxilla, pushing it posteriorly. If the alveolar segments are collapsed, the premaxilla is limited in its remodeling, and proper positioning must await definitive orthodontic realignment of the segments.

Millard Repair of Bilateral Cleft Lip. This technique provides an aesthetically acceptable lip with lengthening of the columella. The technique requires two stages. The lip is repaired at the first operation and the columella is lengthened at a second stage. The Millard bilateral cleft repair is usually performed at 3 months of age. The lip is repaired, and bilateral prolabial flaps are elevated. These flaps may be banked in the nostril sills for future columella elevation or discarded. The lateral lip elements are used to augment the central prolabial vermilion. The prolabium is used to contruct the philtrum. Because the prolabium does not contain any muscle, the muscle of the lateral elements is approximated to the muscle component of the other side behind the prolabium (Fig. 10–8). The columella elevation may be carried out several months later, although it is often delayed for 3 to 4 years. The nostril floor is advanced as a bipedicled flap, lengthening the columella and correcting the abnormal nostril flaring (Fig. 10–9).

Secondary Procedures for Prealveolar Lip Clefts

Unilateral. Secondary procedures may be necessary for the following:

1. Contraction of the skin scar with retraction of the vermilion margin producing an asymmetric Cupid's bow. The skin scar needs to be excised and,

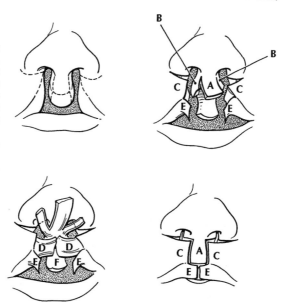

FIGURE 10–8. Millard repair of the bilateral complete cleft lip deformity. A rectangular prolabial flap (A) is elevated for reconstruction of the philtrum. Two lateral prolabial flaps (B) are created. These flaps may be stored in the nostril sill for future columella elevation or discarded. Lateral lip elements (C) are used to reconstruct either side of the lip. Orbicularis muscle (D) is dissected free in these lateral elements to be approximated behind the prolabial flap. Vermilion flaps (E) from the lateral elements are sutured beneath the prolabial flap to provide a full vermilion beneath the philtrum. The mucosa behind the prolabium (F) is used in the mucosal closure to provide a deep lip sulcus.

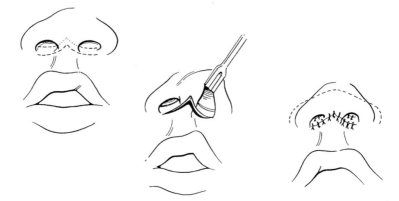

FIGURE 10–9. Columella elevation as described by Cronin for the second-stage reconstruction of a bilateral cleft lip.

after some undermining, the wound edges are approximated. A Z-plasty is marked out with angles of 60 degrees, and the flaps are transposed. If repair is short on the cleft side, the repair may require a complete redo of the rotation advancement.

2. Drooping of the lateral elements of the free border of the lip is easily corrected by excision of a wedge of mucosa and submucosa from the posterior aspect of the lower part of the lip. After undermining the lower margin, the wound is carefully closed.

3. Residual nasal tip deformities are corrected through an open tip rhinoplasty at about 4 years of age. Attention is directed at correction of the slumped ala on the cleft side by repositioning of the alar cartilages (Fig. 10–10).

Bilateral. After repair of the cleft followed by a columella elevation, the nasal tip should be symmetric with a columella of good length. The prolabium usually grows to produce a normal-sized philtrum. Secondary procedures may be indicated as the lip grows during the child's development.

1. Central flattening may occur as a result of the absence of muscle tissue in the prolabial segment. The previously sutured muscle can be approached from the mucosal surface without affecting the skin scar.

2. Deficiency in the central tubercle area may require augmentation with

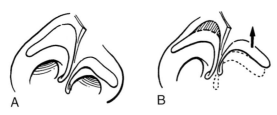

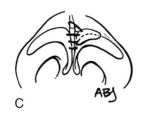

FIGURE 10–10. The slumped alar cartilages of the unilateral complete cleft lip deformity (A) are corrected by repositioning the cleft side lateral alar cartilages (B). Correction may require a columella strut and onlay cartilage grafts from the septum or conchal bowl (C).

local mucosal flaps. Severe deficiency may require complete take-down of the repair and revision with a Millard bilateral lip repair.

3. On rare occasions the upper lip is sufficiently tight and distorted to require a two-stage transfer of a lower lip flap (Abbé flap).

CLEFTS OF THE SECONDARY PALATE

The hard palate is composed of the palatine processes of the maxilla in front and the horizontal plates of the palatal bones behind. Its overlying mucous membrane is intensely dense and is incorporated with the underlying periosteum.

At the junction of the hard and soft palate, the posterior palatine arteries emerge from the palatine canal medial to the last molar tooth and run forward in a shallow groove on the lateral side of the hard palate. In surgical procedures for cleft palate, it is important to avoid injury to the palatine arteries as flaps of mucoperiosteum are elevated.

Behind the alveolus of the last molar tooth is a readily palpable hamular process to which is attached the pterygomandibular ligament, which passes down to be inserted into the posterior end of the mylohyoid line of the mandible, producing a fold in the mucous membrane overlying it, readily visible with the mouth open. Just below this attachment of the pterygomandibular ligament, the lingual nerve may be palpated as it passes down and forward, deep to the mucous membrane.

The soft palate consists of interlacing muscle fibers attached to the posterior border of the hard palate and enclosed in mucous membrane, hanging as a curtain between the nasopharynx and oropharynx. The median elongation of the soft palate is known as the uvula.

The pillars of the fauces pass downward as two folds of mucous membrane from each side of the soft palate, enclosing the tonsil between them. The anterior fold contains the palatoglossus muscle, extending to the side of the tongue, and the posterior fold contains the palatopharyngeus, terminating on the pharyngeal wall.

The sensory supply of the palate is mainly from the maxillary division of the trigeminal nerve, but fibers of the glossopharyngeal nerve supply its posterior part. The motor innervation of the palatal muscles is transmitted by vagal fibers in the pharyngeal plexus derived from the glossopharyngeal nerve, with the exception of the tensor palati, which is supplied by the mandibular division of the trigeminal nerve.

The soft palate closes off the nasopharynx from the buccal cavity during swallowing, blowing, and articulation. Palatal paralysis causes voice impairment, and fluids regurgitate through the nose during swallowing. Its fibromuscular structure is altered in shape and position by five muscles.

1. Tensor palati: Its origin is from the scaphoid fossa at the base of the medial pterygoid plate and the adjacent cartilaginous part of the eustachian tube. It extends anteriorly and inferiorly, turning around the hamulus for insertion into the palatal aponeurosis. The muscle tenses the palate and dilates the eustachian tube orifice.

2. Levator palati: Its origin is from the petrous temporal bone and the medial aspect of the eustachian tube. The muscle spreads downward and extends over the entire portion of the soft palate. It lifts and moves the palate posteriorly.

3. The palatopharyngeus has two heads of origin from the palatal aponeurosis

and descends, to form the posterior tonsillar pillar, for insertion into the thyroid cartilage. Its function, together with that of the palatoglossus, is to narrow the pharyngeal isthmus.

4. The palatoglossus arises from the undersurface of the palatal aponeurosis and inserts into the tongue, forming the anterior tonsillar pillar.

5. Each uvular muscle arises from the posterior nasal spine and inserts into the uvula. In forming the levator eminence, its function is to shorten the palate longitudinally.

Developmental Basis of Palatal Clefts

Medial extensions of the maxillary processes grow downward on either side of the tongue. As the mandible widens and the tongue descends, the palatal processes can swing upward and unite in the midline. The fused palatal processes also unite with the premaxilla and the nasal septum, which extend down as a partition from the roof of the oronasal cavity. The soft palate is formed by the migration of ectomesoderm from two growth centers. The entire process is completed by the twelfth week of intrauterine life.

Cleft palate may take a number of forms:

1. Complete: The cleft extends throughout the entire length between the two palatal processes.
2. Incomplete: As the two processes unite from the front to the back with the two halves of the uvula, the last part to fuse, the incomplete fusion may involve:
   a. Uvula alone, resulting in a bifid uvula
   b. Whole length of the soft palate
   c. Whole length of the soft palate and the posterior part of the whole palate
3. Submucous cleft palate. A bifid uvula, although usually an incidental finding without clinical significance, may be part of the submucous cleft complex. A rare condition, occurring once in 15,000 births, it is due to dehiscence of the levator palati muscles, causing a submucous cleft in the posterior palate and associated hypernasal speech. The mucous membrane in the midline is thin and transparent and is designated a zona pellucida.
   Hypernasal speech unresponsive to speech therapy should be treated by repair of the cleft, or this may be closed in conjunction with a pharyngeal flap procedure. In the mentally normal child the main causes of defective articulation in cleft palate subjects are nasal escape and defective hearing in patients who have not had appropriate middle ear drainage procedures.
4. Pierre Robin syndrome: The syndrome of "sequence" is characterized by:
   a. Micrognathia
   b. Glossoptosis due to the genioglossi muscles having their bony attachment displaced posteriorly. The retroposition of the tongue causes airway obstruction until the mandible grows forward.
   c. Cleft palate, although not invariable, is often present. It is usually incomplete but may extend to the incisive foramen. If a cleft is not present, the palate usually has a high arch.

Effects of Cleft Palate

Phonation. The most important reason for cleft palate repair is to allow the development of normal speech. The production of normal speech depends upon the provision of a sensitive, competent nasopharyngeal sphincter before the child begins to imitate heard speech at 12 to 18 months of age. By this time the child should have a mobile, intact soft palate. As it takes about 6 months after palate repair for scar tissue to resolve and soft palate mobility to be restored, cleft palates should be repaired no later than 12 months after birth.

Eighty per cent of children develop normal to "acceptable" speech after cleft repair, although speech therapy may be required. Occasionally, after cleft repair, a child may develop a nasal quality to his or her speech with associated problems in articulation. This is due to velopharyngeal incompetence with failure of contact betwen the soft palate and the posterior pharyngeal wall at the adenoid pad level.

Velopharyngeal incompetence may be helped by speech therapy, but most cases require a secondary surgical procedure to correct the velopharyngeal mechanism.

Feeding Difficulties. The child with a cleft palate may not develop strong sucking ability, although swallowing remains unaffected. The delivery of milk or soft food to the back of the oral cavity by means of a long nipple with a larger opening generally permits maintenance of good nutrition.

Middle Ear Disease. Malfunction of the eustachian tube in children with palatal clefts leads to the accumulation of thick, sterile fluid behind the ear drum, which in time may become infected. Left untreated, permanent hearing loss develops. Otolaryngologic examination must be carried out in every child with cleft palate and, when indicated, myringotomy is followed by insertion of a Silastic tube that allows the equalization of air pressure which cannot be provided via the eustachian tube. Bilateral myringotomy and insertion of ventilating tubes are usually done at the time of primary repair of lip or palate.

Repair of the Palate

Timing. Most surgeons close soft palatal clefts between 3 and 12 months of age. The hard palate may be closed at the same time, although many proponents prefer a two-staged closure, repairing the soft palate early and delaying hard palate closure until 9 to 12 months. Initial closure of the soft palate narrows the hard palatal cleft, requiring less mucoperiosteal dissection for hard palate repair.

Objective. Whether the palate is closed in one or two stages, the objectives of repair are to create a competent velopharyngeal mechanism and to separate the oral pharynx from the nasal pharynx. Principles of repair regardless of the techniques used include (1) reorientation of the levator palati muscle to provide a sling mechanism across the soft palate; (2) a two-layered closure providing a nasal mucosal surface and an oral mucosal surface for the hard palate and a three-layered closure providing nasal mucosa, muscle, and oral mucosa for the soft palate; and (3) a tension-free closure that lengthens the palate while providing a soft, mobile soft palate.

Debate continues regarding the best technique and timing of repair. Concerns relate to the incidence of postoperative velopharyngeal insufficiency and the effect of surgery on maxillofacial development.

Techniques of Repair

Intravelar Veloplasty. The levator palati muscle is dissected free from the oral mucosa above and nasal mucosa below on either side of the cleft. The malpositioned muscle is freed from its insertion on the hard palate and rotated down. A three-layered closure of nasal mucosa, muscle, and oral mucosa is accomplished in the midline (Fig. 10–11).

Furlow Repair. A double reverse Z-plasty is used to lengthen the soft palate at the expense of width. A posteriorly based Z-plasty flap of oral mucosa and muscle is transposed down while the opposite anteriorly based flap containing oral mucosa is transposed upward. Mirror-image Z-plasties are designed and transposed on the nasal mucosa side. As the posteriorly based flaps lie opposite each other, their transposition realigns the levator palati muscle in a transverse orientation with reconstruction of a sling mechanism (Fig. 10–12).

Complete Clefts. Clefts involving both the hard and soft palate mandate more extensive dissection to close the hard palate. The cleft margin is incised along its entire length, and mucoperiosteal flaps are elevated on both sides of the hard palate. A superiorly based mucoperiosteal flap is elevated on the vomer to aid in closure anteriorly. The soft palate may be closed by the intravelar veloplasty

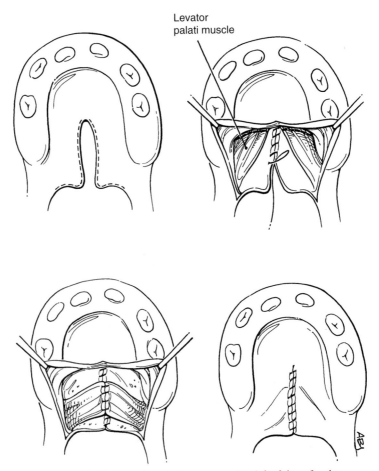

Levator
palati muscle

FIGURE 10–11. Intravelar veloplasty repair of a cleft of the soft palate.

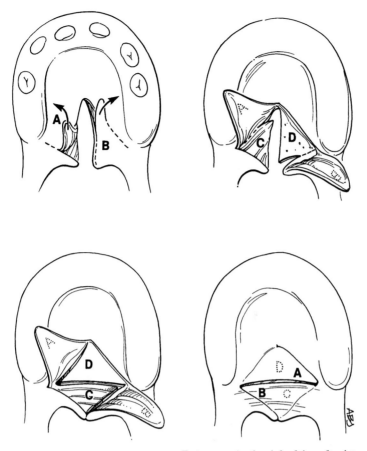

FIGURE 10–12. Furlow double-reverse Z-plasty repair of a cleft of the soft palate.

or Furlow methods, and the hard palate is closed by approximating the nasal mucoperiosteal flap to the vomer flap and approximating the oral mucoperiosteal flaps (Fig. 10–13). Bilateral clefts and wide unilateral clefts require more extensive dissection by the Von Langenbeck or Veau–Wardill-Kilner repair.

VON LANGENBECK PALATOPLASTY. The cleft margins are incised and mucoperiosteal flaps elevated on both the nasal and mucosal surfaces of the palatal shelf. A lateral relaxing incision through mucosa and periosteum begins anteriorly and extends around the maxillary tubercle to the anterior tonsillar pilar. The nasal surface is closed by approximating nasal mucosa posteriorly and suturing nasal mucosa to a superiorly based vomer flap anteriorly. The bipedicled mucoperiosteal flaps are sutured in the midline. The hamulus may be infractured to reduce tension on the closure. The levator palati muscle is dissected from oral and nasal mucosa and repositioned, and the soft palate is closed in three layers (Fig. 10–14).

VEAU–WARDILL-KILNER PALATOPLASTY. The initial dissection is similar to the Von Langenbeck repair, but the relaxing incision joins anteriorly with the incision along the cleft margins. The posteriorly based mucoperiosteal flaps are closed as a V-Y lengthening procedure, leaving a raw space anterolaterally which re-epithelializes within 10 days (Fig. 10–15). The soft palate is closed with an intravelar veloplasty.

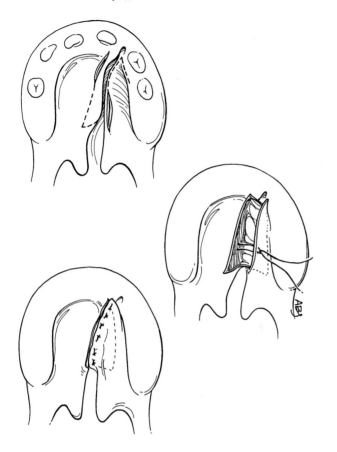

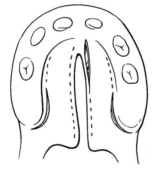

FIGURE 10–13. A vomer mucoperichondrial flap may be used to close the anterior portion of the hard palate cleft.

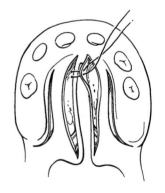

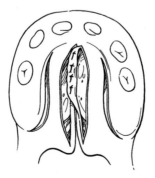

FIGURE 10–14. Von Langenbeck palatoplasty.

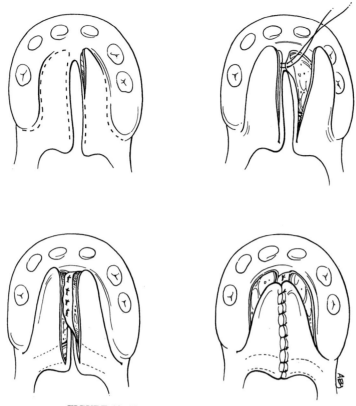

FIGURE 10–15. Veau–Wardill-Kilner palatoplasty.

SECONDARY PALATAL PROBLEMS

Velopharyngeal Insufficiency (VPI)

A competent velopharyngeal mechanism requires a coordinated sphincter effect of the soft palate, posterior pharynx, and lateral pharyngeal walls on phonation. Failure of this mechanism allows air to flow into and through the nasopharynx, resulting in hypernasal speech. Associated articulation problems develop as a consequence of VPI. Primary causes are twofold: (1) poor mobility of the soft palate: short palate, tight scarred palate, or malposition of the levator palati muscle. (2) poor mobility of the pharyngeal wall: primarily neuromuscular pathology of pharyngeal muscles. The degree of VPI is established with the input of a speech pathologist. Cine and video radiographs and direct inspection with fiberoptic nasopharyngoscopy help define the faulty mechanisms in phonation.

Numerous procedures to correct VPI have been described. Procedures have been directed at palatal lengthening, narrowing of the velopharyngeal opening, and re-creation of a functioning velopharyngeal sphincter mechanism.

Palatal Lengthening. This can be done by one of two procedures: (1) V-Y *pushback palatoplasty:* The original palate repair is revised with a V-Y retrodisplacement of the mucoperiosteal flaps, which are isolated on the palatine vessels. Reorientation of the levator palati muscle with an intravelar veloplasty is essential.

(2) *Furlow double reverse palatoplasty*: The soft palate is lengthened and a sling mechanism of the levator palati muscle is ensured.

Narrowing of the Velopharyngeal Opening. Augmentation of the posterior pharyngeal wall is effective for minimal VPI. It is primarily of historic interest. The posterior pharynx is built up by injection or insertion of Teflon or silicone.

Pharyngeal Flap Pharyngoplasty. The most widely used pharyngoplasty is the superiorly based posterior pharyngeal flap. The creation of the flap requires two vertical incisions through the mucosa and muscles down to the prevertebral fascia. A transverse cut well down in the pharynx joins the vertical incisions, and the musculomucosal flap is elevated. The donor area is then closed with interrupted polyglycolic acid sutures. Mucosal flaps are raised from the nasal side of the palate for lining the undersurface of the pharyngeal flap. The pharyngeal flap is sutured as far anteriorly as possible, and the lining flap is then sutured in place (Fig. 10–16). Modifications enable control of the ports between the flap and the pharyngeal wall (Hogan pharyngoplasty).

Dynamic Spincteroplasty. Orticochea described a pharyngoplasty that has since been modified by Jackson. The principle is to create a dynamic functioning sphincter rather than simply to narrow the velopharyngeal space. The posterior tonsillar pillars are elevated carefully, including the palatopharyngeus muscles. They are transposed medially and sutured to an incision in the posterior pharyngeal wall (Fig. 10–17). The innervated palatopharyngeus muscles contract on phona-

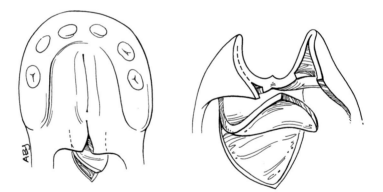

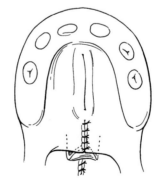

FIGURE 10–16. Superior-based pharyngeal flap for velopharyngeal insufficiency.

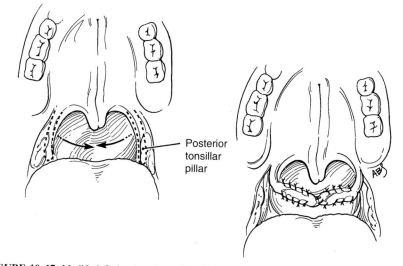

Posterior
tonsillar
pillar

FIGURE 10–17. Modified Orticochea dynamic sphincteroplasty for the correction of velopharyngeal insufficiency.

tion, closing the port created between palate, posterior pharynx, and posterior tonsillar pillars. Velopharyngeal competence is restored without creating a tight, tethered palate.

Palatal Fistulae

Fistulae may occasionally develop in the suture line of the cleft palate repair. The usual sites are at the junction of the hard and soft palates or anteriorly. The leakage of air, fluid, and food particles through the oronasal fistula mandates early repair, which may be difficult because of local scarring. Total excision of the fistula epithelium must be followed by tension-free apposition of the edges and closure in two layers, avoiding any dead space. If the cleft involves the alveolar ridge, a fistula persists anteriorly until the alveolar cleft is closed. Symptomatic palatal fistulae may be obturated with a dental appliance until definitive closure is accomplished.

Alveolar Reconstruction

Several stages of orthodontic treatment may include use of a spreading appliance to correct a collapsed dental arch. Straightening and alignment of teeth are required, and use of a retainer is necessary until the permanent teeth erupt. The final positioning of the permanent teeth requires several years of treatment, during which time a fixed bridge is used for replacement of missing teeth. Time of eruption of adult teeth is important in coordinating appropriate orthodontic management (Fig. 10–18).

Alveolar reconstruction may be necessary between 9 and 11 years of age when the permanent canines erupt. The cleft area can be opened by elevating a

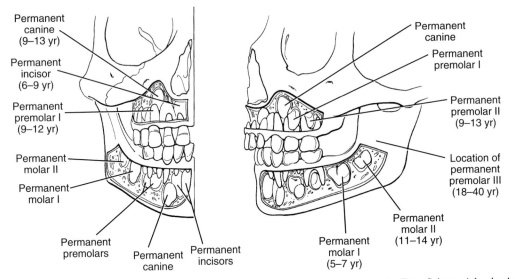

FIGURE 10–18. Dentition of a five year old and the expected eruption of permanent teeth. (From Sobotta, Atlas der Anatomie des Menschen, 2 vols, 20th ed. Baltimore, Urban and Schwarzenberg, 1993.)

gingival flap and autogenous bone packed into the defect. The gingival flaps are then transposed to cover the bone graft.

Dental Malocclusion

Despite early and aggressive orthodontic management, significant malocclusion may occur. The cause of malocclusion probably relates more to the scarring associated with palatal closure than to developmental abnormalities. Surgical correction is delayed until after the adolescent growth spurt, usually around 13 to 14 in female and 15 to 16 in male patients. Le Fort I or II maxillary advancement corrects the retruded hypoplastic maxilla, although mandibular retrusion may also be required in some cases.

Suggested Readings

Furlow LT Jr: Cleft palate repair by double opposing Z-plasty. Plast Reconstr Surg 78:724, 1986
Jackson IT, Silverton JS: Sphincter pharyngoplasty as a secondary procedure in cleft palates. Plast Reconstr Surg 69:518, 1977
Kernahan DA, Stark RB: A new classification for cleft lip and cleft palate. Plast Reconstr Surg 22:435, 1958
McGregor IA: The Abbé flap: Its use in single and double lip clefts. Br J Plast Surg 16:46, 1963
Millard DR Jr: Closure of bilateral cleft lip and elongation of columella by two operations in infancy. Plast Reconstr Surg 47:324, 1971
Millard DR Jr: Extensions of the rotation-advancement principle for wide unilateral cleft lips. Plast Reconstr Surg 42:535, 1968
Millard DR Jr, Latham RA: Improved primary surgical and dental treatment of clefts. Plast Reconstr Surg 86:856, 1990
Oneal RM, Greer DM Jr, Nobel GL: Secondary correction of bilateral cleft deformities with Millard's midline muscular closure. Plast Reconstr Surg 54:45, 1974
Orticochea M: A review of 236 cleft palate patients treated with dynamic muscle sphincter. Plast Reconstr Surg 71:180, 1983

Labels in Figure 10–18: Permanent canine (9–13 yr); Permanent incisor (6–9 yr); Permanent premolar I (9–12 yr); Permanent molar II; Permanent molar I; Permanent premolars; Permanent canine; Permanent incisors; Permanent canine; Permanent premolar I; Permanent premolar II (9–13 yr); Location of permanent premolar III (18–40 yr); Permanent molar II (11–14 yr); Permanent molar I (5–7 yr)

Randall P: A triangular flap operation for the primary repair of unilateral clefts of the lip. Plast Reconstr Surg 23:249, 1959

Trier WC, Dreyer TM: Primary Von Langenbeck palatoplasty with levator reconstruction: Rationale and technique. Cleft Palate J 21:254, 1984

Witzel MA, Clarke JA, Lindsay WK, Thompson HG: Comparison of results of pushback or Von Langenbeck repair of isolated cleft of the hard and soft palate. Plast Reconstr Surg 64:347, 1979.

CHAPTER 11

Head and Neck

OROMANDIBULAR DISORDERS

The Teeth

The dental enamel organ is formed by downgrowth of ectoderm. It is invaginated by the mesodermal dental papilla and dental sac, which provides the vascular pulp, dentine, and peridental membrane (Fig. 11–1).

Persistence of epithelial remnants between the teeth may, in later life, give rise to the formation of a dental cyst or to an epithelial odontoma. If the dental sac fails to disappear, a dentigerous cyst develops. The presence of a tumor of the jaw in association with a missing tooth that has not been dentally removed is strong evidence that the patient has a dentigerous cyst or some other form of odontoma.

ODONTOGENIC CYSTS

Dentigerous cyst: This arises in relation to an unerupted tooth. Usually unilocular, its fluid content is sterile, although secondary infection may occur. It may involve either the mandible or the maxilla. The cyst is ideally managed by enucleation.

Keratocyst: Arising from nests of dental lamina, it most commonly involves the mandible and is either unilocular or multilocular. It may grow large with destruction of adjacent tissue. It is ideally treated with curettage; however, recurrence rate is significant, requiring resection and bone grafting.

ODONTOGENIC TUMORS

Usually benign, odontogenic tumors may also be malignant. Benign lesions may be locally invasive. They are of epithelial or ectomesenchymal origin.

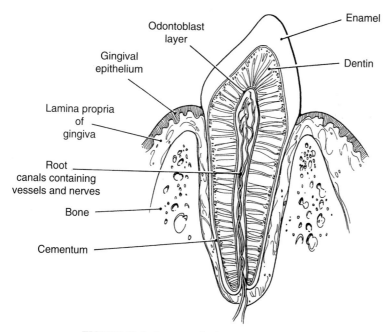

FIGURE 11–1. Anatomy of a human canine tooth.

Odontoma: Complex and compound odontomas are the most common odontogenic tumors. They are benign tumors composed of well-developed tooth elements. The complex odontoma is often associated with an unerupted tooth and consists of a cystic area with contained tooth elements readily managed by local curettage. The compound odontoma is a solid benign tumor found at the root of the incisor-cuspid deciduous teeth. It needs to be removed to permit eruption of the permanent tooth.

Cementoma: This is a benign radiopaque mass arising from the periodontal membrane which gradually enlarges and ultimately ossifies.

Ameloblastoma/adamantinoma: This represents the most common locally malignant tumor. It is an epithelial odontogenic tumor occurring predominantly in the molar area of the mandible, presenting as a multilocular swelling that on radiologic examination gives a "honeycomb" appearance. It may have a variegated histologic pattern with a follicular, plexiform, granular, or acanthomatous pattern. Lymphatic and hematogenous metastatic spread may occur.

Intraoral resection should be accompanied by the removal of a wide margin of clinically healthy bone to prevent local recurrence. The residual defect should be reconstructed by a bone graft.

NONODONTOGENIC TUMORS OF THE JAW

Benign tumors: Relatively uncommon lesions, these include chondroma, giant cell tumor, osteoma, osteoblastoma, and osteoid osteoma. They are managed by enucleation or local excision.

Fibrous dysplasia: This presents as a progressive mass. Radiographs demonstrate a characteristic ground glass appearance with indistinct borders. Mandibular involvement is usually monostotic and is less frequent than maxillary involvement. Treatment requires either recontouring of bone by burring or excision of involved bone and bone graft reconstruction.

Aneurysmal bone cyst: This fast growing lesion presents as a painless swelling. It tends to erode the adjacent cortex and is treated by removal with curettage and cautery.

Malignant tumors: Primary nonodontogenic malignancies are either sarcomas or lymphomas. Sarcomas include chondrosarcoma, fibrosarcoma, osteosarcoma, and Ewing sarcoma. Lymphomas include primary non-Hodgkin lymphoma and Burkitt lymphoma.

Metastatic disease from breast, lung, prostate, and thyroid.

The Tongue

Soon after the development of the branchial arches, a median elevation appears on the ventral wall of the pharynx, named the tuberculum impar. A little later, two projections arise from the floor of the primitive oral cavity which unite and enclose this structure within the primitive oral cavity to form the anterior two thirds of the tongue. The posterior third of the tongue develops separately from a posterior median elevation, the hypobranchial eminence, and the adjoining parts of the second and third branchial arches.

A V-shaped groove, the sulcus terminalis, separates the anterior two thirds of the tongue, which forms the floor of the oral cavity, from the posterior one third, which belongs to the pharynx. The apex of the V points posteriorly and is at the foramen cecum.

A median bud of entoderm grows downward from the foramen cecum in front of the hyoid bone as the thyroglossal duct and then bifurcates to form the isthmus and lateral lobes of the thyroid gland. The lower end of the thyroglossal duct normally forms the pyramidal lobe of the gland. Its proximal part normally disappears, or it may remain as a fibrous cord that attaches that lobe to the hyoid base.

DEVELOPMENTAL ABNORMALITIES

1. The tongue may be bifid, although the deformity is usually localized to the tip.

2. Congenital macroglossia is usually the result of dilation of the lymph spaces, which may affect all or part of the tongue.

3. Lingual thyroid: Failure of descent of the thyroglossal duct may result in ectopic thyroid tissue being situated at the base of the tongue. Thyroid tumors can occur in the ectopic gland. More often, a swelling of the tongue may affect speech, swallowing, or breathing. A thyroid scan confirms the absence of thyroid tissue at any other site. Surgical excision is indicated for the symptomatic ectopic gland, with autotransplantation of the excised thyroid tissue.

4. Thyroglossal duct cyst: This usually presents in childhood as a painless cystic swelling in the region of the hyoid bone. Usually in the midline, it moves on swallowing and protrusion of the tongue. It is excised by the Sistrunk procedure. This involves excision of the cyst and its associated tract as well as the body of the hyoid bone up to the base of the tongue (see Fig. 11–10).

LINGUAL BLOOD SUPPLY

Each lingual artery arises from the external carotid artery opposite the greater corner of the hyoid bone and is directed forward and upward, deep to the hyoglossus, to the tongue. The artery ends at the anterior border of the hyoglossus by dividing into the sublingual branch and the profunda artery of the tongue, which extends forward along the lateral side of the genioglossus toward the tip of the tongue. Other branches of the lingual artery are a small suprahyoid branch and a dorsalis linguae branch.

The abundant vascularity of the tongue permits the raising of anteriorly and posteriorly based flaps to provide mucosal cover to adjacent areas. The donor area is closed by direct suture of its margins.

TONGUE FLAPS

Posteriorly based dorsal tongue flap: This flap can be rotated laterally into a defect in the tonsillar fossa, buccal area, or floor of the mouth.

Anteriorly based dorsal tongue flap: This flap is suitable for coverage of cheek, lip, floor of the mouth, and hard palate.

Bipedicled transverse flap: This is useful for lip reconstruction but needs a second stage for division of the pedicle.

Tip-derived flaps: These use dorsal and ventral components as perimeter flaps for vermilion repairs of the lip.

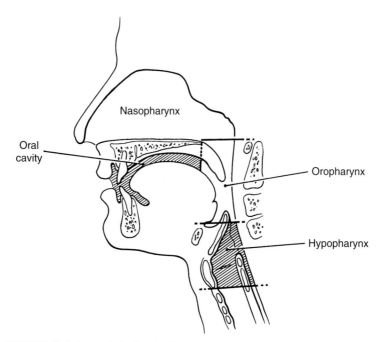

FIGURE 11–2. Anatomic landmarks of the oral cavity, oral pharynx, and hypopharynx.

ORAL AND OROPHARYNGEAL CARCINOMA

The oral cavity extends from the lips to the junction of the hard and soft palates superiorly and the junction of the anterior two thirds and posterior third of the tongue inferiorly. The structures involved include the lips, buccal mucosa, floor of the mouth, alveolar ridge, retromolar trigone, anterior two thirds of the tongue, and hard palate.

The oropharynx extends from the posterior aspect of the oral cavity to the hypopharynx and includes (Fig. 11–2) the soft palate, tonsils, tonsillar pillars, tonsillar fossa, posterior one third of the tongue, and pharyngeal walls cephalad to the epiglottis.

Carcinomas of the head and neck are classified and staged by the TNM classification (Table 11–1).

T: Refers to the primary tumor. The size, location, and degree of invasion of the

TABLE 11–1. TNM Classification of Oral Cavity and Oropharyngeal Carcinoma

T_1	≤2 cm
T_2	>2 cm ≤4 cm
T_3	>4 cm ≤6 cm
T_4	Invades skin, muscle, bone, or >6 cm
N_0	No nodes
N_1	Single ipsilateral node ≤3 cm
N_2a	Single ipsilateral nodes 3–6 cm
N_2b	Multiple ipsilateral nodes ≤6 cm
N_2c	Contralateral or bilateral nodes ≤6 cm
N_3	Any nodes >6 cm
M_0	No systemic metastatic disease
M_1	Systemic metastatic disease

lesion determine its T classification. Oral cavity and oropharyngeal lesions are classified by size, whereas other head and neck lesions are classified by their anatomic extension.

N: Refers to the status of the regional nodes. Classification is determined by number, size, and location of involved nodes.

M: Refers to the absence or presence of distant systemic metastatic disease.

Staging: The disease stage is determined by the classification of the primary lesion, status of the regional nodes, and absence or presence of systemic metastases. The stage predicts prognosis and, in conjunction with anatomic location, determines appropriate management (Table 11–2).

Oral Carcinoma

Squamous cell carcinoma represents 90 per cent of all oral malignancies. Other tumors include intraoral lymphoma, sarcoma, and malignant disease of intraoral salivary tissue.

The cancerous lesion usually presents as an ulcer with indurated edges. Related etiologically to tobacco, alcohol, and lack of oral hygiene, the lesion often commences in an area of leukoplakia and may first manifest itself in one of three ways:

1. An exophytic lesion usually presents in the buccal area as a soft white outgrowth that grows very slowly.

2. A proliferative verrucous lesion presents as a well-differentiated papillary lesion that is locally aggressive but does not metastasize to lymph nodes until very late in the disease process. Usually seen in the mandibulobuccal sulcus, alveolar mucosa, and tip of the tongue, these lesions are not very radiosensitive, making wide local resection the treatment of choice.

3. Ulcerative invasive carcinoma is the most common variety, with deep invasion and tissue destruction, and is classically seen in the floor of the mouth and tongue.

CARCINOMA OF THE LIP

Carcinoma of the lip is the most common of the head and neck malignancies associated with actinic damage and smoking. It is often preceded by leukoplakia. Ninety per cent of lesions involve the lower lip, and more than 90 per cent are squamous cell carcinoma. They typically present as ulcerated or crusted lesions and are best managed by excision. Ipsilateral neck dissection is reserved for

TABLE 11–2. Staging of Disease by the TNM Classification

Stage 1	T_1, N_0, M_0
Stage 2	T_2, N_0, M_0
Stage 3	T_3, N_0, M_0
	T_1, T_2, T_3, N_1, M_0
Stage 4	T_4
	N_2 or N_3 regardless of T
	M regardless of T or N

clinically involved nodes. A contralateral suprahyoid dissection is included if the lesion crosses the midline.

CARCINOMA OF THE ANTERIOR TWO THIRDS OF THE TONGUE

This condition affects the lateral borders or ventral surface of the anterior two thirds of the tongue. It presents as an ulcer with indurated edges, with the gradual development of symptoms. Difficulty with speech and swallowing develops as the tongue muscles are invaded. Pain, both local and referred to the ear via the chorda tympani nerve, is a late symptom. The cancerous process progressively invades the floor of the mouth and mandible. Submandibular, digastric, and jugular lymph node involvement on the ipsilateral side is present in one third of cases.

Cancer of the middle third of the tongue may involve cervical lymph nodes bilaterally once it extends to the midline. It may extend locally with invasion of the palatoglossal fold, the anterior pillar of the tonsil, the retromolar trigone, and the floor of the mouth.

Treatment is by surgery or radiation therapy.

Surgical: Wedge resection may be done for small lesions on the tongue margin. Partial glossectomy may be done for larger lesions. Suprahyoid or radical neck dissection may be indicated, depending on the merits of the situation.

Radiation therapy: After a confirmatory biopsy of the lesion, radiation therapy may cure the primary tumor if it is in an early stage. Radical neck dissection is indicated for lymph node involvement. Neck dissection is followed by postoperative radiation.

CARCINOMA OF THE FLOOR OF THE MOUTH

Representing about 25 per cent of oral cancers, this cancer presents at two main sites: laterally and anteriorly. At the anterior segment of the floor of the mouth, which is the most common site, it commences just lateral to the lingual frenulum. The ulcerative process extends to involve the base of tongue and the genioglossus as well as the mandibular periosteum. Extension to the cervical lymph nodes occurs in almost half the cases.

Surgical treatment is usually the treatment of choice. A preliminary tracheostomy is indicated whenever radical procedures are to be carried out in the oral cavity.

1. En bloc excision of the floor of the mouth plus suprahyoid neck dissection: If the lesion is posterior to the edge of the mylohyoid or is an early lesion of the anterior segment of the floor of the mouth, this limited resection may suffice.
2. Lip-splitting incision: If more extensive resection is required, an incision through the lip down to the chin and then curving around as a submandibular incision permits division of the mandible with a Gigli saw. This approach, with the mandible retracted, provides extensive access to the entire oral cavity. Subsequently, the mandible can be rewired and, if teeth are present, an arch bar may be wired to the incisors.
3. Composite resection (commando procedure): This represents an in-continuity en bloc resection of the primary tumor in its total pathologic extent, together

with radical neck dissection and immediate reconstructive procedures using pectoralis major, trapezius, or free flaps to reconstruct the normal anatomy.

4. Mandibular resection in cancer of the floor of the mouth is not always necessary but, if required, may vary in extent:

   a. Segmental resection of the horizontal ramus: Insertion of a metal spacer, such as a Kirschner wire or stainless steel plate, permits sufficient temporization until assurance that cure of the cancer has occurred before bone grafting is contemplated.

   b. Mandibular involvement posterior to the mental foramen requires mandibulectomy of the lateral arch from the mental foramen to the temporomandibular joint. If adequate soft tissue replacement is provided through use of a flap, then bony replacement is not mandatory, although it is preferable.

   c. Hemimandibulectomy from the symphysis to the temporomandibular joint requires adequate soft tissue replacement with the need for bony replacement. Free tissue transfer of composite flaps including skin, soft tissue, and bone may be indicated at the time of tumor resection in selected cases. Potential free flaps include the iliac flap based on the deep circumflex iliac vessels; the scapular flap based on the circumflex scapular vessels; and the fibular flap based on the peroneal vessels.

Aggressive lesions, including those with histologic features of perineurial invasion and intralymphatic spread or nodal involvement, require postoperative radiation to the site of primary resection. If there is nodal involvement, the neck is also radiated after neck dissection.

Although chemotherapy may cause preoperative reduction in tumor size, these drugs are usually used as adjunctive therapy in a postoperative regimen. In unresectable cases, a combination of radiation and chemotherapy may be helpful.

Oropharyngeal Carcinoma

Posterior one third of the tongue: This is an aggressive lesion in which 70 to 80 per cent of patients have regional nodal involvement at presentation. Localized lesions are usually treated with radiation therapy, whereas invasive lesions require surgical resection with postoperative radiation therapy. External beam radiation may be augmented with implantation of interstitial radium needles or iridium-192 wires.

Soft palate: Patients tend to present early with localized lesions manageable by radiation.

Tonsil and peritonsillar region: Early lesions are managed by radiation alone. However, patients most commonly present with invasive disease requiring surgical excision and postoperative radiation.

Pharyngeal wall: Patients generally present with invasive lesions and regional node involvement requiring combined therapy.

Carcinoma of the Nasopharynx

Relatively uncommon in the West, this cancer is very common in China, where there seems to be a genetic predisposition and an association with the Epstein-Barr virus. Nasopharyngeal carcinoma include squamous cell carcinoma, lymphoma, sarcomas, and highly anaplastic cancers. An early lesion may present with nose bleeds, nasal stuffiness, or otitis media, although initial presentation is often a neck mass representing nodal metastases.

Diagnosis is made by endoscopy and CT or MR scan. Management requires 6000 to 7000 rad of external beam radiation to the primary lesion and the bilateral neck region.

MAXILLARY CARCINOMA

Although the antrum and body of the maxilla may be involved by various forms of sarcoma, Burkitt tumor, lymphoma, adamantinoma, or metastatic disease, squamous cell carcinoma remains the predominant form of malignancy arising from the pseudostratified columnar epithelium lining the sinus. Next in frequency is the adenocarcinoma derived from the mucus-secreting cells of the sinus.

CLINICAL FEATURES

Apart from causing enlargement of the antral cavity, symptoms and signs are related to involvement of adjacent anatomic structures and thus present late in the course of the disease.

1. Forward displacement of the anterior wall leads to retrusion of the malar part of the cheek.
2. Upward extension of the growth compresses the infraorbital nerve with appropriate facial pain, and subsequently anesthesia of the skin over this area develops. Later, proptosis and diplopia develop as a result of displacement of the eyeball.
3. Medial spread causes destruction of the nasal fossa, with blockage of the nasolacrimal duct causing epiphora.
4. Further growth causes extension into the nasopharynx, with epistaxis due to erosion of blood vessels.
5. Inferior extension causes bulging of the palate, and involvement of palatine nerves causes severe pain referred to the upper jaw teeth.

RADIOLOGIC FEATURES

Stereoscopic and CT views are necessary to demonstrate the expansion or destruction of the sinus walls, increased opacity of the sinuses, and irregularity of soft tissue outline.

DIAGNOSIS

Confirmation of the suspected diagnosis of a maxillary tumor requires biopsy and pathologic endorsement. Punch biopsy can be performed via nasoantral, buccal sulcus, or palatal routes. A Caldwell-Luc route provides a direct approach to the sinus, and after pathologic confirmation definitive surgery can be planned.

TREATMENT

Radiation therapy is indicated postoperatively for patients with undifferentiated lesions, lymphoma, and any doubt that the cancer has been totally eradicated.

Surgical management is undertaken by one of three approaches:

1. Total maxillectomy: After anesthesia has been induced and the pharynx packed off, the external carotid artery is ligated. The Weber-Fergusson incision commences below the inner canthus of the eye, skirts the nose and its ala nasi, and divides the upper lip in the midline. At the upper end of this incision, a transverse incision crosses and divides the lower eyelid lateral to the lacrimal punctum, divides the conjunctiva in the lower fornix, and crosses the zygoma (Fig. 11–3). The cheek flap is raised and the mucosa of the gingivolabial sulcus divided. The nasal cartilage is separated from the nasal base. The periosteum along the lower edge of the orbit is divided and the orbital floor exposed. The nasal bone and nasal process of the maxilla are divided. The maxilla is mobilized after all intervening structures have been divided. The central incisor tooth is removed and the periosteum of the hard palate divided; the soft palate is freed, and the alveolar and palatal processes of the maxilla are divided. The maxilla is lifted off the pterygoid plates and removed. After hemostasis has been achieved, the entire soft tissue defect is resurfaced with a split-thickness skin graft. A compressive dressing and a prosthesis are put in place and the skin incision is closed.

2. Total maxillectomy with orbital exenteration: This is necessary if ocular, middle turbinate, or ethmoid involvement is present. The entire floor of the orbit is resected, with en bloc resection of the orbital contents and the maxilla.

3. Radical neck dissection is carried out if enlarged lymph nodes are present.

Carcinoma of the Hypopharynx

The hypopharynx consists of the pyriform sinus, the posterior pharyngeal wall (lower portion), and the postcricoid region.

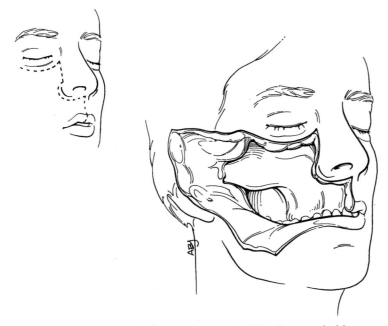

FIGURE 11–3. Exposure of the maxilla by the Weber-Fergusson incision.

Patients usually present with a late invasive squamous cell carcinoma fixed to surrounding tissues. Nodal metastases occur early owing to the rich lymphatic drainage to the midjugular nodes and jugular digastric nodes.

The occasional localized lesion may be managed by radiation, but surgical resection combined with postoperative radiation is generally required. Early lesions of the pyriform sinus and pharyngeal wall are treated with local pharyngeal resection and preservation of the voice. Large invasive lesions and lesions involving the postcricoid larynx require laryngopharyngectomy. The pharynx is reconstructed with a gastric pull-up or free jejunal transfer, whereas significant soft tissue defects require transfer of a pedicled myocutaneous or free flap.

PRIMARY SALIVARY GLAND TUMORS

The parotid gland is the largest of the salivary glands and is the site of about 6 per cent of all head and neck tumors. The parotid, submaxillary, and sublingual glands provide the main salivary flow via their respective ducts. Salivary gland tissue may also be distributed throughout the oropharynx and palate.

Salivary gland tumors present as a mass in the appropriate area. Submaxillary tumors are clearly palpable on bimanual examination with one finger on the floor of the mouth and the other in the submandibular area. Minor salivary gland tumors most frequently present as submucous palatal or pharyngeal masses.

The most common site for neoplasia is the parotid gland. The "rule of eighties" defines the fact that 80 per cent of parotid neoplasms are benign; of these, 80 per cent are pleomorphic adenomas—that is, mixed parotid tumors—and 80 per cent are located in the superficial lobe. Other benign neoplasms of the salivary glands include Warthin tumor (papillary cystadenoma lymphomatosum), oncocytoma, and monomorphic adenoma.

The parotid tumor that presents as a preauricular or intra-auricular mass that is firm and nontender without facial nerve involvement is usually a mixed parotid tumor. Occasionally metastasis to a parotid lymph node from head and neck cancer or melanoma needs to be considered. Rarely, parotid duct calculous disease may be considered but is readily excluded by radiography. Neither sialography nor CT scan is necessary, and biopsy is contraindicated if pleomorphic adenoma is likely.

Parotid Anatomy

The gland occupies the space between the mandibular ramus and the upper segment of the mastoid process. It is irregular in outline, being limited above by the zygoma, where it is situated in close proximity to the external auditory meatus and the temporomandibular joint (Fig. 11–4).

Below, the gland projects into the neck and overlies the posterior belly of the digastric, approaching the submandibular gland, from which it is separated by a process of deep cervical fascia. A horizontal line extending from the angle of the mandible to the mastoid process marks the extent of the gland in its downward direction.

Anteriorly, the gland projects toward the face and overflows the mandible and masseter muscle. Medial to it is the styloid process and its muscles, the styloglossus

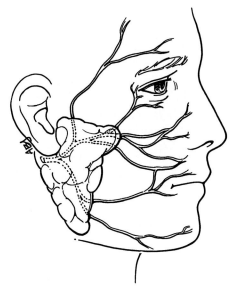

FIGURE 11-4. Relationship of the superficial lobe of the parotid gland to the facial nerve.

and stylohyoid, which separate the gland from the internal jugular vein, the internal carotid artery, the last four cranial nerves, and the lateral wall of the pharynx.

The gland is enclosed in its own capsule derived from the deep cervical fascia. The superficial and most extensive portion of the gland reaches the angle of the mandible, and from its anterior border, situated on the masseter muscle, emerges the parotid duct.

The parotid (Stensen) duct is 2 inches in length. Arising from the anterior border of the gland, it passes forward over the masseter below the small accessory portion of the gland to perforate the buccinator and the mucous membrane of the cheek opposite the second upper molar tooth. Situated about 1 inch below the zygomatic arch, the path of the duct is represented by a line drawn from the external auditory meatus to a point below the nostril. The midpoint of that line is situated opposite the duct's oral opening.

The caliber of the duct permits passage of a probe and the injection of radiopaque material to produce a sialogram, which may provide information regarding calculi, fistulas, or ductal displacement by tumor. It also demonstrates the presence of sialectasis in patients who suffer episodes of recurrent parotitis.

Structures Within the Parotid Gland

1. The external carotid artery runs through the middle of the gland to ascend behind the ramus of the mandible, where it gives off the posterior auricular, superficial temporal, and maxillary branches.
2. The posterior facial vein is formed by the junction of the superficial temporal and maxillary veins. The posterior facial vein receives parotid tributaries and divides within the substance of the gland into two branches. One joins the anterior facial vein, and the other inclines posteriorly over the sternomastoid muscle to join the posterior auricular vein and thereby constitutes the external jugular vein.
3. The facial nerve (Fig. 11-4) emerges from the stylomastoid foramen and runs forward, traversing the parotid gland superficial to the posterior facial vein and

external carotid artery. Situated between the superficial and deep parts of the parotid gland, it reaches the area over the ramus of the mandible where, within the gland, it bifurcates into its two main divisions—the zygomaticotemporal and zygomaticofacial nerves.

a. The zygomaticotemporal nerve divides into temporal, zygomatic, and buccal branches.

b. The zygomaticofacial nerve provides mandibular and cervical branches, which emerge on the anterior aspect of the parotid gland to lie on the masseter and then supply the facial muscles. Because the facial nerve lies between the superficial and deep parts of the gland, resection of the superficial part for benign lesions and tumors can be accomplished without damage to the major facial nerve trunk and its branches. Temporary paralysis may occur in 20 per cent of patients from excessive handling or retraction, but total recovery usually occurs within 3 months.

Non-neoplastic Pathologic Conditions of the Parotid Gland

1. Pyogenic infection of the gland may proceed to acute suppurative parotitis in dehydrated, debilitated individuals or to a granulomatous parotitis complicating ductal obstruction by a calculus.

2. Chronic sialectasis with recurrent episodic sialadenitis

3. Von Mikulicz disease: Granulomatous enlargement of the parotid gland

4. Sjögren syndrome: Granulomatous involvement of parotid, submaxillary, and lacrimal glands associated with uveitis.

Benign Tumors

Pleomorphic adenoma: Consisting of varying proportions of mesenchymal and epithelial components, this mixed tumor may be lobulated or cystic, contained within a thin pseudocapsule from compression of adjacent uninvolved gland. More common in women, it usually presents in the fifth decade. The tumor occurs predominantly in the superficial lobe of the gland, thus permitting cure by lobectomy. Any lesser procedure results in recurrence of the tumor.

Papillary cystadenoma lymphomatosum: Warthin tumor predominates in males and occurs bilaterally in 10 per cent of cases. It is often cystic, and local excision with a wide margin of normal tissue may be sufficient without risk of recurrence. Lobectomy, if possible, is the preferred treatment (Fig. 11–5).

Miscellaneous benign tumors: Oncocytoma, which is an oxyphilic adenoma; monomorphic adenoma; basal cell adenoma; glycogen-rich adenoma; and sebaceous lymphadenoma occur infrequently. In children, lymphangioma and hemangioma are the most common neoplasms, often resolving spontaneously.

Lipoma of the parotid gland: Presents as a multilobulated tumor with a distinctive appearance on CT scans.

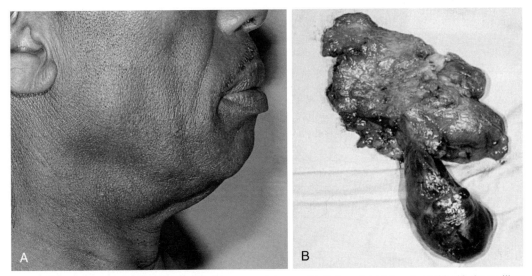

FIGURE 11–5. *A,* A typical location of a Warthin tumor of the parotid. *B,* Superficial lobe of parotid with the papillary cystadenoma lymphomatosum (Warthin tumor) involving the inferior pole of the gland.

Malignant Tumors

Mucoepidermoid carcinoma is the most common malignant tumor of the parotid gland. Although its low-grade form usually remains localized for a long time, its high-grade variety extends rapidly to involve the facial nerve, muscles, and bone. It also metastasizes to lymph nodes and, hematogenously, to the lungs.

Other malignant salivary gland tumors are (1) *cylindroma:* This adenocystic carcinoma is the most common malignant tumor affecting the submaxillary and other minor salivary glands. Local invasion and metastatic spread to lungs and brain occur slowly but relentlessly. (2) *Adenocarcinoma,* a slow-growing, locally invasive tumor. (3) *Acinic cell carcinoma,* with its origin in the acinic cells of the salivary gland and a tendency to low-grade malignancy. (4) *Malignant transformation* of a mixed tumor. (5) *Squamous cell carcinoma,* representing about 7 per cent of malignant parotid and submaxillary gland tumors. It grows rapidly, with early local fixation and extension to involve the facial nerve and overlying skin. Metastasis to lymph nodes and by hematogenous spread results in a surgical 5-year cure rate of less than 50 per cent.

Surgical Treatment

Superficial Parotidectomy. Benign tumors of the parotid gland are best managed by lobectomy, with identification and preservation of the facial nerve and its branches. The nerve trunk is best identified as it issues from the stylomastoid foramen in the space bounded by the mastoid process and anterior border of the sternomastoid muscle. The superficial lobe is dissected anteriorly off the facial nerve and its branches. Alternatively, the facial nerve branches may be identified anteriorly, using nerve stimulators if necessary, and the gland dissected posteriorly, using the normal anatomic landmarks. Access to the parotid gland is provided by a preauricular incision that extends around the ear lobule and along the upper end of the mandible into the neck and elevation of the flap.

Total Parotidectomy. If the nerve can be spared, it should be conserved if it is not surrounded by tumor. The nerve must be sacrificed if it is involved in tumor, and any contiguously involved muscle or bone must also be resected in a monobloc manner. Radical neck dissection must also be completed if lymph node involvement is suspected.

After resection of the facial nerve, restoration of nerve continuity may be possible by direct suture. If the gap cannot be closed, even after freeing up the nerve proximally and distally, nerve grafts using the greater auricular nerve should be used.

Frey Syndrome. This is gustatory sweating that occurs several months later in up to 20 per cent of patients who have undergone parotid surgery. Mild to profuse perspiration occurs over the cutaneous distribution of the auriculotemporal nerve.

Transposition of the Parotid Duct. Excessive drooling may be corrected by transposition of the parotid duct in conjunction with removal of the submaxillary glands (Wilke procedure). First described for treating drooling associated with cerebral palsy, it is also effective for drooling due to loss of oral lip sphincter following trauma or surgery. A buccal mucosal flap is elevated to include the opening of the parotid duct. It is tubed and tunneled behind the anterior tonsillar pillar. Saliva is diverted from the oral cavity into the oropharynx.

The Submandibular Salivary Gland

ANATOMY

The submandibular salivary gland is situated under cover of the mandible and the insertion of the internal pterygoid muscle and partly in the submandibular triangle, where it overlaps both bellies of the digastric. It lies under cover of the platysma and deep fascia and consists of a large superficial and a small deep lobe, which communicate around the posterior border of the mylohyoid muscle (Fig. 11–6).

Its deep aspect lies against the mylohyoid and rests posteriorly against the hyoglossus muscle, where it is in intimate contact with the lingual and hypoglossal nerves, both of which run along the hyoglossus muscle as they pass toward the tongue.

The facial artery is intimately related to the gland, approaching it posteriorly before arching over its superior aspect to reach the inferior border of the mandible before it ascends on the face.

The submandibular (Wharton) duct emerges from the medial surface of the gland and runs forward between the mylohyoid and hyoglossus muscles to pass forward over the genioglossus and deep to the sublingual gland to open into the floor of the mouth on each side of the frenulum of the tongue. The lingual nerve, which first lies above the duct, crosses it superficially and then turns upward on its deep surface while pursuing its course along the hyoglossus muscle. The submandibular lymph nodes are embedded within the gland as well as between it and the mandible.

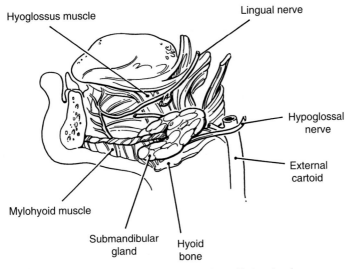

Hyoglossus muscle

Lingual nerve

Hypoglossal nerve

External cartoid

Mylohyoid muscle

Submandibular gland

Hyoid bone

FIGURE 11–6. Anatomy of the submandibular triangle.

CLINICAL DISORDER

Calculous disease is more common in the submaxillary than in the parotid gland. It may be located in the gland or impacted in the duct. In the latter case, the calculus can be palpated manually between a finger in the mouth and a finger below the angle of the jaw. Intermittent enlargement of the submandibular gland occurs. An incision in the floor of the mouth over the stone permits its ready removal.

Tumors of this gland are much less common that parotid tumors, but the presence of a tumor requires removal of the gland. The gland may also need to be removed because of an impacted stone.

After an incision through skin, platysma, and cervical fascia, two finger-breadths below the mandible, the submandibular salivary gland is mobilized, taking cognizance of its anatomic relationships, with exposure and ligation of the facial vessels and identification and preservation of the hypoglossal and lingual nerves.

THE NECK

Anatomy

The Platysma. This is a thin subcutaneous muscular sheet lying across the side of the neck, extending from the shoulder to the face and covering the anterior and posterior triangles of the neck. The platysma belongs to the muscles of expression and is supplied by the facial nerve. The muscle helps to draw the corners of the mouth downward and laterally while the skin of the upper part of the chest and shoulder is raised.

Incisions in the neck generally gape because of contraction of the platysma. In order to provide cosmetic healing, it is important to suture the edges of the platysma separately from the skin.

Sternomastoid Muscle. The sternomastoid muscle divides the neck into two triangular spaces. The anterior triangle is enclosed between the sternomastoid, the anterior and median line of the neck, and the mandible above. The posterior triangle is between the sternomastoid, the trapezius, and the clavicle below.

The muscle arises by a medial or sternal head and a lateral clavicular head. It is directed upward and backward to be inserted into the outer aspect of the mastoid process. Innervated by the spinal accessory nerve and a motor branch of the second cervical nerve, the two head muscles acting together flex the head at the atlanto-occipital joint. Each muscle, acting alone, turns the face to the opposite side.

Lymphatic Drainage. Lymphatic drainage from the head and neck is to one of five levels: the submandibular nodes, upper jugular nodes, midjugular nodes, lower jugular nodes, and posterior triangle nodes (Fig. 11–7).

Developmental Disorders

Congenital Torticollis. Shortly after birth, a tumor-like mass may be noted in the lower segment of the sternomastoid muscle, which may be short and tight. Owing to birth trauma, contraction of the muscle develops. The mass disappears after some months and the head becomes displaced toward the affected side, with the chin tilted upward and the mastoid process drawn downward (Fig. 11–8). By the end of a year these changes are irreversible, and the face on the affected side becomes smaller and flatter. The cervical spine develops a curve with a concavity to the affected side and a compensatory curve in the opposite direction in the dorsal region.

Treatment is surgical. Through an adequate skin incision, the upper or lower

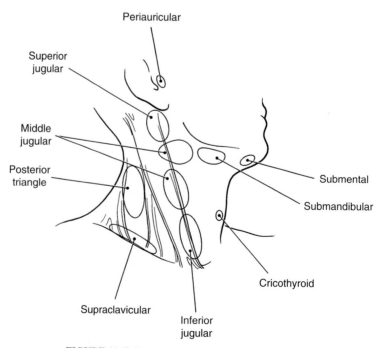

FIGURE 11–7. Lymphatic drainage of the head and neck.

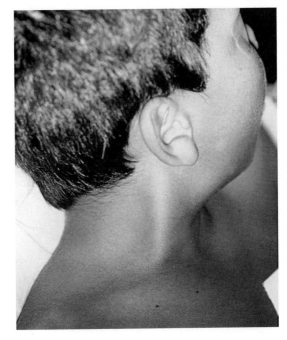

FIGURE 11–8. Congenital torticollis.

end of the muscle and its sheath is divided and mobilized. A subcutaneous tenotomy is usually inadequate and inadvisable.

Lower tenotomy: Through a collar incision 2 inches above the clavicle, the platysma is divided and the external jugular vein ligated. The clavicular head of the muscle is transected. If there is residual muscle tightness, the sternal head should also be divided.

Upper muscle release: An incision over the mastoid process permits detachment of the muscle from its insertion by sharp dissection and rugine, avoiding damage to the underlying occipital artery and posterior belly of the digastric. After closure of the incision in layers, the head and neck are splinted in a slightly overcorrected position.

Congenital Midline Web. The congenital deformity presents as a vertical midline web between the submental region and the cricoid cartilage, limiting extension of the head. A single large Z-plasty with transposition of two large flaps or a series of lesser Z-plasties corrects the condition.

Lateral Cervical Webs. The Turner syndrome, as part of this congenital disorder of females, is characterized by a chromosomal aberration with an XO pattern instead of the normal XX pattern. The neck webbing is associated with hypertelorism, a broad shieldlike chest, ovarian dysgenesis, and frequently cardiovascular abnormalities. In the *Klippel-Feil syndrome*, if functional improvement is necessary, excision of the web can be repaired by transposition of hairless skin.

Branchial Cysts and Fistulae

The lower part of the face, neck, and pharynx are formed from six visceral or branchial arches (Fig. 11–9). These arches constitute a series of rounded projections

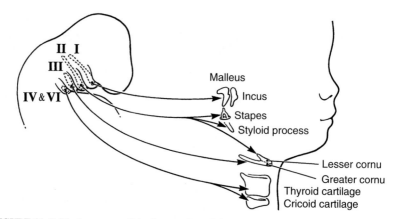

FIGURE 11–9. The lower part of the face, neck, and pharynx are formed from six visceral or branchial arches. The fifth arch does not develop in humans. (From Moore KL, Persaud TVN: The Developing Human, 5th ed. Philadelphia, WB Saunders, 1993.)

that protrude into the entodermal wall of the pharynx and also elevate the overlying ectoderm. Between the arches are clefts or furrows where the entoderm and ectoderm come into direct contact. They are lined internally by columnar epithelium and externally by squamous epithelium.

Each arch has a plate of cartilage, a muscle mass, a nerve, and an artery.

First (mandibular) arch: Its nerve is the mandibular branch of the trigeminal nerve; its artery is the facial artery.
Second (hyoid) arch: It is subserved by the facial nerve and the external carotid artery.
Third (thyrohyoid) arch: This is supplied by the glossopharyngeal nerve and the internal carotid artery.
The fourth and fifth arches are unnamed.

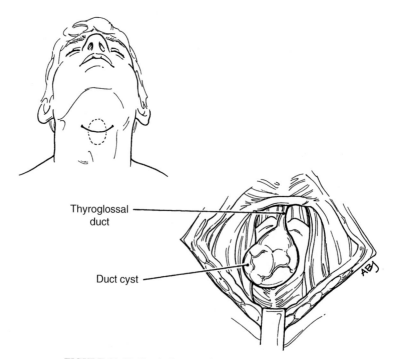

FIGURE 11–10. Surgical approach to a thyroglossal duct cyst.

The second arch grows more rapidly than the lower arches so that it soon overhangs them, forming a deep groove called the cervical sinus. With fusion of the second and fifth arches, the cervical sinus becomes a buried space, lined by squamous epithelium, that normally disappears. If it persists, it forms a branchial cyst. If fusion between the second and fifth arches fails, a persistent opening on the exterior of the neck forms a branchial fistula along the line of the anterior border of the sternomastoid.

The branchial cyst is situated deep to the upper part of the sternomastoid, appearing in the adolescent or young adult as a fluctuating swelling that projects forward from beneath the anterior border of the muscle in the region of the mandibular angle. There may or may not be an opening in the pharynx which represents the visceral pouch and is situated just behind the tonsil.

The cyst, lined by squamous epithelium, and the fistula, as a remnant of the cervical sinus, are situated between the internal and external carotid arteries as well as between the facial and hypoglossal nerves anteriorly and the glossopharyngeal nerve deeply. These anatomic relationships need to be kept in mind in the course of excision of the cyst and sinus, which are approached through a collar incision centered on the mass.

Swellings of the Neck

The clinical implications of the many anatomic structures in the neck relate to the differential diagnosis of neck masses.

1. Lymph node enlargement: This may be due to acute inflammatory reactions, granulomatous disease, a reticuloendothelial disorder such as Hodgkin disease or lymphoma, or metastases from melanoma of the head and neck or carcinoma of the tongue, floor of the mouth, nasopharynx, or thyroid gland. The disease process may involve the superficial glands arranged circularly around the base of the head and face or may spread to the deep cervical chains along the internal jugular vein.
2. Swellings due to causes other than lymph node involvement
   A. Midline swellings
      1. Thyroglossal duct cyst (Fig. 11–10)
      2. Subhyoid bursa
      3. Dermoid
      4. Plunging ranula
      5. Adenoma of the isthmus of the thyroid gland
      6. Aneurysm of the innominate artery
   B. Lateral swellings
      1. Congenital causes
         a. Branchial cyst
         b. Cystic hygroma
         c. Sternomastoid tumor
      2. Acquired disorders
         a. Salivary glands
            i. Parotid gland
            ii. Submaxillary gland
         b. Thyroid enlargement: goiter, thyroiditis, or cancer
         c. Pharyngeal (Zenker) diverticulum

    d. Sternomastoid mass: hematoma, fibrosarcoma
    e. Neurofibroma: cutaneous or vagus nerves
    f. Vascular tumors
       i. Aneurysm of the carotid artery
       ii. Carotid body tumor (chemodectoma)

Evaluation of the Solitary Neck Mass

Thorough history and physical examination exclude most of the previously outlined causes of a neck mass. If a malignancy is suspected, fine-needle aspiration may provide a diagnosis. Endoscopy under anesthesia with biopsies of the hypopharynx is warranted, as this is the most common site of occult malignancy. The nasopharynx may also be a site of occult malignancy, although much less frequently. If the neck lesion is a squamous cell cancer, radical neck dissection with postoperative radiation is warranted even if a primary tumor is not identified.

TUMORS OF THE THYROID GLAND

The solitary thyroid nodule is usually a benign lesion. Radioactive scanning of the thyroid with ^{131}I or ^{99}Tc defines the nodule as "cold" or "hot." Absence of isotope concentration in a nodule characterizes it as "cold," with a 10 per cent likelihood that the nodule represents a thyroid cancer. Ultrasonography identifies the presence of a benign cystic lesion.

Fine-needle aspiration of a solid lesion permits histologic identification of the disease process, with categorization of whether thyroiditis or neoplasia is present.

Benign adenomas: These encapsulated tumors may vary histologically and represent an embryonal adenoma, fetal adenoma, Hürthle cell tumor, or follicular adenoma.

Malignant tumors: Thyroid cancer is often associated with previous irradiation to the head and neck in infancy and childhood, with up to a 30-year hiatus before the cancer appears. Thyroid tumors seem to have a higher incidence in areas of endemic goiter.

Differentiated Tumors

Papillary carcinoma is the most common form of thyroid cancer, presenting in late childhood or early adulthood. It presents as a solitary nodule and grows very slowly. It spreads primarily to the cervical lymph nodes. This generally nonaggressive tumor is best treated by removal of the appropriate lobe and isthmus of the gland if it is unicentric. If nodes are involved, they should be removed without radical neck dissection. If the tumor is multicentric, then total thyroidectomy is the appropriate treatment. The tumor is not usually responsive to radioactive iodine.

Follicular carcinoma, presenting usually as a solitary nodule, occurs predominantly in the fourth decade and most often in females. It metastasizes by hematogenous spread to lungs and bones. Diagnosis is established by fine-needle aspiration. The sensitivity of metastases to radioactive iodine mandates that total thyroidectomy be performed for removal of tumor and all functioning thyroid tissue. Suppressive doses of thyroxine are subsequently administered.

Hürthle cell carcinoma is characterized by its pale acidophilic cells. This rare well-differentiated thyroid cancer does not take up radioiodine and is treated by total thyroidectomy. It has a 50 per cent 10-year survival rate.

Undifferentiated anaplastic carcinoma occurs in women over 60 years of age. This rapidly growing infiltrative neoplasm presents with a large neck mass, hoarseness, and pressure effects on the trachea and esophagus. Radiation therapy may be helpful, and tracheostomy may be necessary for tracheal compression.

Medullary carcinoma occurs sporadically. These lesions are usually familial, with embryologic origin from the parafollicular, calcitonin-producing cells of the thyroid gland. They are derived from the neuroectodermal cells and may have associated adrenal pheochromocytoma representing the Sipple syndrome. As its cells are part of the amine precursor uptake decarboxylation (APUD) system, medullary thyroid carcinoma may be part of the type II multiple endocrine neoplasia syndrome. The lesions are usually bilateral, requiring total thyroidectomy and neck dissection if nodal involvement is present. Calcitonin level elevation in these tumors provides a tumor marker in members of the family before a thyroid nodule becomes apparent. A provocative calcium or pentagastrin injection that elevates the calcitonin level is indicative of the presence of medullary cancer in an otherwise asymptomatic family member.

Metastatic cancer of the thyroid from a primary in the kidney, pancreas, or bronchus and occasionally from melanoma may present as a large single nodule in the thyroid.

Lymphoma may present in elderly women as a rapidly enlarging, diffuse thyromegaly, often on a background of Hashimoto thyroiditis. Radiation therapy following total thyroidectomy may provide a 5-year survival rate greater than 80 per cent.

RADICAL NECK DISSECTION

The cure of cancer of the head, neck, and pharynx must incorporate a curative resection of the sites of secondary spread, that is, the cervical lymphatics. This requires, after cure of the primary site, a monobloc resection of the draining lymph node–bearing tissues of one side of the neck. The procedure is carried out under general endotracheal anesthesia. The extent of the operation depends upon the natural lymphatic drainage of the neoplasm, which may be confined to the upper cervical area or involve the descending jugular chain. It also depends on whether the procedure is performed "prophylactically" or "curatively."

Suprahyoid neck dissection: In cancer of the tongue, which may have been cured by wedge resection, hemiglossectomy, or radiation therapy and in cancer of the floor of the mouth, similarly cured by excision or radiation therapy, this procedure may suffice. In the procedure, the submandibular gland and adjacent lymph nodes and the submental and facial vessel lymph nodes are resected in monobloc fashion.

Supraomohyoid neck dissection: This procedure may suffice in patients with papillary carcinoma of the thyroid and in prophylactic operations in head and neck cancer. The tissue removed includes the lymph nodes within a block of tissue situated between the mandible extending to the contralateral mental triangle above and the omohyoid between the strap muscles medially and the retracted sternomastoid muscle laterally, with resection of the jugular lymph nodes up to the base of the skull.

Modified neck dissection: This procedure amends the radical procedure by conserving the sternomastoid muscle, the spinal accessory nerve, and the internal jugular vein. It may be justified in the performance of a one-stage bilateral neck dissection where, on the side contralateral to the primary lesion, the modified procedure is done while a radical neck dissection is done on the ipsilateral side.

The radical neck dissection: First devised in 1906 by George Crile, Sr, the procedure entails a monobloc excision of the cervical lymph nodes extending from the lower border of the mandible above to the clavicle below and from the midline to the anterior border of the trapezius. Within this perimeter the only structures conserved are the carotid arteries, the vagus, phrenic, and hypoglossal nerves, the trunks of the brachial plexus, and the sympathetic chain.

Resected are the sternomastoid, omohyoid, stylohyoid, and digastric muscles, the carotid sheath and internal jugular vein, the spinal accessory and ansa hypoglossi nerves, and the contents of the submental, submandibular, and posterior triangles of the neck.

Among the many incisions available for exposure of the area, two are in common use (Fig. 11–11): (1) *The Crile incision*: A curved collar submandibular incision is turned into a T incision by an oblique incision from the midpoint of the collar incision, ending at the midclavicular point with appropriate raising of the flaps. (2) *The MacFee incision*: Two parallel transverse cervical incisions provide adequate access and a good cosmetic result and heal well, even if the area has been previously irradiated.

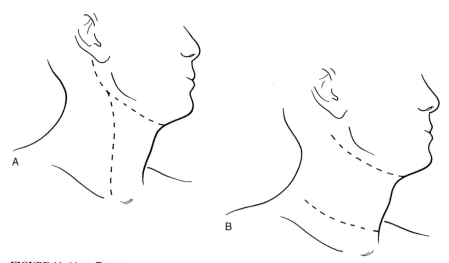

FIGURE 11–11. *A*, T incision for radical neck dissection. The vertical limb courses along the anterior border of the sternocleidomastoid muscle. *B*, The MacFee incision: Two parallel transverse incisions provide a good cosmetic result. It avoids a T incision in a pre-irradiated field.

Suggested Readings

Beahrs OH: Surgical anatomy and technique of radical neck dissection. Surg Clin North Am 57:663, 1977

Beahrs OH, Adson MA: The surgical anatomy and technic of parotidectomy. Am J Surg 95:885, 1958

Bocca E, Pignataro O, Sasaki CT: Functional neck dissection. A description of operative technique. Arch Otolaryngol 106:524, 1980

Candela FC, Kothari K, Shah JP: Patterns of cervical node metastases from squamous carcinoma of the oropharynx and hypopharynx. Head Neck 12:197, 1990

Gorlin RJ, Chaudhry AP, Pindborg JJ: Odontogenic tumors: Classification, histopathology and clinical behavior in man and domesticated animals. Cancer 14:73–101, 1961

Mashberg A, Samit AM: Early detection, diagnosis, and management of oral and oropharyngeal cancer. CA 39(2):67, 1989

Spiro RH: Salivary neoplasms: Overview of a 35-year experience with 2,807 patients. Head Neck Surg 8:177, 1986

Woods JE, et al: Pathology and surgery of primary tumors of the parotid. Surg Clin North Am 57:565, 1977

CHAPTER 12

Maxillofacial Trauma

SOFT TISSUE INJURY

Soft tissue injuries of the head and face may represent focal wounds or may be part of a conglomerate of life-threatening injuries that require priority management in order to save life. In any case of multiple trauma, an assessment is made whether life is endangered and injuries that affect function and aesthetic appearance can safely be left for later.

Immediate Priorities

1. Maintain the airway: The upper airways may be obstructed by blood, vomitus, or dentures. Finger clearance of foreign bodies and aspiration of trachea and bronchi often dramatically improve the previously depressed level of consciousness. The presence of penetrating chest wounds or flail chest can be managed by immediate endotracheal intubation and positive-pressure ventilation. Tracheostomy may be necessary if fracture of the larynx or trachea is present.

2. Control hemorrhage: Open wounds of the scalp and face may cause profuse hemorrhage, but pressure hemostasis and suture readily control it.

3. Control shock: The presence or subsequent development of shock indicates injuries other than facial should be sought. In the meantime, intravenous fluid administration is commenced, an indwelling urethral catheter is inserted, and vital signs are monitored.

4. Examine for associated injuries: Clinical and radiologic examinations are carried out to ascertain the presence or absence of intracranial, cervical, thoracic, intra-abdominal, or retroperitoneal injury. Examination of the extremities for fracture or vascular impairment is completed and appropriate treatment for such injuries initiated.

Before suture of any obvious scalp or facial lacerations, the presence or absence of facial skeletal injury should be established, as the reduction of facial fractures may require prolonged surgical management, leaving formal skin suture for a later stage after placement of a few key skin sutures.

Although craniofacial fractures may occur without significant injury to the overlying soft tissue, the presence of soft tissue injury suggests two possible groups of patients: (1) those with wounds involving the soft tissues only, and (2) those with soft tissue wounds associated with underlying skeletal fractures. Fracture is suggested by the presence of (a) ecchymosis or contusion over a bony prominence; (b) subconjunctival hemorrhage or periorbital ecchymosis, indicating possible fracture of zygoma or frontal or nasal bones; (c) maxillomalar deformity in fracture of the zygoma; (d) malocclusion of teeth or open bite due to maxillary or mandibular displacement; (e) trismus due to mandibular or zygomatic fracture; and (f) excessive mobility of the midface.

A CT scan accurately delineates cranial and facial fractures and their degree of displacement or comminution. Both axial (sagittal) and coronal images should be obtained (Fig. 12–1). Plain radiographs are useful as a cost-effective means of evaluating isolated fractures. The most informative views include the following:

Waters view: Posteroanterior oblique projection of the face to evaluate the maxilla, maxillary sinuses, zygoma and zygomatic arch, orbital floor, and inferior orbital rim (Fig. 12–2).

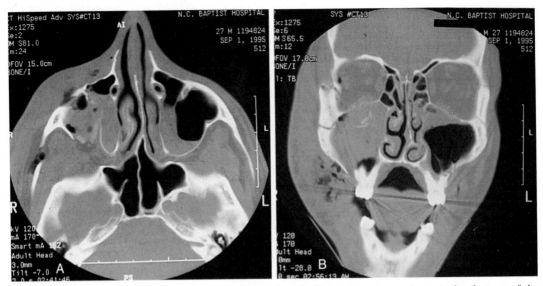

FIGURE 12–1. CT scan of the face. *A*, Axial (sagittal) cut through the maxillary sinuses demonstrating fractures of the anterior and posterior walls of the right maxillary sinus. *B*, Coronal cut through the orbit demonstrating fractures of the right orbital floor with fragments of bone in the opacified right maxillary sinus.

Caldwell view: Posteroanterior projection to evaluate the frontal bone and sinuses, orbital margins, and zygomatic frontal suture.

Submentovertex view: Submentovertex projection to evaluate the zygomatic arches and base of the skull.

Towne's view: Anteroposterior projection to evaluate the mandibular condyle, occipital bone, and posterior cranial fossa.

Lateral facial view: Lateral projection to evaluate the frontal sinuses, lateral orbital wall, maxilla, and mandible.

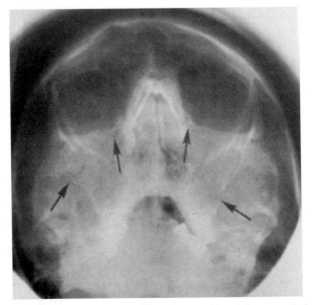

FIGURE 12–2. Waters view of a maxillary fracture with a right zygomatic fracture.

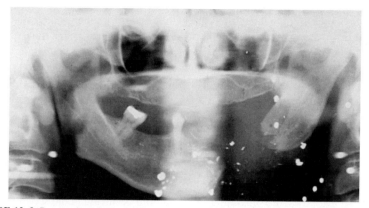

FIGURE 12–3. Panoramic radiograph of the mandible following a shotgun wound with a loss of bone from the angle to the symphysis.

Panorex view: A panoramic view of the mandible providing the best plain radiographic images of the entire mandible (Fig. 12–3).

Treatment of Craniofacial Soft Tissue Injury

THE SCALP

The anatomic layers of the scalp, from outside in, in the fronto-occipital region are (a) skin, (b) superficial fascia, (c) fronto-occipital muscle and epicranial aponeurosis (galea aponeurotica), (d) subaponeurotic connective tissue, and (e) pericranium.

Injuries of the Scalp. An open wound of the scalp may be incised, punctured, lacerated, or avulsed. Gaping of the wound implies that the galea has been divided, and although such a wound may resemble an incised wound, it is more likely to be due to a blow with a blunt instrument.

Hemorrhage is frequently profuse due to the dense subcutaneous tissue around the scalp vessels. Their ligation is often difficult, but control is best obtained with mattress sutures.

Neglect of a scalp wound may lead to cellulitis and suppuration. If the wound involves the pericranium, then osteitis and involvement of the intracranial contents may ensue, with serious sequelae from meningitis or brain abscess, due to extension via emissary veins.

The force of the blow that produces the scalp wound may cause a linear or depressed fracture of the skull as well as intracranial hemodynamic disturbances with concussion, cerebral edema, and laceration or cerebral compression by extradural or subdural hemorrhage.

Closed Wounds of the Scalp. A blow on the head may be severe enough to cause contusion of the scalp without lacerating the skin. Its effects may be any of the following:

1. Superficial hematoma: This is an extravasation of blood superficial to the aponeurotic layer with formation of a small localized hematoma that generally resolves spontaneously.

2. Subaponeurotic hematoma: This is the result of a more severe blow and is associated with extravasation of blood beneath the epicranial aponeurosis. It forms a large fluctuant mass that tends to gravitate toward eyebrows, zygoma, or occiput. The soft center of such a hematoma contrasts with its firm periphery and may be readily mistaken for a depressed skull fracture.

3. Cephalohematoma: This is a collection of blood between the pericranium and one of the cranial bones.

Avulsion of the Scalp. This may be partial or total, depending on whether the avulsed scalp retains connection with the intact scalp. It usually follows industrial or motor vehicle accidents. A tear usually occurs above the ears and through the eyebrows, the separation from the skull occurring in the subaponeurotic layer, leaving the pericranium intact.

If avulsion is partial, the attached scalp should be cleansed and, after control of hemorrhage, should be sutured back into place and drains placed. After total avulsion, if it is not too mangled, the scalp should be débrided and reattached using microvascular techniques.

Scalp Defects. Scalp defects may result from deep burns, traumatic avulsion, and tumor resection. Defects less than 5 cm can usually be closed primarily with wide undermining and scoring of the galea from below. Large defects may be grafted if periosteum is intact or closed with local flap transfer if necessary for aesthetic appearance or lack of periosteum. Local flaps include rotation flaps, transposition flaps, and multiple advancement flaps with primary closure of the donor defect (Fig. 12–4). A defect may also be closed with a local flap and the donor site grafted because flaps are elevated above the periosteum. Large defects may require coverage with a distal flap such as the trapezius or with a free flap. Exposed bone may be burred down to the diploic layer and allowed to granulate and then secondarily grafted. Exposed bone may also be resurfaced with an adjacent galeal flap, which is immediately covered with a skin graft.

Secondary reconstructions may be facilitated by tissue expansion of a planned flap, which is then transferred at a later procedure.

SKULL DEFECTS

Indications for the removal of parts of the skull vault include osteomyelitis and malignant disease. In order to protect the brain and restore contour, proper reconstitution of the area must be achieved.

Available materials fall into two groups:

Autogenous bone, which is harvested from the cranial vault, iliac crest, or ribs. Split rib grafts can cover large calvarial defects and are easily harvested through a short anterolateral thoracotomy. Iliac bone grafts are useful in covering moderate-sized defects. Calvarial bone may be readily harvested from the parietal area, providing the advantage of proximity and contour.

Alloplastic material, the most popular of which currently is methyl methacrylate. The use of acrylic should be delayed for 1 year in an area where infection has been present. In the interim, a lightweight protective shield can be worn under a wig.

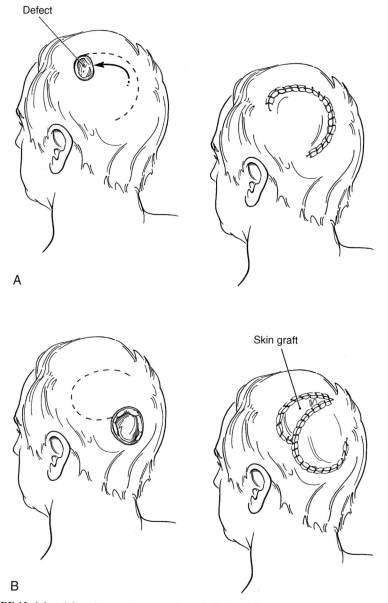

FIGURE 12–4. Local flaps for reconstruction of a scalp defect. *A*, Local rotation flap. *B*, Transposition flap with skin graft to the periosteum of the donor defect.

Illustration continued on following page

FACIAL SOFT TISSUE WOUNDS

Irrigation of these wounds removes clotted blood, debris, gravel, dirt, and most foreign bodies. Deeply ingrained tar and similar embedded particles must be thoroughly removed by brush scrubbing or débridement to prevent tattooing of the wound. Once exogenous particles become fixed in the tissues, surgical abrasion may become necessary.

Although devitalized tissue should be débrided, all well-vascularized skin and tissue should be conserved. The excellent facial blood supply determines survival of skin that is attached only by small pedicles.

Facial lacerations may involve muscles, nerves, salivary glands, or their ducts.

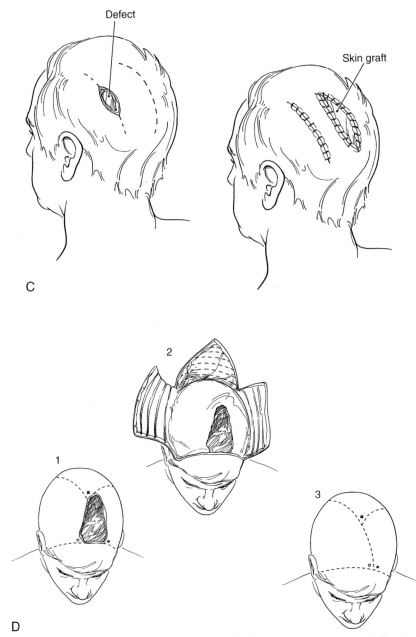

FIGURE 12–4 *Continued C,* Bipedicle flap closure with skin graft to donor defect. *D,* Closure of a large defect with a modified Orticochea flap. The galea has been scored to increase the amount of the flap advancement.

Anatomic repair of muscles, fascia, and skin results in a well-healed scar with normal muscular function.

Division of the facial nerve or its major branches should be identified at the time the wound is explored and the ends identified by faradic stimulation. The ends are approximated by careful suture using a magnifying loupe or by microneural technique. Facial nerve injuries should be explored and repaired within 72 hours, during which time the distal end of the cut nerve can still be stimulated with faradic impulses. It is not necessary to suture divided terminal branches of the facial nerve because approximation of the adjacent tissues leads to nerve regeneration within 1 year.

The subcutaneous position of the parotid gland and its duct makes them vulnerable to injuries in this area. The gland itself does not need to be sutured, but damage to the Stensen duct can result in a parotid fistula, with leakage of saliva. A fistula from the parotid gland itself usually closes spontaneously within 1 week, but one from the duct should be prevented by its repair. The Stensen duct extends along a line from the tragus of the ear to the philtrum of the upper lip, traversing the middle third of that line. Its intraoral buccal opening is opposite the second upper molar tooth. A probe or silicone tube can be passed through this opening and, after the proximal end is identified, the silicone tube is maneuvered into it to act as a splint while the duct is sutured over the splint. The intraoral segment of the splint is fixed to the buccal mucosa to prevent it from becoming dislodged. The splint can be removed by the seventh postoperative day.

PERIORBITAL INJURIES

Attention should be given to eyelid lacerations only after one has ensured that the cornea and globe have not suffered injury or foreign body penetration and that visual activity is unimpaired. Lacerations that involve the lid margin should be anatomically approximated. The lid margin must be perfectly aligned and the skin, muscle, tarsal plate, and conjunctiva anatomically approximated (Fig. 12–5). If the levator muscle mechanism is injured in the upper lid, it must be repaired to prevent lid ptosis. If loss of skin cannot be repaired primarily, the defect should be covered with a preauricular or postauricular full-thickness graft. Large tissue loss may require temporizing procedures with secondary formal eyelid reconstruction. Medial canthal injuries may lacerate the lacrimal sac or the canaliculus. The divided ends of the canaliculus should be repaired over a silicone tube (Fig. 12–6). Delayed development of dacryocystitis or epiphora may require a dacryocystorhinostomy. Injury to the medial or lateral canthal tendon is repaired primarily, or the tendon is reattached to the appropriate orbital rim.

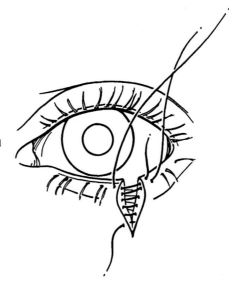

FIGURE 12–5. Layered closure of a lower lid defect.

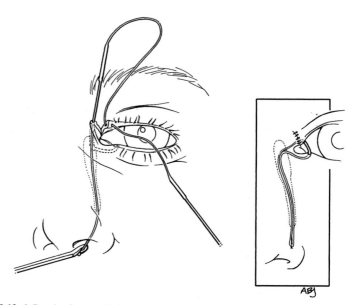

FIGURE 12–6. Repair of a canalicular injury is stented with silicone tubing, which is passed into the lacrimal sac and down the lacrimal duct into the nose. The other end of the tubing will be passed into the nose through the lower canaliculus. The silicone tubing is removed in 10 to 12 weeks.

NASAL LACERATIONS

Injury to the nose may affect the skin, the lining of the nasal vestibule, or the mucous membrane of the nasal cavity, usually at the junction of bone and cartilage. Accurate tissue approximation generally results in good healing as long as the underlying bony framework is properly reconstructed.

A septal hematoma should be evacuated through a small mucosal incision because, if it is untreated, chondromalacia may lead to loss of the septal cartilage with development of a saddle-nose deformity. Avulsion of the nasal ala or tip should be treated by its replacement as a composite graft, if available, with good prospect of primary healing.

EAR INJURY

Hematoma, if untreated, undergoes fibrotic change with the development of "cauliflower ears." This injury is common in those engaging in physical contact sports. Direct early evacuation of the hematoma via a small incision is essential. Compressive dressings should then be applied for at least 1 week.

Abrasions and lacerations of the ear generally heal well after simple repair due to good blood supply, even with laceration of the underlying cartilage. Small avulsed segments may be replaced as a composite graft. Large avulsed segments may be de-epithelialized, buried in a retroauricular subcutaneous pocket, and elevated at a later time. Total avulsions may be reattached using microvascular techniques. Delayed chondritis after ear burns may respond to local antibiotic therapy, but chondrectomy with subsequent auricular reconstruction may be necessary.

LIP INJURY

Lacerations of the lips are repaired in layers. If tissue is missing after a dog bite, even if contaminated, normal parts should be approximated and a free graft applied to replace any missing skin. Restoration of a normal lip configuration is the primary objective. A step-off at the vermilion-cutaneous junction is to be avoided. The mucocutaneous junction is precisely re-approximated, followed by repair of the muscle layer, skin, and mucosa.

FACIAL FRACTURES

Fractures of the facial bones represent fractures below the supraorbital ridges.

1. Fractures affecting the bones between the supraorbital ridges and the maxillary teeth represent the facial "middle third."
   A. Central components
      1. Nose
      2. Nasoethmoid complex
      3. Maxillary block
   B. Lateral components
      1. Zygomatic arch
      2. Malar bone
2. Mandibular fractures (Fig. 12–7)
   A. Body of mandible
      1. Canine: Through the cuspid teeth
      2. Main body: Between cuspid teeth and angle
      3. Angle: Through the angle of the mandible behind the second molar tooth
   B. Ramus of mandible: Fracture is between the angle of the mandible and the sigmoid notch.
   C. Mandibular processes
      1. Coronoid process
      2. Condyle
      3. Alveolus

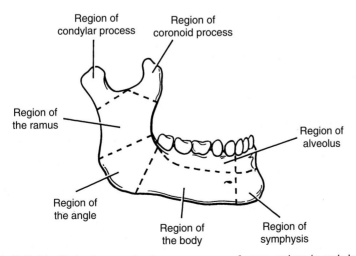

FIGURE 12–7. Mandibular fractures involve one or more of seven regions in each half of the mandible. (Reproduced with permission from Dingman RO, Natvig P: Surgery of Facial Fractures. Philadelphia, W.B. Saunders, 1964.)

ETIOLOGY

Although pathologic fracture due to a cyst or neoplasm of bone may result from minimal trauma, a forceful blow is the usual cause. A fracture at the site of the blow usually causes discontinuity and displacement of the bone. A contra-coup effect on the side opposite the blow results in a condylar fracture. Bilateral condylar fractures may result from a blow to the mandibular symphysis.

A fracture associated with discontinuity of the overlying skin or mucosa represents a compound fracture, as the fracture site communicates with the external environment. Absence of such communication represents a simple fracture. A comminuted fracture is reflected in the presence of many small fragments. If the bone ends are driven together in displaced position, it is defined as an impacted fracture.

GENERAL MANAGEMENT

1. Maintain airway.
2. Attend to serious associated injuries with control of shock, neurosurgical problems, and cerebrospinal rhinorrhea.
3. Give prophylaxis against tetanus and sepsis.
4. Delay attention to soft tissue wound until underlying fractures have been reduced and immobilized under general anesthesia. In comminuted fractures, all bone fragments with periosteal attachment should be retained.
5. Priorities in fracture reduction
   a. Maxillary fractures: These have the highest priority, as the fragments become firmly united within 10 days. Floating fractures with gross displacements are easier to reduce.
   b. Mandibular fractures are often compound, requiring reduction as soon as possible. The development of infection may lead to delayed or non-union of the fracture.
   c. Simple nasal and malar fractures may be reduced after a few days delay, by which time most of the edema and swelling have resolved.

FACIAL BUTTRESSES

The transverse and vertical buttresses provide the structural pillars supporting the three-dimensional architecture of the facial skeleton (Fig. 12–8). Reconstruction of facial fractures is directed at stabilization of the buttresses, with rigid fixation and bone graft reconstruction when necessary. This ensures stability of facial height, width, and projection.

There are three vertical buttresses of the maxilla:

The *nasofrontal* buttress extends anteriorly from the alveolar process of the maxilla, along the pyriform aperture.
The *zygomatic* buttress extends through the zygoma to the frontal bone.
The *pterygomaxillary* buttress lies posteriorly, extending through the pterygoid plates.

The transverse buttresses of the face include the mandibular body, zygomatic arch, infraorbital rims, and frontal bar.

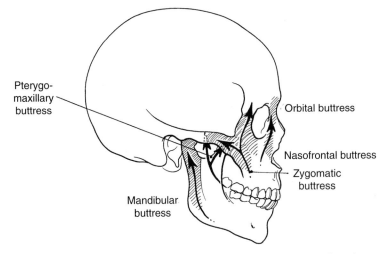

Pterygo-
maxillary
buttress

Orbital buttress

Nasofrontal buttress

Zygomatic
buttress

Mandibular
buttress

FIGURE 12–8. The vertical buttresses of the face include the nasofrontal, zygomatic, and pterygomaxillary buttresses of the maxilla, the orbital buttress, and the mandibular buttress.

Fractures of the Maxilla

The midface is formed by the midline junction of the paired maxillae, forming part of the orbit, nose, and palate. Each consists of the following:

1. A *pyramidal body* that contains the maxillary sinus
2. The *frontal process*, that extends upward to the medial orbital wall and nasal bones
3. The *zygomatic process*, which joins the zygoma to form the malar prominence
4. The *palatine process*, which forms the anterior three fourths of the hard palate, meeting the horizontal plates of the palate bones posteriorly
5. The *alveolar process* with its upper jaw teeth, which provides the strong buttress that supports and protects the horizontal processes

The posterior surface of the maxilla contains the alveolar canals for the posterosuperior alveolar vessels and nerves, which pass through the anterior wall of the bone to the teeth. The infraorbital nerve passes through the infraorbital canal of the maxilla to innervate the soft tissues of the upper lip and the lateral aspect of the nose.

The palatine branches of the maxillary division of the trigeminal nerve pass through the palatine canal between the maxilla and palatine bone to innervate the palatal mucosa. The nasopalatine nerves pass from the nose through the incisive foramen to supply the mucosa over the front of the hard palate.

Fractures of the maxilla result from a direct blow to the bone, with fractures developing through the thinner portions of the maxilla. Fractures through these areas of structural weakness provide the Le Fort classification of maxillary fractures.

Maxillary fractures may affect adjacent structures: (1) the nasolacrimal system: The nasolacrimal duct passes through the groove that is partially formed by the maxilla and may be damaged in midface fractures; (2) the anterior cranial fossa: High maxillary fractures may damage the cribriform plate and the ethmoid sinuses with cerebrospinal rhinorrhea, dural laceration, and brain damage.

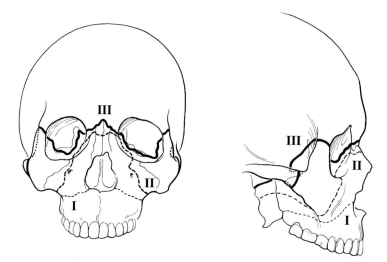

FIGURE 12–9. Le Fort classification of maxillary fractures.

CLASSIFICATION OF MAXILLARY FRACTURES

Tranverse Fractures. Central middle-third facial fractures should be suspected in any patient involved in an accident who has a bruised, swollen face. The type of fracture can be categorized by the classification of Le Fort (Fig. 12–9):

1. Le Fort I (Guerin fracture): A transverse fracture above the teeth includes the alveolar process, the vault of the palate, and the pterygoid process in a single block.
2. Le Fort II: This is a pyramidal fracture due to a blow to the upper maxilla which involves the frontal process and extends laterally through the lacrimal bones, the floor of the orbits, the zygomaticomaxillary suture lines, and the lateral maxillary walls to involve the pterygoid plates in the pterygomaxillary fossa. The inevitable posterior displacement may cause damage to the nasal septum and ethmoidal and lacrimal areas, with widening of the interorbital space.
3. Le Fort III: Craniofacial dysfunction occurs when a high fracture runs across the roof of the nose, extending through the zygomaticofrontal and nasofrontal sutures and across the orbital floors. The facial bones and structures of the middle third of the face become totally separated from the base of the skull, continuity being maintained only by the soft tissues.

Vertical Fractures. A sagittal fracture may occur through the thin portion of the hard palate and extend unilaterally through the lateral maxillary wall and the thin portion of the orbital floor.

Alveolar Fractures. These are localized to the dentoalveolar segment of the maxilla as a result of a direct blow or by transmission from a blow to the mandible, which forces the maxillary alveolar fracture.

MECHANISM OF INJURY

The degree of force and the direction of the forces at the moment of impact of the middle third of the face against the immovable object determine the type of fracture and the degree of skeletal displacement. (1) A blow on the maxilla at tip level causes an alveolar or Le Fort I fracture. (2) A sustained violent force at a higher level causes a Le Fort II fracture, often with some comminution of the maxilla. (3) An upward force transmitted through the mandible tends to cause a vertical fracture, whereas lateral forces may cause displacement of maxillary segments into the maxillary sinus or the palatal region.

The posterior and downward displacement of the midface provides a "dish-face" appearance, with elongation of the facial structures which is partially aggravated by the action of the pterygoid muscle.

CLINICAL FEATURES

Swelling of the face develops rapidly with epistaxis, periorbital, conjunctival, and scleral ecchymosis, and obliteration of the bony contours. In dentulous patients, a malocclusion occurs when the unfractured mandible is apposed to the maxilla. In edentulous patients, malalignment of the dentures results.

The maxilla may be either impacted or mobile. The mobility is assessed by holding the head steady with one hand while rocking the maxilla with the other. A step-down deformity may be palpable at the infraorbital margins of the zygomaticomaxillary suture and is indicative of a Le Fort II fracture.

Radiologic examination may provide difficulty in identification of fracture of the maxilla. The occipitomental and posteroanterior (Waters position) projections provide the best views for identifying fractures of maxilla and the sinuses, the zygomatic arches, and the orbital regions. Opacification of the maxillary sinuses due to contained blood suggests a maxillary fracture. CT scans define the facial fracture and degree of displacement.

The fractured, displaced maxilla should be reduced as soon as possible because thin, splintered bone consolidates rapidly, making it difficult to move after 10 to 14 days. If no displacement of the fractured segments has occurred, no specific treatment is necessary. If the maxilla is impacted under a displaced molar, this must be reduced before disimpaction of the maxilla can be accomplished.

MANAGEMENT

Although prolonged delay should be avoided, reduction of middle-third, transverse, and Le Fort fractures is often successful up to 3 weeks after injury using Rowe disimpaction forceps. It is important to establish and maintain good functional dental occlusion. Fractures are exposed through incisions in the buccal sulcus, lower eyelids, and lateral brow and a transcoronal incision (Fig. 12–10).

Le Fort I or Le Fort II Fractures
1. Intermaxillary fixation with internal wire suspension: Intermaxillary fixation is accomplished with arch bars and rubber bands or wire. This requires a stable mandible with teeth and a complement of teeth in the fractured segment. The maxillomandibular unit is suspended by wires to either the zygomatic process, frontal bone, or infraorbital rim above the fracture.
2. Plate and screw fixation: After intermaxillary fixation is established, fractures at the nasofrontal junction, orbital rims, and zygomaticomaxillary levels are exposed, and direct fixation is achieved by plate and screw fixation. Maxillary

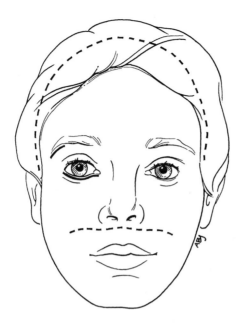

FIGURE 12–10. Common surgical approaches to the facial skeleton.

buttress disruptions are reduced and immediate bone grafts incorporated to replace missing bone. This approach has minimized malunions and is the preferred method of management (Fig. 12–11).

Le Fort III Fractures. The presence of nasoethmoidal, zygomaticofrontal, and supraorbital wall fractures requires open operation and reduction through a transcoronal approach while a gingivobuccal incision provides exposure of associated lower maxillary fractures. Interfragment plate and screw fixation with appropriate bone grafts provides the necessary stability.

Management of Malunion

1. Le Fort I fracture: Through an oral vestibular incision, the fracture site is exposed and mobilized by transecting the fracture line. After replacing the fractured

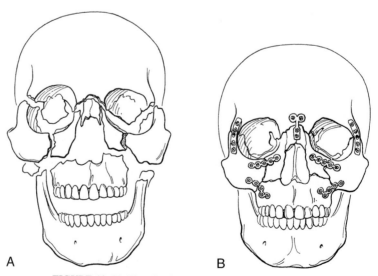

A   B

FIGURE 12–11. Plate fixation of a complex maxillary fracture.

segment in the correct occlusal relationships, it is fixed in the corrected position with plate and screws.

2. Le Fort II and III fractures: An infraorbital approach with either transcoronal, intracranial, or extracranial exposure permits osteotomy and repositioning of the fragment with appropriate fixation. Cranial bone grafts may be needed to minimize postreduction relapse.

Fractures of the Nose

In a simple fracture, the direction of the blow determines the nature of the injury. A lateral shift of the bony skeleton is attributable to a blow from the side, whereas a frontal blow drives the nose back into the ethmoid cells and buckles the septum.

Manipulative reduction of the bony skeleton is possible for about 2 weeks after injury. Walsham forceps can be used to disimpact the nasal bones, and the fragments can then be molded into shape. The central nasal forceps can be used to disimpact and straighten the septum. It can also be used to reduce a nasoethmoid fracture by disimpacting the nasal skeleton from the ethmoid cells. Internal silicone splints are sutured to either side of the septum to maintain the septum in the midline. They are left in place for 2 weeks.

Comminuted fractures can be treated by threading a mattress suture of stainless steel wire through the fragments and tying it over lead plates to prevent it from cutting into the skin. The suture can be cut by the fifth day and removed on the tenth day.

A malunited nasal fracture requires a corrective rhinoplasty.

Zygomatic Fractures

The zygoma or malar bone is a quadrilateral bone with four processes (Fig. 12–12). The *frontal process* articulates superiorly with the frontal bone at the zygomaticofrontal suture. The *maxillary process* articulates with the maxilla at the zygomaticomaxillary suture. The *temporal process* articulates with the temporal

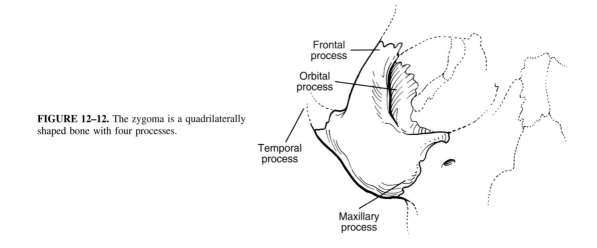

FIGURE 12–12. The zygoma is a quadrilaterally shaped bone with four processes.

bone at the ear. The *orbital process* articulates with the greater wing of the sphenoid in the lateral orbit.

The zygoma is a prominent bone forming the malar eminence and thereby determines cheek projection. It is the major buttress between the cranium and maxilla. Despite the zygoma's sturdy nature, its prominence subjects it to frequent injury.

Fractures may involve the zygomatic arch or zygomatic body.

Zygomatic Arch. An isolated fracture of the zygomatic arch causes a visible depression of the cheek. Sufficient displacement may cause the arch to impinge on the coronoid process, impairing mandibular mobility (Fig. 12–13). The fracture is readily corrected through a small temporal incision. The incision is carried down through the temporal fascia and an elevator passed deep to the temporal fascia and beneath the zygomatic arch. The medial and lateral arch segments are reduced, and the elevator is withdrawn. Unless the fracture is comminuted, the reduction is stable without the need for internal fixation. The procedure may also be accomplished through a lateral brow incision. Dissection is continued down to the lateral orbital rim, and an elevator is passed behind the zygomatic arch and the fracture reduced.

Zygomatic Body. Fractures of the zygomatic body may be nondisplaced, displaced with medial or lateral rotation, or comminuted. Displacement is downward, inward, and backward, causing the malar prominence to become flattened (Fig. 12–14). The lateral wall of the antrum is broken so that the sinus fills with blood, and there may be nasal bleeding. The fracture line usually involves the infraorbital canal, resulting in facial anesthesia. Posterior displacement of the inferior orbital rim may result in disruption of the orbital floor. There may be an uncomplicated linear fracture or a comminuted fracture with prolapse of the orbital contents through the defect into the maxillary sinus.

Physical examination demonstrates some or all of the following:

Periorbital swelling and bruising
Displacement of the lateral canthal tendon with mongoloid slant to the eyelids
Flattening of the cheek
Restriction of mandibular mobility
Numbness in the infraorbital nerve distribution
Step deformity of the inferior orbital rim

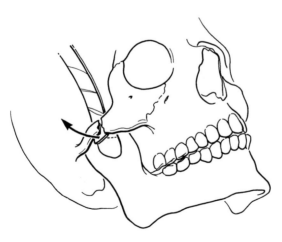

FIGURE 12–13. Isolated fracture of the zygomatic arch may be elevated with an elevator passed through a temporal incision. Rigid fixation is rarely necessary.

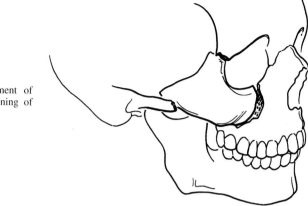

FIGURE 12–14. Displacement of the zygoma results in flattening of the malar prominence.

Tenderness or irregularity of the zygomaticofrontal suture

Tenderness or irregularity between the maxilla and malar eminences on intraoral examination

Enophthalmos, diplopia, or entrapment of orbital contents due to orbital floor fracture

Diagnosis may be confirmed with plain films, the best of which are the Waters, Caldwell, and submentovertex views. CT scan accurately defines the fracture and degree of displacement and is necessary to fully evaluate orbital floor involvement.

Nondisplaced fractures do not require surgery. If the malar bone is displaced, open reduction and internal fixation are accomplished. The zygomaticofrontal suture is exposed through a lateral brow incision, the inferior orbital rim through a lower lid incision, and the zygomaticomaxillary buttress area through a buccal sulcus incision. The orbital floor may be exposed and inspected through the lower lid incision. The fractures are anatomically reduced and miniplates secured at multiple points (Fig. 12–15). A significant orbital floor disruption is reconstructed by insertion of a Teflon or silicone sheet, bone graft, or conchal cartilage graft.

Orbital Fracture

A fracture of the orbital walls unassociated with other facial bone fractures is termed a *blow-out fracture*. The mechanism of injury is a blow to the orbit which displaces the orbital contents posteriorly into the narrower unyielding bony orbit. The increased intraorbital pressure is transmitted to the orbital walls, causing a blow-out in the orbital floor or medial or lateral orbital wall. The classic blow-out fracture involves the weak posteromedial region of the orbital floor (Fig. 12–16). Displacement of the orbital soft tissues through the fracture into the maxilla may result in one or more of the following:

Diplopia: Diplopia or double vision results from contusion of the extraocular muscles and orbital soft tissues. Contusion of the inferior rectus may cause diplopia on downward gaze, whereas contusion of the inferior oblique causes diplopia on upward gaze.

Entrapment: Prolapsed orbital soft tissues, particularly the inferior rectus muscle, may become incarcerated, limiting upward rotation of the globe. It is demon-

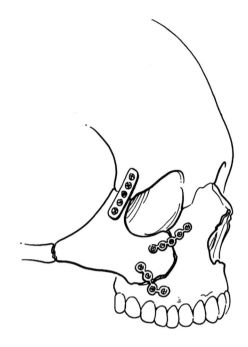

FIGURE 12–15. Displaced zygomatic fracture requires reduction and rigid fixation. The fracture must be fixed at two of these three locations.

strated by the forced duction test. The globe is grasped with forceps at the insertion of the inferior rectus 6 or 7 mm from the lower limbus. Rotation of the globe is absent or limited if it is entrapped.

Enophthalmos: This refers to a backward and downward displacement of the globe. It results either from an increase in skeletal orbital volume or atrophy of fat surrounding the globe. The eye has a hollow, sunken appearance with secondary ptosis of the upper lid.

CT scan is accurate in diagnosing the degree of orbital wall displacement. Surgical intervention is indicated for CT scan demonstrating significant orbital floor disruption, nonreducible entrapment, enophthalmos, and persistent diplopia after swelling subsides.

A ciliary or conjunctival incision through the lower eyelid provides good access to the orbital floor. All incarcerated orbital tissue is dissected off the fracture site, and a rigid support is provided by a bone graft from the outer calvarium or iliac crest which is wired or screwed to adjacent bone. Alternatively, orbital floor reconstruction may be achieved with an alloplastic implant such as silicone or Teflon. Conchal cartilage graft can be used for small defects. Any residual minor degree of diploplia may be adjusted by orthoptic exercises or by ophthalmologic extraocular muscle length adjustments.

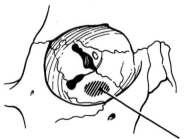

Site of
blowout fractures

FIGURE 12–16. The blowout fracture occurs inferiorly and medially at the weakest point of the orbital floor.

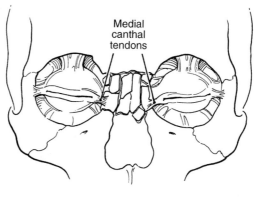

FIGURE 12–17. Comminuted nasoethmoid fracture with displacement of the medial canthal tendons.

Nasoethmoid Fracture

These fractures result from a blow to the glabella or nasofrontal area. They may occur as isolated fractures but are commonly seen in conjunction with maxillary fractures. A nasoethmoid fracture (Fig. 12–17) includes fractures of the frontal process of the maxilla, the medial orbital wall, the nose, and the nasofrontal area.

Often associated with a nasoethmoid fracture is a frontal cranial or anterior cranial fossa fracture with a dural tear and cerebrospinal fluid leak. Clinical evaluation demonstrates comminuted and depressed nasal fracture resulting in a flat nasal dorsum, orbital hematoma with subconjunctival hemorrhage, increased intercanthal distance (telecanthus), and mobility and crepitation on palpation of the medial canthal ligament.

Plain radiographs are not helpful, and CT scan is necessary to evaluate the frontal sinus, cribriform plate, and orbits. Exploration is through a transcoronal incision and any associated lacerations in the nasofrontal area. A subperiosteal dissection exposes the nasofrontal skeleton and medial orbit. The medial canthal tendon insertions are carefully preserved, and the bone fragments to which they are attached are reduced and sequentially wired to surrounding bone fragments. This network of fragments is wired or plated to the frontal bone and a cranial bone graft onlayed to reconstruct the nasal dorsum. The bony and cartilaginous nasal septum is replaced in the midline if necessary, and internal silicone splints are sutured to each side of the septum to maintain its reduction.

Neurosurgical correction is directed toward reduction of the depressed frontal skull fracture and related intracranial injuries.

Frontal Sinus Fracture

The frontal sinus develops by 10 years of age. It is composed of two cavities separated by a septum, each cavity draining through nasofrontal ducts passing from the sinus floor into the nose. Fractures may involve the floor of the sinus, the anterior table, or both the anterior and posterior tables.

An anterior table fracture is isolated to the anterior table or associated with nasoethmoid or supraorbital rim fractures.

Anterior and posterior table injury may be either a transverse or a vertical linear fracture or a comminuted fracture. Comminuted fractures may be isolated to the frontal sinus or associated with a nasoethmoid fracture. Frontal sinus fractures are explored through a coronal incision. Isolated floor fractures usually do not require treatment. Depressed fractures of the anterior table are managed by irrigation of the sinus and elevation and wiring of plates to maintain reduction. If it is associated with a nasoethmoid fracture, the orifices of the nasofrontal duct are inspected. If the ducts are damaged, the sinuses are obliterated. Mucosa is removed and the sinus packed with a galea frontalis flap or cancellous bone. If the anterior table is severely comminuted, it is reconstructed with a cranial bone graft. If the posterior table is fractured, the area is inspected for a cerebrospinal fluid leak and dural tears are repaired. If the posterior table is severely comminuted, the sinus may be cranialized by removal of the posterior table and sinus mucosa. The sinus cavity is filled by brain with its overlying dura. Nasofrontal ducts are packed with bone graft or a galeal flap, and the anterior table is reconstructed.

Mandibular Injury

The mandible or lower jaw consists of a body and two rami fusing by the second year of life at the symphysis menti. From the posterior part of the body, at the angle, projects the vertical ramus surmounted by an anterior coronoid process and a posterior condyle. Between these two processes is the mandibular notch.

The mandibular foramen is situated on the medial aspect of the ramus, giving entry to the inferior alveolar nerve, which passes within the substance of the body along the mandibular canal, emerging as the mental nerve through the mental foramen on the lateral surface of the body, just below and between the two premolar teeth.

The medial surface of the body of the mandible is divided into two parts by an oblique mylohyoid line that gives attachment to the mylohyoid muscle. The ramus is a four-sided plate with a lateral and a medial surface.

The masseter muscle, which arises by a flattened tendon from the lower border and deep surface of the zygoma and the zygomatic arch, is inserted into the whole of the lateral surface of the ramus.

The temporal muscle, after arising from the floor of the temporal fossa of the skull, converges to a tendon that is inserted into the borders and inner surface of the coronoid process.

The lateral pterygoid muscle arises by two heads opposite the pterygomaxillary fissure and passes backward to be inserted into the hollow in front of the neck of the mandible and into the articular disk of the mandibular joint.

The medial pterygoid muscle arises in the pterygoid fossa from the inner surface of the lateral pterygoid plate and descends to be inserted on the inner aspect of ramus of the mandible, extending from the mandibular foramen to the angle.

These four muscles of mastication pull the mandible upward, forward, and medially and determine the degree and direction of displacement of fractured segments of the mandible (Fig. 12–18).

Factors in addition to muscle pull determine the extent and direction of fragment displacement in mandibular fracture. These include the direction and intensity of the force and the site of the fracture. The mandibular muscles that depress or open the mandible tend to displace the fractured segment downward, posteriorly, and medially.

Mylohyoid muscle: A fan-shaped muscle that supports the floor of the mouth, it

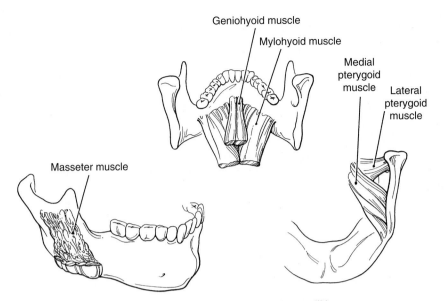

FIGURE 12–18. Muscle insertions of the mandible.

arises from the mandibular mylohyoid line and inserts into a median raphe and the hyoid bone. It can elevate the hyoid and depress the mandible.

Digastric muscle: This consists of two fleshy bellies united by an intervening tendon. The posterior belly is larger, arising from the mastoid notch on the inner side of the mastoid process. The anterior belly arises from a depression on the lower border of the mandible close to the midline. From these origins the muscle fibers are directed to their insertion into an intervening tendon, which is bound to the hyoid bone by a strong loop of fibrous tissue.

The mylohyoid branch of the mandibular nerve supplies the anterior digastric belly and the mylohyoid muscle. The posterior digastric belly is supplied by a branch of the facial nerve. With the mandible fixed, the two bellies acting together elevate the hyoid bone. If the hyoid bone is fixed, the digastrics depress the mandible.

Genioglossus Muscle: This thick, fan-shaped muscle has its apex at the mandible and its base at the tongue and hyoid bone, taking origin from the genial tubercles of the mandible and helping to protrude the tongue, elevate the hyoid, and depress the mandible.

Geniohyoid Muscle: Arising from the mandibular inferior medial spine, the geniohyoid inserts into the body of the hyoid and can elevate the hyoid and depress the mandible.

MANDIBULAR FRACTURE

Patients usually have a history of direct trauma to the mandible with localized pain on mastication. Clinical examination demonstrates local swelling, bruising, and tenderness. Dental malocclusion may be present.

Fractures of the mandible may be unilateral, in which case the smaller posterior fragment tends to be displaced forward and outward by the temporal muscle, overlapping the larger anterior fragment.

If a bilateral fracture occurs, the central fragment is driven downward and backward by the impact of the blow and by the action of the mandibular depressor muscles, whereas the other fragments are displaced forward and outward. The most common fracture is situated in the vicinity of the canine tooth, as the bone is relatively narrow in this area, where it is weakened by the presence of the mental foramen and the depth of the canine socket.

Less frequently, fractures of the ramus and angle occur with little displacement because of the presence of the masseter and medial pterygoid muscles, which splint the bone.

Fractures of the coronoid process are rare and again, owing to the extensive temporalis muscle attachment, little displacement occurs.

Fractures of the neck of the bone generally occur below the insertion of the lateral pterygoid insertion so that the upper fragment is drawn medially and forward by this muscle and the larger lower fragment is elevated and drawn to the opposite side. Teeth in the line of fracture should be retained if possible, but if they are loose or interfere with fracture reduction, they should be removed.

Factors Influencing Displacement

1. Direction and angulation of fragments (Fig. 12–19)
   a. Horizontally favorable: Fractures directed downward and forward are stable because of the antagonistic pull of the two muscle groups.
   b. Horizontally unstable: Fractures directed downward and backward are subject to medial displacement.
   c. Vertically unstable: Fractures running from posteriorly forward and medially suffer medial displacement because of the pull of the masticatory elevator muscles.
   d. Vertically favorable: The fracture passes from the lateral surface of the mandible posteriorly and medially. The muscle pull tends to prevent displacement.
2. Presence of teeth in fractured segments: The occlusal contact between upper and lower teeth minimizes displacement of the posterior segment.
3. Splinting action of muscles prevents displacement in fractures of the ramus.

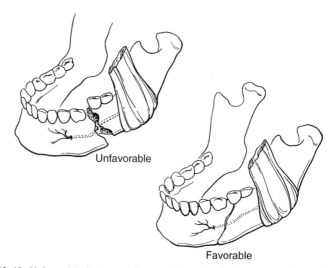

Unfavorable

Favorable

FIGURE 12–19. Unfavorable fracture of the mandible with displacement and favorable mandibular fracture without displacement.

Reduction of Mandibular Fractures

Restoration of masticatory function and occlusal alignment are the primary considerations in reducing the fragments to their normal anatomic relationships and holding them in position until healing occurs. Antibiotic prophylaxis against infection is advisable. Clinical union is usually complete within 6 to 8 weeks, although radiologic evidence of complete healing may take up to 1 year.

Methods of Fracture Fixation

1. Interdental eyelet wiring: This is the simplest method of fixing the mandible to the maxilla. Enough teeth must be present to hold at least one pair of wires on each side. Six-inch lengths of 0.35-mm stainless steel wire are passed close to the necks of the teeth from without in. The ends are brought out, and one end is threaded through the eyelet. The ends of the wire are twisted and tightened, leaving room to pass a tie-wire through the eyelet. Pairs of wires are joined directly or obliquely by tie-wires. The procedure can be done under local anesthesia, but general anesthesia is required if fracture reduction is necessary.

2. Cap splints: Cast in a dental laboratory, the silver cap splints are cemented to the teeth and may be retained for a long time, providing accurate and rigid fixation. Alternatively, an easily fabricated transparent thick, strong, acrylic splint can be made by an orthodontist.

3. Arch bars made of semirigid pliable metal can be contoured to the dental arch and used for intermaxillary fixation. Cable arch wires and banded arch wires can also be used for the fixation of mandibular fractures.

4. Gunning splints can be used in edentulous jaws. They are made from impressions or modified from the patient's own dentures. They can be fixed to the upper and lower jaws by perialveolar or circumferential wiring.

5. Open reduction and internal fixation may be necessary in complex fractures when teeth cannot be used as points of fixation, in fractures with a displaced posterior fragment, and in edentulous patients. Internal fixation is achieved with interosseous wires or plate fixation. Plate fixation provides a rigid fixation, often avoiding the need for intermaxillary fixation.

Guidelines to Type of Treatment

Class I fractures: A tooth is present on each side of the fracture, permitting intermaxillary fixation or dental appliances. Open reduction and internal fixation are not necessary except for symphyseal and parasymphyseal fractures.

Class II fractures: Teeth are present on one side of the fracture site only. Open reduction and direct fixation are necessary if displacement is present.

Class III fractures: Fractures of the edentulous mandible are treated by intraoral appliances, circumferential wiring, interosseous wiring, and plate or lag screw fixation.

Condylar neck fracture: A unilateral condylar fracture is the most common fracture of the mandible. It may go unrecognized unless radiologic examination is carried out on all patients struck on the chin. No treatment is necessary if the jaw moves normally. If occlusion is abnormal, the jaws should be wired together for 3 weeks. In fracture dislocation of the condyle, the jaws should be wired for 3 to 5 weeks and then attain normal occlusion with active movement. Bilateral condylar fractures usually respond to wiring the jaws together for 5 weeks to avoid development of an open bite. Lateral pterygoid pull may cause significant medial and forward displacement with dislocation of the condyle outside the glenoid fossa, coming to rest on the articular eminence.

Open reduction with replacement of the condyle from the pterygoid space into the glenoid fossa is achieved via a preauricular incision with careful retraction of the facial nerve branches. The lateral pterygoid muscle is left intact to avoid avascular necrosis of the condyle. The articular disc is conserved and replaced to prevent delayed ankylosis of the temporomandibular joint. Fixation of the restored condyle is achieved by the use of either a 28-gauge wire threaded through the condylar fragment and the ramus for immobilization in an end-to-end position or plate fixation of the fracture segments.

Ramus fracture: Displaced ramus fractures below the condylar neck require open reduction and internal fixation. These fractures may be approached through either an intraoral or an external incision.

Angle fracture: Displaced angle fractures are managed by open reduction and internal fixation. The angle may be exposed through an intraoral incision, but an external approach provides better exposure and facilitates the procedure.

Body fracture: Class I fractures may be treated by reduction and intermaxillary fixation without the need for internal fixation. Displaced Class II fractures are reduced and plated through an intraoral buccal sulcus incision. The inferior alveolar nerve exits the mandible adjacent to the premolars, and care must be exercised to avoid injury to it.

Symphyseal and parasymphyseal fractures: These fractures are generally displaced, and both Class I and II fractures are reduced and plated through a buccal vestibular incision.

Complications of mandibular fracture: Antibiotic therapy is used to prevent respiratory complications as well as infection of the mandible. Late complications include delayed union, malunion, or non-union. Bone plating or bone grafting may be indicated.

MANDIBULAR DISLOCATION

This occurs when the condyle of the mandible passes over the summit of the articular eminence to enter the zygomatic fossa, where it is retained by contraction of the temporal and masseter muscles. Dislocation is usually bilateral, although it may occur unilaterally. It may be precipitated by wide opening of the mouth, as in yawning, or may be the result of a blow on the chin. Dislocation is readily reduced by placing protected thumbs over the lower molar teeth and pressing the mandible downward and backward to overcome the contraction of the masseter and temporal muscles. The chin is then raised and the mandible pushed backward to make the condyle pass over the articular eminence.

TEMPOROMANDIBULAR JOINT

The joint is formed between the mandibular condyle and the articular fossa and eminence of the temporal bone, these surfaces being separated by an articular disc.

The articular capsule is lax, permitting forward movement of the head of the mandible. The articular disc fuses with the capsule and divides the joint into an upper and lower part, each part retaining a separate synovial membrane. The sphenomandibular ligament provides an accessory ligament to the joint, extending from the spine of the sphenoid to the lingula on the inner margin of the mandibular foramen. Between the ramus of the mandible and the sphenomandibular ligament pass the auriculotemporal nerve, the maxillary vessels, and the inferior alveolar nerve.

Internal Derangement of the Temporomandibular Joint

Resulting from malocclusion and long-term microtrauma, the triad of preauricular pain, clicking of the joint, and limitation of joint movement is not uncommon in young to middle-aged females. Muscle spasm is noted clinically.

Radiographic examination in selected cases not responding to conservative treatment and splinting include tomography, CT scanning, MR imaging, and arthrography.

Possible findings include disorder of the meniscus—displacement with or without perforation; degenerative joint disease; loose bodies in the joint; and synovial chondromatosis.

Surgical treatment may be indicated in a small group of patients, and the procedure selected depends on the pathologic findings (meniscectomy, condylar molding, or condylectomy with condylar head replacement).

Ankylosis of the Temporomandibular Joint

Intra-articular (true) ankylosis represents fibrous or bony fusion between the condyle and fossa. Extra-articular (false) ankylosis consists of periarticular adhesions or bony impingement.

Difficulties with mastication and speech are often accompanied by pain. Although joint infection and congenital deformities may provide a cause, trauma is the most common agent, leading ultimately to destruction of the meniscus, atrophy of condylar and fossa cartilage with bony erosion, lipping, and finally bony ankylosis.

Effective treatment includes condylectomy with gap arthroplasty, condylar molding, and condylectomy with condylar head replacement.

Suggested Reading

Barton NW, Miller SH, Graham WP III: Managing lacerations of the parotid gland, duct, and facial nerve. Am Fam Physician 13:130, 1976

Gruss JS: Fronto-naso-orbital trauma. Clin Plast Surg 9:577–589, 1982

Gruss JS, Mackinnon SE: Complex maxillary fractures: Role of buttress reconstruction and immediate bone grafts. Plast Reconstr Surg 78:9–22, 1986

Gruss JS, Mackinnon SE, Kassel EE, Cooper PW: The role of primary bone grafting in complex craniomaxillofacial trauma. Plast Reconstr Surg 75:17–24, 1985

Luce EA: Frontal sinus fractures: Guidelines to management. Plast Reconstr Surg 80:500–508, 1897

Manson PN, Crawley WA, Yaremchuck MJ, et al: Midface fractures: Advantages of immediate extended open reduction and bone grafting. Plast Reconstr Surg 76:1–10, 1985

Manson PN, Hoopes JE, Su CT: Structural pillars of the facial skeleton: An approach to the management of Le Fort fractures. Plast Reconstr Surg 66:54–61, 1980

Paskert JP, Manson PN, Iliff NT: Nasoethmoidal and orbital fractures. Clin Plast Surg 15:209–223, 1988

Schultz RC, Oldham RJ: An overview of facial injuries. Surg Clin North Am 57:987, 1977

CHAPTER **13**

Reconstructive Procedures of the Face

PERIORBITAL RECONSTRUCTION

The Eyelids

The eyelids are essential for protection of the cornea. The upper eyelid is larger and more important in this protective function. The essential structures of both eyelids are similar, being composed of five layers (Fig. 13–1).

1. *Skin*: Thin and elastic, the skin is fairly adherent to the orbicularis muscle over the tarsus but more mobile and loose nearer the orbital rim. The eyelashes arise at the mucocutaneous junction. Large sebaceous glands, known as meibomian glands, have their openings behind the lashes and, if blocked, they distend and give rise to meibomian cysts. Along the free border of the lids are the glands of Moll and Zeiss: These are modified sweat glands and obstruction and infection of the gland ducts give rise to a stye (hordeolum).
2. *Loose connective tissue*
3. *Muscle layer*
   a. The orbicularis oculi muscle surrounds the palpebral fissure and is responsible for closure of the lid. Each muscle in the upper and lower lid consists of three concentric components defined as orbital, preseptal, and pretarsal portions. Medially the pretarsal muscle divides into deep and superficial segments. Fusion of the upper and lower superficial segments creates the medial canthal tendon, which inserts above and anterior to the anterior lacrimal crest. The deep components of the pretarsal muscle fuse and, as Horner's muscle, insert behind the posterior lacrimal crest. It tenses the tarsal plate. The orbicularis oculi is innervated by the facial nerve, and its action is to close the palpebral fissure.
   b. Levator palpebrae superioris: Arising posteriorly from the undersurface of the lesser wing of the sphenoid, this muscle is inserted by a broad tendinous

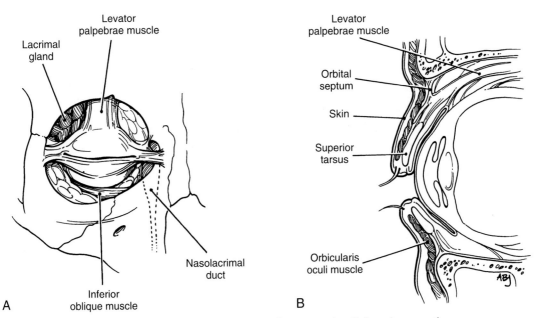

FIGURE 13–1. Anatomy of the eyelid. *A*, Anterior cross-section. *B*, Lateral cross-section.

aponeurosis into the anterior surface of the tarsus and the skin of the upper eyelid. Innervated by the oculomotor nerve, it elevates the upper lid.

   c. Muller's muscle: Arising from the aponeurosis of the levator, this is inserted into the upper border of the tarsus. Its smooth, unstriated muscle is innervated by a branch of the cervical sympathetic system.

4. *Tarsal plates*: These are thin, elongated plates of connective tissue which provide form and support to the eyelids. The semilunar upper tarsal plate is larger than the thinner, elliptical inferior plate.

5. *Conjunctiva*: This delicate membrane consists of a palpebral portion that lines the ocular surface of the lids and a bulbar portion that covers the cornea and adjacent sections of the sclera. Although firmly adherent over the tarsal plates, it is loose and movable in all other respects. The bulbar conjunctiva is continuous with the palpebral portion along the conjunctival fornices and is firmly applied to the cornea but loosely applied to the sclera.

The palpebral fissure is the area enclosed within the eyelids and is bounded by a medial and lateral canthus. The upper and lower lids meet directly at the lateral canthus, but medially they enclosed a shallow recess named the lacrimal spot in which lies a small elevation known as the caruncle. Internal to the caruncle a small fold marks the extremity of the bulbar conjunctiva.

Subconjunctival hemorrhage may be the result of a local injury but may also be due to fracture of the anterior cranial fossa, presenting as a fan-shaped subconjunctival hemorrhage on the medial segment of the eyeball.

The Lacrimal Apparatus. The lacrimal gland occupies a fossa on the frontal bone and is situated in the upper outer part of the orbit. The gland consists of two parts, orbital and palpebral, the latter being a small extension beneath the upper eyelid to the superior fornix of the conjunctiva.

Fifteen to 20 ducts from both portions of the gland open into the superior fornix, and tears pass across the conjunctiva to reach the lacrimal puncta. These are minute openings on the summit of the lacrimal papillae which, in turn, are situated on the margins of the eyelids close to the inner canthus of the eye. These puncta open into the lacrimal canaliculi, which open by a common canal into the lateral part of the lacrimal sac. If the puncta are blocked or excessive tears are produced, they tend to flow over the lower lid onto the cheek. This condition is known as epiphora.

The two canaliculi, superior and inferior, open into the lacrimal sac, which may be considered the dilated upper extremity of the nasolacrimal duct. The lacrimal sac is situated in a small depression on the medial surface of the orbit under the tarsal ligament. An abscess of the lacrimal sac, if unrelieved surgically, discharges spontaneously through the skin below the internal tarsal ligament.

The nasolacrimal duct is three fourths of an inch in length, pursuing a downward course within its bony canal to open into the inferior nasal meatus.

Regional Anesthesia

Anesthesia of the orbital regions requires understanding of the sensory innervation of the area, which is derived from the ophthalmic and maxillary divisions of the trigeminal nerve. Innervation of the mandibular teeth and lower lip is from the mandibular branch of the trigeminal nerve (Fig. 13–2).

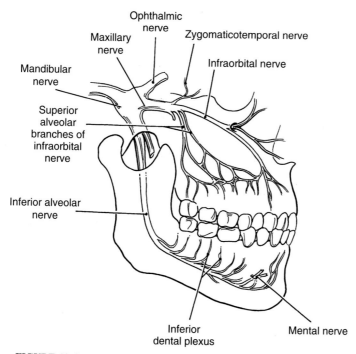

FIGURE 13–2. Maxillary and mandibular branches of the trigeminal nerve.

Ophthalmic Nerve. The ophthalmic nerve is the first subdivision of the trigeminal (fifth cranial) nerve. Entirely sensory, it is distributed in the orbit to the upper part of the face and front part of the scalp. After leaving the trigeminal ganglion, in its middle cranial fossa site, the nerve runs forward in the lateral wall of the cavernous sinus and, just before reaching the orbit, it divides into three branches, which pass separately through the superior orbital fissure. The branches are the following:

The *frontal nerve*, gives off a supraorbital and a supratrochlear branch, both of which turn around the supraorbital margin and appear as cutaneous nerves in the forehead.

The *lacrimal nerve* enters the orbit above the extraocular muscles and runs laterally to supply the lacrimal glands before its terminal branch supplies the skin over the lateral half of the upper eyelid.

The *nasociliary nerve* passes over the optic nerve and between the medial rectus and superior oblique muscles to give sensory branches to the globe, anterior ethmoid, and infratrochlear nerve.

Maxillary Nerve. As the second subdivision of the trigeminal nerve, the maxillary nerve leaves the cranium via the foramen rotundum. It pursues a course to the face across the pterygopalatine fossa, through the infraorbital canal, to the maxilla along the floor of the orbit. There it becomes the infraorbital nerve issuing at the infraorbital foramen to provide branches to the face which radiate to the lower eyelid and upper lip.

The branches of the maxillary nerve include ganglionic branches to the sphenopalatine ganglion; the zygomatic nerve, which ascends along the lateral wall of the orbit and divides into the zygomaticofacial and zygomaticotemporal branches; the posterior superior dental nerves; and the middle and anterior superior dental nerves.

Regional anesthesia of the eyelids can readily be achieved by strategic infiltration of local anesthesia agents at points along the superior orbital rim and infraorbital foramen and at the lateral zygomatic area in the region of the zygomaticofacial foramen. Protection of the cornea during periocular surgery by the application of a protective ointment prevents damage from the heat of the overhead lights, from desiccation, from gauze irritation, and from instrumental trauma. A plastic protective shell over the orbit is advisable.

Mandibular Nerve. The third branch of the trigeminal nerve divides into the lingual and inferior alveolar nerves. The terminal branches of the inferior alveolar nerve become the mental and inferior incisor nerves.

RECONSTRUCTIVE SURGERY OF THE EYELIDS
Lower Lid
Small defects: These can generally be closed primarily. Adequate excision of a lid neoplasm should, if possible, be done as a pentagonal wedge excision. If undue tension occurs as the opposing raw surfaces are approximated, lateral cantholysis relaxes the lower lid sufficiently. The lateral canthus is incised laterally after exposure of the lateral canthal ligament. Incision of the lower crus of the ligament releases enough lower lid tension to enable closure of defects up to 10 mm in width. The tarsoconjunctival layer is closed with interrupted fine absorbable sutures, but the tarsocutaneous layer is approximated with nonabsorbable sutures.

Intermediate defects: Closure of defects equivalent to loss of one half of the lid's horizontal dimension may be repaired by several methods: (1) Lateral canthal semicircular flap (Tenzel procedure). This is a one-stage repair in which a lateral upwardly convex canthal semicircular flap of skin and muscle is raised. The lower crus of the canthal ligament is divided, thereby mobilizing the flap so that it can be advanced medially and the edges of the defect approximated and sutured. The raw advancement flap posterior surface may be covered

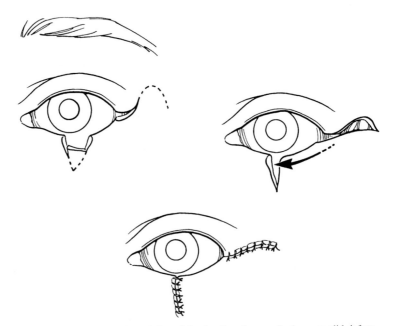

FIGURE 13–3. Lateral canthal semicircular flap closure of a lower eyelid defect.

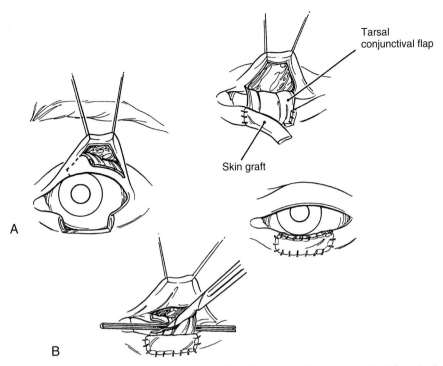

Tarsal conjunctival flap

Skin graft

A

B

FIGURE 13–4. Tarsoconjunctival advancement flap from upper lid to lower lid defect. *A*, A tarsoconjunctival flap is transferred into the lower lid defect and covered with a skin graft. *B*, The pedicle is divided at 2 to 3 weeks and inset to complete the reconstruction.

with a free conjunctival graft, readily available as a wedge excised at the base of the defect. The lateral canthus is then reconstituted (Fig. 13–3). (2) Tarsoconjunctival advancement flap: A tarsoconjunctival flap is fashioned from the everted upper lid to conform to the size of the lower lid defect. The flap is mobilized in a downward direction in the plane of the pretarsal fascia until it fits into the defect. The flap is sutured to the base of the defect with interrupted fine absorbable sutures (Fig. 13–4). A skin graft, derived from the opposite upper lid or postauricular or supraclavicular area, is then placed over the raw tarsal surface. About 2 to 3 weeks later the flap is opened along the line of the palpebral fissure as a blepharotomy and any residual trimming accomplished. Using the upper lid to reconstruct lower lid defects is probably best avoided if possible.

Large defects: Defects larger than one-half the lower lid are best reconstructed with a cheek rotation flap (Mustarde flap). The larger the defect, the more cheek is transposed. A chondromucosal graft from the nasal septum is sewn to the posterior aspect of the flap to provide lining and support (Fig. 13–5).

Upper Lid

Small defects: These defects are closed in layers, including a lateral cantholysis if there is tension on the primary closure.

Intermediate defects: These defects consist of loss of up to half of the upper lid. (1) Lower lid advancement flap (Cutler-Beard procedure): A full-thickness skin-orbicularis tarsoconjunctival flap is fashioned in the lower lid, 4 mm below the lid margin, corresponding to the upper lid defect, and the flap is advanced beneath the bridge of lid margin and sutured to the conjunctiva-levator aponeurosis and attached structures of the upper lid. The second (release) stage is carried out about 2 to 3 weeks later. The flap is opened along the line of the palpebral fissure and any necessary trimming is completed.

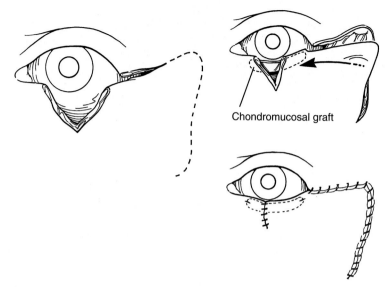

Chondromucosal graft

FIGURE 13–5. Closure of a large eyelid defect with a Mustarde cheek flap and a nasal chondromucosal flap.

(2) Lower lid transposition flap: A full-thickness flap of lower eyelid based on the marginal vessels is transposed into the upper lid defect. The flap need be only about one-half the size of the defect, which is reduced initially by lateral cantholysis (Figs. 13–6 and 13–7).

Large defects: Defects larger than half the upper lid are reconstructed with appropriately wide transposition flaps from the lower lid. The lower lid is then reconstructed by techniques previously described.

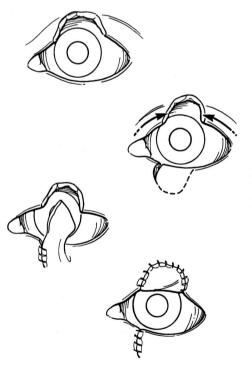

FIGURE 13–6. Lower lid transposition flap to an upper eyelid defect. The flap is divided and inset 2 to 3 weeks following initial transposition.

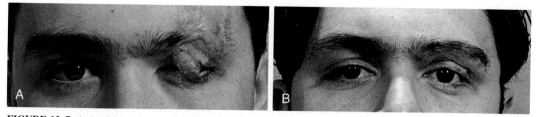

FIGURE 13–7. *A,* Avulsion injury to the upper eyelid and brow corrected with a lower lid switch flap and partial thickness scalp graft. *B,* Two years following inset of lower lid flap and brow reconstruction with a superficial temporal scalp island flap.

The Medial or Lateral Canthus. Displacement of the medial or lateral canthus due to laceration of the canthal ligaments is difficult to correct. Medial canthal repair is complicated by the anatomic presence of the nasolacrimal system. A suture is fastened to the medial canthal tendon, passed through a drill hole in the nasal bones, and tied over a toggle or screw on the contralateral side. The lateral canthal tendon may simply be sutured to the periosteum on the lateral orbital wall. Placement must be exact.

The Lacrimal Apparatus. In eyelid lacerations, the lower lacrimal canaliculus may be divided and should always be probed and, if the ends are located, repaired.

Nasolacrimal duct obstruction, whether it occurs early or late after periorbital or nasal injury, causes epiphora. Repeated dilatation of the obstruction may be helpful. Stagnation of the lacrimal sac contents leads to its distention by a mucocele, with subsequent abscess formation as a result of infection. An early anastomosis of the lacrimal sac to the nasal mucous membrane through an opening in the base of the lacrimal fossa as a dacrocystorhinostomy prevents these complications (Fig. 13–8).

Ectropion. Eversion of the eyelid margin may vary in degree and may be due to various causes. It more commonly affects the lower lid because its tarsal plate is smaller.

Causes of ectropion include (1) congenital tissue deficiency in the outer layers of the eyelid (coloboma); (2) spastic ectropion in exophthalmos due to pull of the

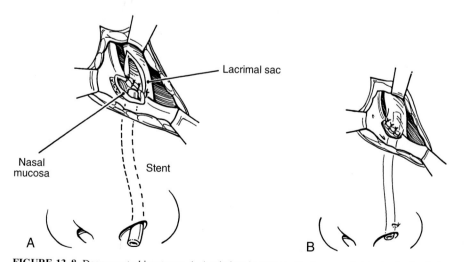

FIGURE 13–8. Dacryocystorhinostomy: *A,* A window is made in the bone medial to the lacrimal sac and the lacrimal sac is opened. *B,* The mucosa of the sac is then sutured to the adjacent nasal mucosa. The anastomosis is stented with a catheter, which is removed in 3 months.

orbicularis oculi muscle; (3) senile ectropion due to loss of muscle tone; (4) paralytic ectropion in facial nerve paralysis; and (5) cicatricial ectropion due to traumatic loss of tissue.

Treatment is surgical. Cicatricial ectropion may be amenable to repair by Z-plasty, although skin loss requires a full-thickness skin graft. Senile ectropion requires an infraciliary incision with tarsal tightening. After segmental tarsectomy in the lateral third of the eyelid, it is tightened in horizontal manner, excess skin is excised, and skin is pulled up laterally for support. Coloboma may be repaired with composite cartilage and skin graft or local flap transposition.

Entropion. Inversion of the lid margin causes corneal irritation by the lashes. Trichiasis refers to inturning of the lashes with normally aligned lid margins. Entropion may be congenital, due to lack of a normal tarsal plate, or spasmodic, due to hypertrophy of the orbicularis oculi muscle. Secondary entropion may result from lack of lid support or follow scarring of the conjunctiva which pulls on the lid margin. Cicatricial entropion may result from adhesions of the lids to the globe secondary to symblepharon. It may also be a sequel to eyelid reconstruction when too much lining has been borrowed from the normal lid. Correction is by shortening the tarsus and conjunctiva with an inverted triangular excision. Closure of the triangle prevents return of the tarsus to the inverted position. Excision of skin and orbicularis muscle prevents reinversion.

Symblepharon. Obliteration of the conjunctival fornices may result from conjunctival adhesions that prevent movements of the orbital globe. This may follow chemical burns, fire burns, or penetrating lacerations. After adhesions are freed, mucosal grafts are sutured to the edges of scleral and conjunctival defects.

Orbital Exenteration and Socket Contraction. Following ocular enucleation for trauma, neoplasm, or a blind painful eye, contraction of the eye socket results in a poorly fitting prosthesis. Shortening of the lower fornix and narrowing of the interpalpebral fissure occurs with loss of upper lid support. Ptosis becomes apparent.

Treatment is reconstructive. (1) Fornix reconstruction: Under local infiltration anesthesia, an incision extending the length of the lower half of the socket is made, the conjunctiva is undermined, and scar tissue is excised. A buccal mucous membrane graft is then transposed to the prepared bed in the socket and sutured in position with fine interrupted absorbable sutures. (2) Total socket reconstruction: This requires removal of granulation tissue and scar. The conjunctiva is dissected from the underlying tissues. A conformer is properly shaped and a hole cut in its center. The socket conformer is covered with a split-thickness skin graft with the raw surface facing outward and a new socket with a larger cavity created. The conformer is kept in position by wiring it to the upper and lower orbital rims using two previously constructed drill holes. The mold is left in place for 3 months, when it is removed and a glass shell inserted, which is finally replaced by an artificial eye.

Lining may also be provided by transfer of flaps if no bed is available for a skin graft. A temporoparietal flap pedicled on the superficial temporal vessels covers exposed bone and provides a noncontracting surface for a skin graft.

Ptosis. Ptosis of the upper eyelid is designated blepharoptosis. The edge of the upper eyelid is normally at the level of the upper limbus. Drooping of the lid

TABLE 13–1. Severity of Ptosis

1–2 mm	Mild
3 mm	Moderate
4 mm or more	Severe

below this level represents ptosis and is due to insufficient action of the levator muscle or stretching of the levator aponeurosis.

Congenital Ptosis. Poor levator function is associated with dystrophy of the levator palpebrae superioris. The muscle is usually present but is attenuated so that it cannot take up the slack and elevate the lid. Congenital ptosis may be simple or associated with blepharophimosis, ophthalmoplegias, or Marcus Gunn syndrome.

BLEPHAROPHIMOSIS. The upper eyelid deformity is characterized by epicanthal folds and the absence of a supratarsal fold. Levator function is usually poor or absent.

OPHTHALMOPLEGIAS. Ptosis may be associated with weakness of the superior rectus muscle or may be one manifestation of a congenital third nerve paralysis.

MARCUS GUNN SYNDROME. Misdirection of the oculomotor nerve results in a synkinetic ptosis of the upper lid when the mandible is moved to the contralateral side or depressed (jaw-wink phenomenon).

The droop may be noted at birth and may improve slightly during the first few years and then remain static. Serious interference with vision may require early operative repair, but delay until 3 to 4 years of age is justified otherwise.

Ptosis may be bilateral, and repair should be done bilaterally at the same session so as to match the degree of lid elevation. In designing the proper surgical procedure for ptosis correction, a decision must be made regarding the degree of ptosis and the adequacy of levator function (Tables 13–1 and 13–2). The normal lid sits at the level of the upper limbus with 12 to 15 mm of levator function. Levator function is determined by the distance the upper lid moves from the downward to upward gaze position of the eye. The exact surgical procedure depends upon levator function: (1) Presence of levator function: For mild ptosis, the Fasanella-Servat procedure may be used. A segment of conjunctiva, tarsus, and Müller's muscle is resected within a clamp. A running cross-over pullout stitch is inserted above the clamped area and tied after the composite segment has been resected. Alternatively, the Mustarde split-level tarsectomy is used. A segment of skin and muscle is resected at one level and a segment of tarsus and conjunctiva at another level. Closure of the skin excision corrects the lack of anterior skin fold. For moderate ptosis with fair to good levator function, the procedure requires a levator advancement procedure. Through an anterior skin incision, the levator muscle at its attachment to the tarsus is clamped and transected below the clamp.

TABLE 13–2. Levator Function

>12 mm	Excellent
7–12 mm	Good
5–7 mm	Fair
<5 mm	Poor

It is advanced and sutured to the tarsal plate so as to achieve the desired lid position. Redundant levator muscle is then resected. (2) Absence of levator function: The frontalis suspension procedure using the double triangular or rhomboid suture is recommended. It is performed with autogenous fascia or a synthetic strip after ensuring that the frontalis muscle is functional. Two 4-mm incisions are made 3 mm from the lid margin through the skin, subcutaneous tissue, and orbicularis muscle to expose the anterior tarsal plate. Three linear incisions are made above the eyebrow, with the middle incision over the midline of the lid, down to the frontalis aponeurosis. The suspensory strip passes through the epitarsus subcutaneously, and each end is brought through the lateral and medial eyebrow incisions. The strip is then brought from each end through the frontalis aponeurosis and tied in the middle eyebrow incision. The five skin incisions are then closed.

Acquired Ptosis. Ptosis may be due to (1) neurogenic cause: Paralysis of oculomotor nerve due to head injury or compression by intracranial lesion. Ptosis also occurs in Horner syndrome owing to loss of sympathetic innervation to Müller's muscle; (2) myasthenia gravis; (3) trauma to eyelid with disruption of the levator muscle insertion on the tarsus. Compound fractures of the orbital roof may impinge on the levator mechanism; (4) pseudoptosis due to blow-out orbital fracture with enophthalmos.

Surgical improvement of acquired ptosis requires improvisation of established techniques to deal with the appropriate anatomic deficiency. The basic procedure usually requires skin and orbicularis excision with shortening of the levator aponeurosis and supratarsal fixation. If associated ptosis of the lacrimal gland is present, the capsule of the orbital portion of the gland may be plicated or suspended from the gland under the orbital rim. An associated upper lid blepharoplasty may need to be integrated into the procedure.

LIP RECONSTRUCTION

The lips are composed of the orbicularis oris muscle covered internally by oral mucosa and externally by skin. The vermilion forms the free border of the lip with a distinct white roll at the vermilion-cutaneous junction of the upper lip. The orbicularis oris muscle interfaces with the buccinator muscle fibers and other muscle bundles at the modiolus lateral to the commissures. The levator labii superioris lies superficial to the orbicularis oris; it elevates the lateral lip and contributes to the lower philtral columns. The depressor anguli oris and depressor labii inferioris draw the lip inferiorly. Action of the bucinnators widens the mouth aperture.

Upper Lip

Full-thickness defects comprising one fourth to one third of the lip may be closed primarily. Larger defects require transfer of adjacent lip tissue.

Abbé Flap. A switch flap composed of full-thickness lip is transposed on the marginal labial vessels from the opposite lip (Fig. 13–9). The pedicle is divided

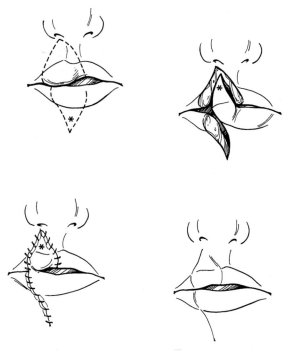

FIGURE 13–9. Reconstruction of an upper lid defect with an Abbé switch flap from the lower lip.

and the flap inset at a second stage 2 to 3 weeks later. If the switch includes the commissure, it is an Estlander flap.

Lip Advancement. Upper lip defects may be closed by advancement of lateral lip tissues with excision of a perialar crescent at the nasolabial junction (Fig. 13–10).

Reverse Karapandzic Flap. A flap of orbicularis oris and overlying lip skin is rotated into the defect. The vessels and nerve branches to the orbicularis oris are carefully preserved. This provides a sensate, animated reconstruction flap.

Fan Flap. Bilateral fan flaps may be used for total upper lip reconstruction. Full-thickness flaps of skin, muscle, and mucosa are transposed from each nasolabial area.

Lower Lip

Defects of one third to almost one half of the lower lip may be closed primarily. Larger defects are closed with one of the following:

Abbé Flap. A reversed Abbé flap is transposed on the marginal labial vessels. The pedicle is divided at 2 to 3 weeks and the switch flap inset.

Karapandzic Flaps. This is the best method for reconstructing defects of 75 to 80 per cent of the lower lip. Bilateral flaps of skin and orbicularis oris are transposed into the defect (Fig. 13–11). Branches of the facial nerve and the

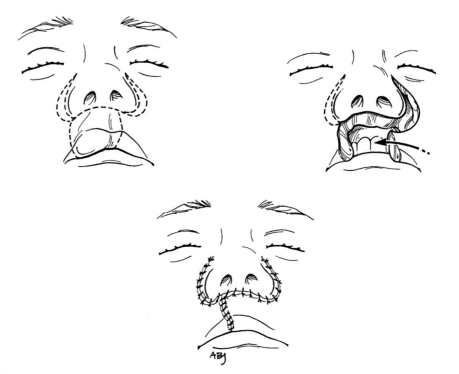

FIGURE 13–10. Closure of a lip defect by advancement of lateral lip tissue and excision of a perialar crescent.

vessels supplying the muscle are teased out from the muscle fibers, preserving them as the muscle is incised. The mucosa is incised enough to mobilize the flaps. The reconstruction provides a sensate, dynamic lip with a competent oral sphincter. If used for total lip reconstruction, the oral appeture is significantly compromised, requiring secondary commissure reconstructions.

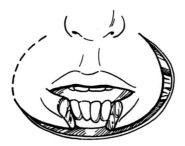

FIGURE 13–11. Karapandzic flap closure of a lower lip defect.

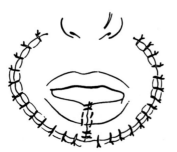

Fan Flap. Bilateral fan flaps reconstruct a total lower lip defect. Full-thickness flaps from the nasolabial area are rotated on each commissure and approximated in three layers at the midline. Free margin can be reconstructed with a ventral tongue flap. This reconstruction does not provide acceptable oral competence.

Oral Commissure

Deformity of the oral commissure is seen in children following a burn after chewing through an electrical cord. It also may result from thermal burns to the face and tumor resection. Repair is difficult, requiring opening of the oral commissure with full-thickness incision through the scar and resurfacing with buccal mucosal flaps. Repair is delayed until the scar has matured. Following commissure reconstruction, the repair must be splinted with a dental device to prevent contracture and recurrence of the deformity.

THE EAR

The auricle is composed of skin closely applied to the underlying cartilaginous framework (Fig. 13–12). Its intrinsic and extrinsic muscles are of no great surgical importance.

The auricle or external ear develops from six tubercles which, from one through six, form the tragus, the crus helicis, the helix, the antihelix, the antetragus, and the lobule. Failure of fusion of any of these tubercles may result in the formation of a preauricular fistula, which may intermittently discharge or ulcerate. The frequent association between auricular and genitourinary congenital malformations should be kept in mind and appropriate clinical and pyelographic examination instituted.

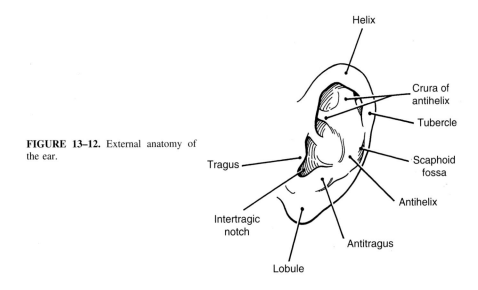

FIGURE 13–12. External anatomy of the ear.

Congenital Abnormalities

1. Normal development of the first and second pharyngeal arches fails to occur.
   a. Congenital absence of the pinna. This may be accompanied by absence of the condyle and ascending ramus of the mandible. Congenital facial paralysis may also be present. The bilateral deformity occurs in patients with the Treacher Collins syndrome.
   b. Congenital absence of the external auditory meatus: The middle and internal ear components are present.
2. Microtic ear: The external ear is represented by a malpositioned lobule to which is attached a piece of skin-covered cartilage that bears little or no resemblance to a pinna.
3. Accessory auricle: A small piece of skin-covered cartilage is situated in front of the external auditory meatus.
4. Preauricular sinus: If repeated infection occurs, the track should be laid open in its entirely and allowed to granulate and epithelialize. If the track is well defined without any ramifications, it may sometimes be amenable to excision and primary suture of the wound.
5. Misshapen ears
   a. Protruding ears: These ears may lack an antihelix and require construction of an antihelix fold, or they may have a deep conchal fossa that requires correction by the excision of conchal cartilage.
   b. Lop or cup ears: A shortened helix margin requires lengthening in order to provide correction. Rearrangement of skin and cartilage is necessary with excision of a strip of cartilage from the concha for replacement of the missing helix margin, which is then covered by a flap of skin from the postauricular area.
   c. Cleft lobes: A cleft in the lobe is readily repaired, creating a Z-plasty at the free border of the split in the lobe.
   d. Radial folds may run from the antihelix to the helix or across the conchal fossa. Flaps can be raised via a W- or Z-plasty. After the skin is elevated, triangular flaps of cartilage are made to interdigitate in a flattened state and the skin is closed over it.
   e. Cryptotia: The upper pole of the ear cartilage is buried beneath the scalp skin. The superior crus of the antihelix may be absent and the inferior crus folded by fibrous tissue. Utilizing a Z-plasty approach on the postauricular skin, the upper pole cartilage is released from the side of the head, and excision of the fibrous tissue releases the inferior crus. The flaps are then transposed and sutured into place.
   f. Macrotia: Excessively large ears can be reduced by excision of a full-thickness triangular wedge of tissue. Small triangles resected at right angle to the main triangle permit restoration of continuity of the ear as a radial suture line. Lobe reduction may be accomplished by appropriate resection and recontouring.

EAR RECONSTRUCTION

Protruding Ear. Ideally, operative treatment should be delayed until ear growth is 80 per cent complete at 4 or 5 years of age and before commencing school.

An ellipse of skin is excised from the posterior auricular surface. Skin and soft tissues are freed off the pinna, and dissection is continued down to the mastoid area. Excess soft tissue in the mastoid area, including the postauricular muscle, is resected. Projections on the posterior conchal bowl are resected. The sutures are then placed so that when they are tied, the conchal bowl is pulled back toward the mastoid. Care must be taken so that when the concha is pulled posteriorly, no constriction of the external auditory meatus occurs.

Dissection is carried around at the tail of the helix onto the anterior conchal surface. Soft tissues are freed from the anterior surface, where the anterior helical fold will be created. Perichondrium is abraded so as to weaken the cartilage. Landmarks on either side of the planned antihelical fold are transferred from front to back of the pinna by needle puncture marks defined with methylene blue. Sutures are placed so that when they are tied, an anterior helical fold with a well-formed superior crus is created. Sutures may also need to be placed to pull the tail of the helix into a better position. Following wound closure, a circumferential dressing is placed and maintained for 7 days.

The Microtic Ear. Because costal cartilage provides the framework for the ear, operative treatment is usually delayed until the child is about 6 years of age. Any contemplated middle ear surgery should await completion of the auricular construction.

The first step in patients in whom the malplaced lobule represents the pinna should be the conservation of the lobule and its placement in a position matching that of the normal side. At this time the distorted mass of skin-covered cartilage is excised and any worthwhile tissue conserved for contouring of the lower helical margin.

At the next stage the supportive framework is implanted. Although homogeneous, heterogeneous, and alloplastic materials have all been tried with variable degrees of success, autogenous costal cartilage provides the best results with the fewest complications.

A template from the pinna of the healthy side is prepared to represent the shape of the required cartilage implant. A block of cartilage is removed from the right costal margin for the left pinna and vice versa and is carved to the shape of the template. A narrow strip of cartilage to contour the helix margin is then fixed to the main cartilage block by stainless steel sutures.

The entire complex is then placed through a preauricular incision, which is undermined so that the composite segment of cartilage is in a position that matches the ear on the other side. The covering skin is then anchored to the implant by transfixion sutures that create prominent ridges in the pinna.

At a subsequent stage, construction of the tragus can be accomplished using a chondrocutaneous composite graft. The postural groove can be created by staged free skin grafts and any remaining raw areas covered by skin grafts.

If necessary, reconstruction of an external auditory meatus is done after completion of the pinna reconstruction by means of a split-thickness skin graft that is fashioned in the form of a sac. This is then placed into a precarved channel in the mastoid so that the sac is placed in contact with the middle ear ossicular tissue. The hairline may need to be rearranged to improve the local relationships.

Although well-constructed latex ear prostheses may be preferable in adults whose ear loss is due to excision of a cancerous lesion, in children a well-constructed auricle is vastly preferable.

Acquired Deformities

Small defects are repaired by direct approximation of the edges after excision of a lesion as a triangular wedge. Larger defects require transfer of local tissue as a flap or cartilage from the contralateral ear as a graft. Tissue and skin may be obtained from the following areas:

Helical rim: The remaining helical rim is dissected off the scapha and each rim advanced into the defect. A V-Y advancement in the helical crus increases the amount of helical rim advancement.

Auriculocephalic sulcus: A tubed flap may be transferred in two stages to replace a large helical rim defect. A banner flap transposes skin from behind the ear to resurface large defects of the scapha.

Concha: An ipsilateral chondrocutaneous flap may be transferred into an upper auricular defect. The donor conchal wound is resurfaced with a skin graft.

Contralateral concha: A cartilage graft from the contralateral ear replaces missing cartilage. The skin defect is resurfaced with a transposition flap from behind the injured ear.

Temporoparietal flap: The temporoparietal fascia may be turned down as a flap based on the temporal vessels to replace missing soft tissue. The flap must be covered with a skin graft and is reserved for total ear reconstruction.

Ear Avulsion

A total ear avulsion may be replanted. Vessels of sufficient caliber can be identified in the lobule for salvage by microvascular technique. If the avulsion is subtotal or replantation is not possible, the ear is buried in a pocket over the mastoid. Skin is first removed from the avulsed ear, and holes are cut in the cartilage. The mastoid pocket is elevated 14 to 21 days later and the donor defect skin is grafted.

Total ear loss is reconstructed with a rib cartilage framework, as for microtia. Mastoid soft tissue may be pre-expanded to provide sufficient skin to cover the reconstructed frame. If mastoid soft tissue is inadequate, the cartilage graft is resurfaced with a temporoparietal flap and skin graft.

RECONSTRUCTION OF NASAL DEFECTS

Surface defects of the nose that cannot be closed by suture should be repaired by a full-thickness skin graft, local flaps, or a median forehead flap. Loss of the columella or nostril margin can be replaced by transfer of a composite graft of cartilage lined by skin on both sides, if the defect is not unusually large. Larger defects may be reconstructed by one of the following methods (Fig. 13–13): local nasal flap, banner flap, bilobed flap, glabellar flap, nasolabial flap, and median forehead flap.

In general, the skin of the forehead provides the best material for nasal reconstruction in view of the good match in color and texture. Pre-expansion of forehead flaps, using skin expanders, has facilitated the use of the forehead in reconstructing total nasal defects.

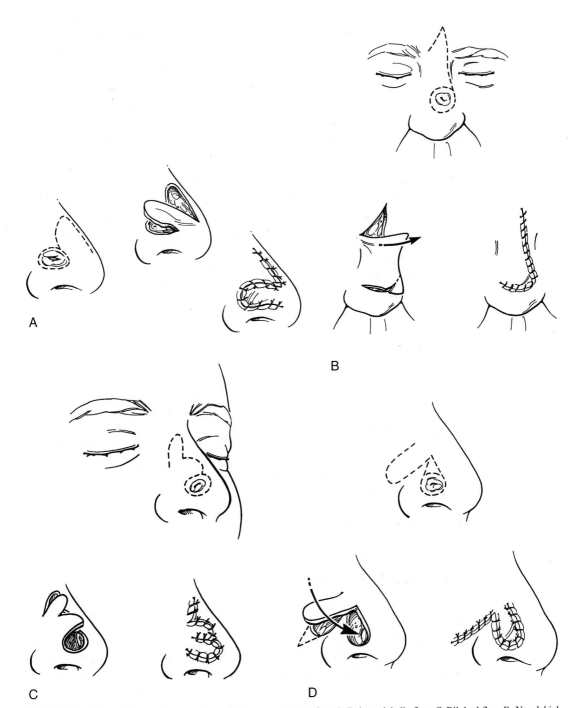

FIGURE 13–13. Local flaps for closure of nasal defects. *A*, Banner flap. *B*, Reiger glabella flap. *C*, Bilobed flap. *D*, Nasolabial transposition flap.

Forehead Flaps for Nasal Reconstruction

Past objections to the use of forehead flaps were generally related to the occasional unsightly effects of scarring and damage to the frontalis muscle and the need for coverage of the secondary forehead defect with well-matched full-thickness skin from the retroauricular or supraclavicular region. If large forehead flaps are required, pre-expansion of the area avoids these problems, leaving the donor area with a very acceptable aesthetic appearance after the forehead defect is closed by direct approximation of the edges without tension.

In nasal reconstruction it is important that skeletal support to the nose be provided at the same time as soft tissue coverage. If only one side of the nose is missing, the skin of the intact side may be used to provide nasal lining and an unbroken external coverage for the entire nose with the forehead flap.

When the normal lining of the nose is deficient, it is important to restore it to the internal surface of the nostril. Other sources of lining include nasal skin turned down from the defect margin, distal advancement of residual nasal lining, chondromucosal flaps from the nasal septum, tunneled skin from the nasolabial area with its raw surface to the outside, and infolding of the end of the reconstructive flap.

Forehead flaps are of three main types:

Median flap: This receives its blood supply from both supratrochlear arteries and is well vascularized. Two parallel incisions are made on either side of the midline and extended through skin, soft tissues, and periosteum. The length of the flap between the glabella and the hairline is joined at the hairline by a transverse incision. Situated between the frontalis muscles, the flap does not disturb the muscles' expressive function. The flap includes periosteum over the frontal bone, inferiorly so as not to injure its blood supply. The flap is sufficiently long that it can reach the nasal tip and restore the columella (Fig. 13–14). If necessary, a composite cartilage graft can be incorporated for reconstruction of the nasal dorsum or its alae. The design of the medial flap may be amended to a "gull-shaped" one for reconstructing the columella and the nasal alae.

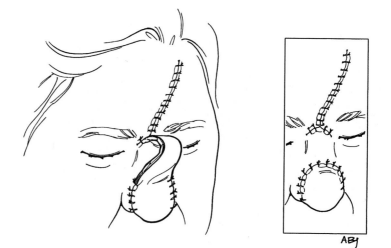

FIGURE 13–14. Forehead flap reconstruction of a nasal tip defect.

Island forehead flap with a subcutaneous tissue pedicle: This flap provides greater mobility because the subcutaneous pedicle is more amenable to twisting and is more readily adjusted to the recipient site. The island of skin, whose size has been predetermined to match the size of the recipient area, is totally detached from the surrounding skin but retains connection via a subcutaneous pedicle that contains the supratrochlear vessels.

The scalping flap: This flap may have a place in patients with a low hairline and a narrow forehead. With a very good blood supply from all the scalp vessels, this flap can be mobilized from the cranium so that sufficient length is provided and the flap rolled on itself as a tube. The flap to be transposed is raised from the frontalis muscle. The rest of the "carrying" flap is raised from the pericranium via a transcoronal incision behind the hairline until enough length is obtained for transfer to the nose. A full-thickness retroauricular skin graft is placed over the area of the permanent donor defect over the frontalis muscle. The "carrying" flap pedicle can usually be divided in 3 weeks and is returned to the forehead, where the dressing is removed and the forehead flap sutured back into position.

FACIAL PARALYSIS

The role of reconstructive surgery in permanent, irreversible paralysis of the facial muscles is based upon the hope that the paralyzed facial muscles may be re-innervated or that the paralysis can be camouflaged by procedures that provide static support to the weakened muscles or dynamic procedures using muscle transposition.

Proper assessment of facial nerve conduction requires monitoring of response to faradic stimulation with electrodes placed over the stylomastoid foramen and along the course of the facial nerve. Electromyography aids in deciding whether the nerve injury has resulted in (a) neuropraxia with retention of nerve conduction, as in Bell's palsy; (b) axonotmesis, in which conduction is lost but nerve continuity is still present; or (c) neuronotmesis, in which the nerve has lost continuity.

Unless it is known that the nerve has been severed or divided, a period of 6 to 9 months should be allowed to elapse before a decision of irreversibility is made. If nerve regeneration occurs, clinical signs of muscle recovery become apparent within 6 months.

The facial nerve, or seventh cranial nerve, provides the total motor nerve supply to the superficial muscles of the face and scalp. In addition, it supplies a small sensory root that provides taste fibers from the tongue.

The facial nerve leaves the medulla oblongata at the lower border of the pons and upper end of the inferior cerebellar peduncle and immediately enters the internal auditory meatus, which it traverses in company with the auditory or eighth nerve. The facial nerve then enters the bony canal, which carries it through the petrous temporal bone to the stylomastoid foramen, its aperture of exit from the skull. During its passage in the bony canal, the nerve runs outward and then bends sharply backward to pass along the inner wall of the tympanic cavity. At this bend a swelling on the nerve occurs which is known as the ganglion of the facial nerve.

From the stylomastoid foramen, the nerve runs forward through the parotid gland, superficial to the posterior facial vein and external carotid artery. Opposite the ramus of the mandible, within the gland, the nerve divides into terminal branches for the facial muscles.

CENTRAL NUCLEI OF THE FACIAL NERVE

Ventral nucleus: The fibers that innervate the facial muscles originate in the ventral part of the lower pons.
Superior salivary nucleus: This nucleus provides the secretomotor fibers for the salivary and lacrimal glands.
Facial ganglion: This provides the cells of origin for the sensory fibers.

BRANCHES OF THE FACIAL NERVE

1. Great superficial petrosal nerve conveys the secretory fibers for the lacrimal gland via the nerve of the pterygoid canal.
2. Nerve to the stapedius
3. Chorda tympani nerve, which joins the lingual nerve, contains taste fibers from the anterior two thirds of the tongue and carries secretory fibers for the submandibular and sublingual salivary glands.
4. Nerve to the posterior belly of the digastric nerve
5. Nerve to the stylohyoid muscle
6. Posterior auricular nerve supplies the occipital belly of the occipitofrontalis and auricularis posterior muscles.
7. Terminal branches at the anterior edge of the parotid gland
   a. Temporal branch to muscles above the eye
   b. Zygomatic branch to muscles below the eye
   c. Buccal branch to the buccinator and muscles at the side of the mouth
   d. Mandibular branch runs along the mandible to the muscles below the mouth
   e. Cervical branch descends below the mandible to supply the platysma

Causes of Facial Paralysis

CONGENITAL

Developmental anomalies of the first and second pharyngeal pouches (mandibulo-otic syndrome) are the most common cause of congenital facial paralysis, as the seventh cranial nerve is the second arch nerve. This condition may, on occasion, be bilateral.

ACQUIRED

1. Supranuclear: Paralysis of the facial muscles may be due to lesions in the supranuclear segment of the nerve. This is usually associated with hemiplegia from a cerebrovascular cause. Only the lower part of the face is paralyzed, as the upper part of the face receives bilateral cortical innervation.
2. Infranuclear lesions of the facial nerve affect all the muscles of the appropriate half of the face. Lesions above the origin of the nerve to the stapedius may cause hyperacusis, whereas those above the origin of the chordae tympani affect the sense of taste. Underlying causes include the following:
   a. Intracranial nerve damage may be due to acoustic neuroma or operative injury during its removal.

b. Bell's palsy represents an inflammatory swelling of the nerve in its bony canal.

c. Fractures of the base of the skull

d. Deep facial lacerations may divide facial nerve branches.

e. Mastoiditis or middle ear and mastoid surgery may damage the nerve.

f. Malignant tumors of the parotid gland or damage to the nerve during parotid gland operations

Clinical Features of Facial Paralysis

When all branches of the nerve are paralyzed, the eye cannot be closed and epiphora may occur. The forehead on the affected side cannot be wrinkled. The mouth is drawn to the opposite side with a characteristic droop on the affected side and dribbling of saliva. Because the buccinator muscle is paralyzed, food tends to collect on the side of the mouth. The affected side of the face develops an expressionless quality.

Operative Treatment of Facial Paralysis

The selection of proper operative procedures in a given case is motivated by the desire to restore normal facial symmetry at rest and during voluntary motion and to restore oral, nasal, and ocular muscular and sphincteric tone. Whenever possible, neural reconstitution and dynamic reconstitution, rather than static procedures, should be used.

RESTORATION OF NEURAL PATHWAY

1. Direct nerve suture: Repair of a transected facial nerve trunk is best done at the time of its traumatic division or ablation during parotidectomy if the ends can be approximated without tension. Although early re-innervation of the facial musculature represents the ideal, the paralyzed muscles have the capacity to respond even after a 12-month delay in the re-innervation procedure.

2. Nerve grafting

   a. Cervical plexus graft: After resection of a segment of facial nerve and its branches, a nerve autograft can be harvested from the ipsilateral neck. If metastatic nodes preclude it, then the contralateral neck can provide a trunk at the C2–C3 level, with its greater occipital, lesser occipital, and great auricular branches available for suture of the peripheral facial nerve branches. After successful re-innervation, recovery of facial muscle activity may take 6 to 18 months, depending on the length of the graft.

   b. Cross-facial graft: Autogenous grafts of sural nerve are brought from facial nerve branches on the intact side of the face to distal branches of the facial nerve, on the paralyzed side, lost in trauma or parotid surgery. The grafts are brought through subcutaneous tunnels created across the upper and lower lips and forehead connecting the incision on both sides (Fig. 13–15).

   c. Faciohypoglossal and facioglossopharyngeal anastomosis: When the facial nerve has been divided above the stylomastoid foramen, as in removal of an

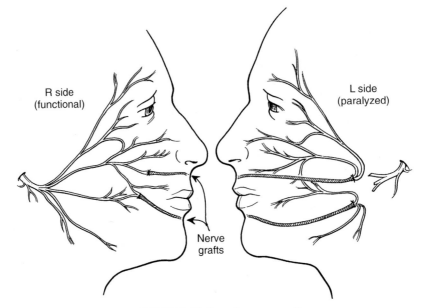

R side
(functional)

L side
(paralyzed)

Nerve
grafts

FIGURE 13–15. Cross-face nerve graft.

acoustic neuroma, the distal part of the facial trunk can be anastomosed to the proximal segment of an adjacent cranial motor nerve. If the hypoglossal nerve is used, its division results in atrophy and paralysis of half the tongue, which may cause occasional difficulty. Half the nerve may be used to maintain motor innervation of the tongue.

The facial and hypoglossal nerves are approached by a submandibular incision between the mastoid process and hyoid bone. The facial nerve trunk is located as it emerges from the stylomastoid foramen, where it is divided and the distal end brought down over the digastric muscle. The hypoglossal nerve is located below the digastric as it crosses the carotid sheath and is divided as near to the tongue as possible. The proximal end of the donor cranial nerve is anastomosed to the distal end of the facial nerve under magnification and without tension. The anastomosis of the twelfth and seventh cranial nerves is generally used as a "babysitter" to maintain facial muscle tone until definitive cross-nerve grafting is accomplished.

DYNAMIC RECONSTRUCTION

Although muscle transplant procedures may have limited usefulness as primary procedures, they may be very beneficial as supportive procedures in the management of facial paralysis. The use of masseter muscle can help lift the angle of the mouth by clenching the teeth and improves the natural expression of the affected side.

Masseter muscle transfer: Under general anesthesia, via either an intraoral or extraoral incision, the anterior two thirds of the masseter is detached from its mandibular insertion and, with its innervation intact, transferred to the angle of the mouth, where it is sutured to the facial musculature so as to overcorrect the mouth droop.

Temporalis muscle transfer: Transposition of the muscle with its coronoid process insertion can be accomplished through a preauricular incision and sutured into the angle of the mouth. The temporalis muscle may be detached from its origin in the temporal fossa with a strip to the epicranium; after mobilizing the fan-shaped muscle, it is separated into four muscle slips. Muscle slips are transposed to the upper and lower eyelids, where they are sutured at the medial canthal ligament, and at the upper lip, commissure, and lower lip as well as the mesolabial fold, where overcorrective sutures are placed. The residual depression in the temporal fossa can be corrected by replacing the muscle mass with cranioplast.

Free muscle grafts: Two to three stages are necessary. The extensor digitorum brevis muscle on the dorsum of the foot is suitable because of its several muscle bellies. The muscle needs to be denervated 2 weeks before it is used as a free muscle graft. These procedures have been abandoned for the most part with the advent of microvascular muscle transfer.

Microneurovascular muscle transfer: This two-stage procedure is designed to provide re-animation of the paralyzed face in conjunction with neural pathway reconnection. It provides new vascularized facial muscles that have been re-innervated and can pull in different directions. The most commonly used muscles include the gracilis, pectoralis minor, and serratus anterior muscles. A cross-face nerve graft is placed initially. Once the axons have regenerated across the graft, as determined by a Tinel sign, the muscle flap is transferred. The nerve innervating the muscle is anastomosed to the cross-face graft. The muscle vessels are anastomosed and the muscle slips sutured into position.

STATIC RECONSTRUCTION

The procedure creates fascia lata slings. Support of the sagging face may be remedied by removing three strips of fascia lata from the thigh, each 0.25 inch in width, and passing them to three separate sites:

Hemicircumoral loop: The strand of fascia passes subcutaneously from the angle of the mouth on the paralyzed side beyond the midline on the sound side and is re-formed subcutaneously after passing through the lip musculature. The two ends are tied at the angle of the mouth.

Zygomatic loop: A second fascial strip connects the mouth loop to the anterior part of the zygomatic loop, where it is tied so as to provide a fair degree of overcorrection.

Mandibular loop: The third fascial strip connects the mouth loop to the posterior border of the ascending ramus of the mandible, where the loop is tied so that overcorrection occurs.

Paralysis or excision of muscles of expression on the intact side, although it has its adherents, is not recommended in most cases.

Suggested Reading

Brent B: The correction of microtia with autogenous cartilage grafts: I. The classic deformity. Plast Reconstr Surg 66:1, 1980

Burget GC, Menick FJ: The subunit principle in nasal reconstruction. Plast Reconstr Surg 76:239–247, 1985

Carraway JH: Surgical anatomy of the eyelids. Clin Plast Surg 14:693, 1987

Furnas DW: Correction of prominent ears with multiple sutures. Clin Plast Surg 5:491, 1978

Jabaley ME, Clement RL, Orcutt TW: Myocutaneous flaps in lip reconstruction. Applications of the Karapandzic principle. Plast Reconstr Surg 59:680, 1977

May M: Facial nerve disorders. Update 1982. Am J Otol 4:77–88, 1982

McCarthy JG, et al: The median forehead flap revisited: The blood supply. Plast Reconstr Surg 76:866, 1985

McCord CD Jr: The evaluation and management of the patient with ptosis. Clin Plast Surg 15:169–184, 1988

McGregor IA: Reconstruction of the lower lip. Br J Plast Surg 36:40–47, 1983

Mustarde JC: Reconstruction of eyelids. Ann Plast Surg 11:149–169, 1983

Wells MD, Manktelow RT: Surgical management of facial palsy. Clin Plast Surg 17:645–655, 1990

CHAPTER 14

Aesthetic Facial Surgery

THE NOSE

A median septum divides the nasal cavity into two fossae, which extend from the anterior nares to the choanae, where they communicate with the nasopharynx. Each triangular fossa has an apex that provides the roof, composed of the nasal bones, the cribriform plate of the ethmoid, and the body of the sphenoid. The base or floor is formed by the palatal process of the maxilla and the horizontal plate of the palatal bone. The nasal septum forms the median wall and is represented by the perpendicular plate of the ethmoid, the vomer, and the septal cartilage, covered on each side by mucous membrane.

The nasal framework consists of an upper and lower part. The upper part is formed by the two nasal bones—the frontal processes of the maxillae and the lateral cartilages, which are firmly attached to the lower border of the bony skeleton and fuse in the midline with the dorsal border of the septal cartilage. The lower part consists of the alar cartilages, which are covered by the skin of the nasal tip and lined by the hairy skin of the vestibule. Each alar cartilage has a lateral and medial crus. The lateral crura provide the outline of the nostril, and the medial crura meet, in the midline in the intercrural angle or dome, at the level of the columella (Fig. 14–1).

Lateral to each nasal fossa are the lacrimal bone, the lateral mass of the ethmoid, the maxilla, the vertical plate of the palate, the inferior turbinate bone, and the medial pterygoid plate of the sphenoid.

FACIAL PROPORTIONS

The nose as the most prominent facial feature should normally harmonize with the rest of the face. The distance from glabella to columella should equal the distance between forehead and glabella, and from columella to chin.

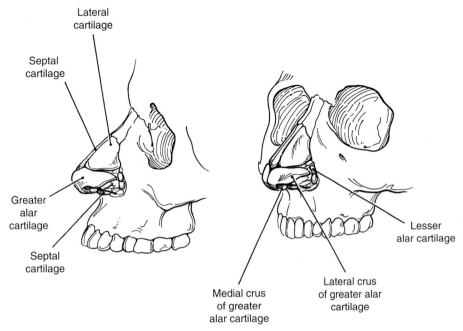

FIGURE 14–1. Anatomy of the nasal architecture.

During childhood the nasal septum is generally in the midline, but adults often have some asymmetry with lateral deflection. The deviation usually affects only the septal cartilage, being maximal where the ethmoid and vomer meet. If this deviation is excessive and affects the nasal airway, then submucous septal reconstruction may be indicated.

NASAL RECESSES

The anterior part of each nasal fossa, just above the opening of the nostril, is called the vestibule and is lined with skin that is continuous with that of the external integuments and contains numerous sebaceous glands and hair.

The nasal cavity is divided into three recesses by three turbinate bones, which are processes of the lateral mass of the ethmoid. These processes create the superior, middle, and inferior meatuses. The superior meatus is a short, narrow recess between the superior and middle turbinate bones into which open the posterior ethmoidal air cells. Above the superior turbinate bone is a small spheno-palatine recess into which drains the sphenoidal sinus. The middle meatus is situated between the middle and inferior turbinate bones. The frontal sinus, the maxillary sinus, and the middle ethmoidal air cells empty into the recess. The inferior meatus, situated between the inferior turbinate bone and the floor of the nasal fossa, receives the opening of the nasolacrimal duct.

Congenital Anomalies of the Nose

Absence of the nose is usually associated with absence of the nasal passages and sinuses. It results from failure of normal development of the embryologic nasal placode on either side of the frontonasal process above the stomodeum, with formation of nasal pits.

Cyclops: Presenting with a single midline orbital fossa, the nose either is absent or presents as a tubular structure attached above the central eye.

Ethmocephaly: Two closely set orbits with replacement of the nose by a proboscis with one or two nares.

Cebocephaly: Two closely set orbits with a normally situated but rudimentary nose with a single nasal cavity.

Bilateral proboscis: The external nose and nostrils are absent and replaced by two supraorbital proboscises.

Choanal atresia: If atresia is unilateral, nasal discharge and obstruction are present. Bilateral atresia causes neonatal respiratory distress requiring an oral airway, as babies are normally nose breathers.

Nasal meningoceles and encephaloceles.

Dermoid cysts and fistulae occur along the dorsal line of the nose.

Rhinoplasty

Plastic or reconstructive operations with the intent of altering the shape of the nose require an understanding of the abnormal anatomic component and a surgical plan to provide the patient with a well-proportioned, natural-looking nose. The alteration may be directed toward the upper and/or lower parts of the nose. Although general anesthesia may be used, more often local anesthesia is used. After blocking of the infratrochlear nerve at the glabella, the needle proceeds to infiltrate 1 per cent xylocaine with epinephrine along the walls of the nasal pyramid to the columella, alar bases, and anterior area of the nasal floor and septum. The infraorbital and anterior palatine nerves are similarly blocked, and the mucosa at the roof of the nasal cavities and alar cartilages is anesthetized. The nasal cavity is packed with cotton or gauze soaked in 4 per cent cocaine.

INCISIONS (Fig. 14–2)

The intercartilaginous incision: The incisions are made bilaterally in the outer wall of the vestibule between the lower border of the lateral cartilage and the upper border of the lateral crura of the alar cartilage. The two incisions meet at the membranous septum, where a transfixion incision through the septum is carried down to the nasal spine. This approach provides good access for

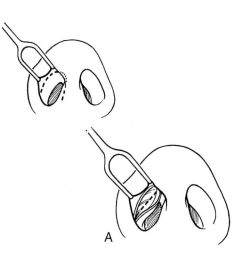

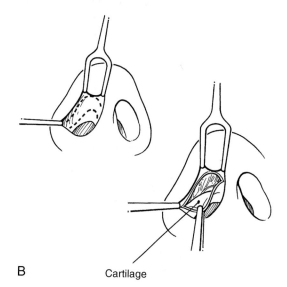

A   B   Cartilage

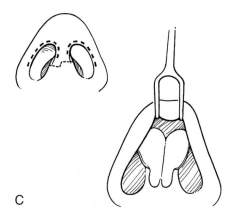

FIGURE 14–2. Incision to expose the nasal tip. *A,* Intracartilaginous incision at the level of the planned cartilage resection. *B,* Rim and intercartilaginous incisions, allowing delivery of the tip cartilages. *C,* Transcolumella incision connecting the rim incisions, providing exposure for the open rhinoplasty technique.

C

alteration of both the upper and lower parts of the nose, which can be undermined as far as the glabella with a periosteal elevator.

Intracartilaginous incision: The mucosal incision is made at the level at which the lateral crural cartilage is to be incised and resected. The incision is extended to the membranous septum to gain access to the nasal dorsum.

The rim incision: The incisions are placed inside the nostril rim along the margin of the tip cartilages. The tip cartilages may be "delivered" for sculpting.

Open rhinoplasty: The bilateral rim incisions are connected across the columella, and the skin is elevated off the underlying nasal skeleton, providing access to the nasal tip and dorsum. The correction of a bifid tip or suture revision of tip cartilages is facilitated by this approach. This technique provides a means of precise sculpting and suture alignment of the tip cartilages.

The central columellar incision: The midline columellar incision permits the introduction of bridge supports, including cartilage or bone grafts.

CORRECTIVE RHINOPLASTY

Proportionate reduction in the dimensions of a nose that is too large represents the most common objective of rhinoplasty. The entire operation consist of four interrelated procedures: (1) altering the shape of the nasal tip, (2) removing a nasal hump or lowering the bridge line, (3) shortening the nose, and (4) narrowing the bony skeleton.

The Tip. The shape and projection of the tip are determined by sculpting of the alar cartilages. Resection of the cephalic margin of the lateral crus of the alar cartilage should leave a minimum of 4 to 7 mm of cartilage (Fig. 14–3). Tip anatomy is further defined by scoring, incising, and suturing techniques as appropriate. Grafting of precisely sculpted septal and conchal cartilage is used as necessary (Fig. 14–4).

Bulbous Tip. These tips have a broad or boxy appearance due to an increased angle between the medial and lateral crura or a wide divergence between the two alar domes. Correction may include appropriate resection of the cephalic margins of the lateral crura, narrowing of interdomal distance with sutures and dome scoring, and incision or suture techniques to control the angle between medial and lateral crura.

Projecting Tip. Referred to as the "Pinocchio" deformity, it is corrected by

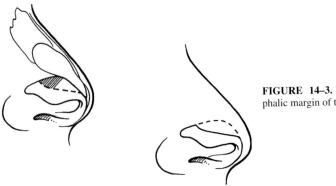

FIGURE 14–3. Resection of the cephalic margin of the lateral alar cartilage.

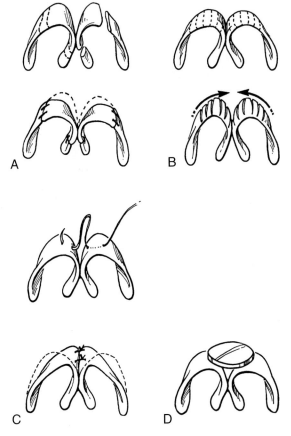

FIGURE 14-4. Techniques to change the appearance of the nasal tip. *A,* Resection of a wedge of lateral and medial crura to correct overprojecting tip. *B,* Scoring tip cartilages to decrease the angle between the inferior and lateral crura in a boxy tip. *C,* Suture technique to narrow the interdomal distance and increase tip projection. *D,* Onlay graft to increase tip projection.

a wedge excision of the lateral crura, medial crura, or both, with precise suture technique to realign the cartilages.

Inadequate Projection. Lack of tip projection is generally corrected with onlay conchal or septal cartilage grafts. Typically, cartilage is added to the dome area, to the junction of the columella and lobule as a shield-shaped graft, or between the medial crura as a columellar strut graft.

Removing the Nasal Hump. The upper part of the hump is osseous and the lower part is cartilaginous. The dorsal aspects of the upper lateral cartilages and of the septum are reduced by cutting the excess with straight scissors or a No. 11 blade. The osseous hump is reduced with a fine osteotome at the desired level and direction and removed, free of mucosa. Any residual irregularities of the resected edges of bone can be smoothed with a rasp.

The same technique is applied in lowering the bridge line in patients with the "Greek" or "Roman" nose by removing the segment of bone that extends upward to the glabella, fracturing it off at the nasofrontal junction and smoothing the nasal bones with a rasp.

Shortening the Nose. In shortening the nose, an aesthetic relationship of the columella, which is visible below the nostril margin, to the lobule, nostrils, and lips must be maintained. Resection of the caudal aspect of the septum and nasal spine affect cephalic tip rotation, tip projection, columella lip angle, upper lip length, and nasal length.

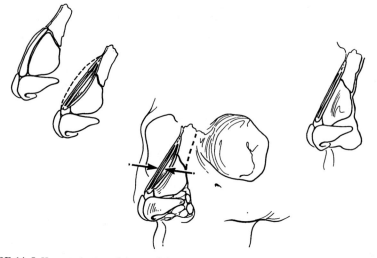

FIGURE 14–5. Hump reduction of the nasal dorsum. Lateral osteotomies narrow the widened dorsum that results from hump removal.

Narrowing the Bony Skeleton. Removal of the hump leaves the dorsum of the nose flat. The side walls of the nose need to be moved medially in order to correct this (Fig. 14–5). Correction requires a small incision in the outer vestibular wall over the lower part of the pyriform margin. A subperiosteal channel is created on the outer surface of the nasal process of the maxilla, where it merges with the cheek. An angled saw is introduced into the channel, and the nasal process is sawn through. Alternatively, a 2-mm osteotome is introduced through a stab wound in the skin over the nasal process of the maxilla and the osteotomy accomplished.

If a broad dorsum is to be narrowed without hump reduction, a medial osteotomy should be performed. The nasal bone is detached from the septum above the level of hump removal, and the side wall of the nose is levered outward with the osteotome. This "outfracture" results in a clean separation at the frontal suture line. This maneuver is repeated on the opposite side, and then the side walls of the nose are molded together by firm digital pressure that results in "infracture" and causes narrowing of the nose in the midline. Preliminary straightening of the bent nasal septum must be achieved to permit the replacement of the nose to the midline.

Septal Straightening. With the intent of restoring a normal nasal airway, good judgment must be used in deciding how much septal cartilage to remove. Excessive removal of septal cartilage may cause the bridge line to fall in, resulting in a saddle-nose deformity. Parts of the perpendicular plate, such as the ethmoid, vomer, or septal cartilage near the floor of the nose, can be removed in order to straighten a deviated nose without risk of a saddle-nose deformity.

Resection of septal cartilage near the dorsum does involve risk of deformation, and any problems in this area are best treated by cross-hatching and manipulation rather than excision. If the septum is straight but is deflected to one side by the nasal deviation, a submucous division of the vomer along the floor of the nose with an osteotome allows the whole septum to be moved.

Nasal Bridge Depression or Saddle-Nose Deformity

Children. A traumatic septal hematoma is the usual cause. Unless the hematoma is evacuated, secondary infection or atrophy of the septal cartilage results in gradual broadening of the bony bridge and a short nose because of failure of septal growth.

Treatment should be delayed until the nose is fully grown. After the nasal tip is improved, the broad nose is narrowed by making longitudinal saw cuts through each nasal bone close to its septal attachment, with removal of small bone segments. A corresponding segment of the medial border of each lateral cartilage is excised. Appropriate lateral osteotome cuts, outfracture, and infracture rearrange the nasal skeleton.

Elevation of the nasal bridge is accomplished by the placement of an implant through a central columellar incision. Our preference is irradiated cartilage, which may be replaced by a cancellous bone graft at maturity.

Adults. Saddle nose results from trauma or submucous resection of the septum. The broad bony bridge is often humped and deviated, with the saddle deformity below the bony skeleton. In the absence of a previous septal resection, nasal obstruction is a problem. The nose is best approached through an open rhinoplasty incision. After reconstructive rhinoplasty and required septal reconstruction, the saddle is corrected with septal or conchal cartilage in mild cases and bone graft in more severe cases (Fig. 14–6).

ILIAC CREST AUTOGRAFT. A 2-inch block of cancellous bone is removed from the iliac crest. Through a midline columellar incision, the skin of the dorsum and sides of the nose is undermined and the bed prepared for reception of the graft by raising the periosteum and rasping the nasal bridge. This is accomplished via the routine intercartilaginous rhinoplasty incision. The piece of bone is carved to reproduce a pattern previously prepared according to the degree of the deformity. The graft is tried and adapted with further trimming to provide the desired size, contour, and profile.

An L-shaped strut may be fashioned if associated columellar support is necessary. It is inserted through an external midcolumellar incision so as to be in contact with the nasal bones and the denuded nasal spine.

Alternatively, such a graft may be harvested from the seventh to eighth ribs as a cartilage autograft.

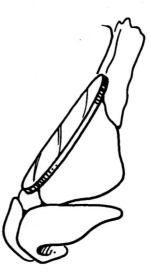

FIGURE 14–6. Onlay bone graft to correct a saddle deformity.

SPLIT CALVARIAL GRAFT. The outer table of the skull provides membranous cancellous bone with the advantage of a relatively pain-free donor site, with camouflage of the scar in patients with hair. Depending on the severity of the saddle deformity, two layers of split cranial graft may be required to achieve correction.

SECONDARY RHINOPLASTY

Secondary rhinoplasty may be necessary to improve an overoperated nose, an undercorrected nose, or a nose compromised by postoperative complications. The corrective procedure should be delayed for about 12 months to allow complete resolution of edema, softening of scar tissue, and optimal revascularization of all tissues. The deformities must be carefully evaluated and surgical correction well planned. The common problems noted after rhinoplasty include the following:

Supratip deformity (parrot beak): Insufficient removal of dorsal septum in the supratip area or excessive hump and tip resection may cause this deformity. Corrective techniques may be as simple as removal of excess supratip fullness or as complicated as onlay grafting of the nasal dorsum and tip. Precise evaluation and understanding of the anatomic deformity are essential.

Saddle and ski-jump deformities: Overresection of the septum may result in loss of dorsal support with a saddle deformity. Excessive resection of the nasal dorsum may also result in a saddle deformity or a nose shaped much like a ski jump. The deformities may be corrected with cartilage or bone grafts.

Tip deformities: Tip deformities may result from overresection of septal or tip cartilage with loss of tip projection, undercorrection of a projecting tip with persistent "Pinocchio" tip, and fibrosis and scar retraction of soft tissues or vestibular lining. The tip is approached through an open rhinoplasty and corrected by an appropriate refinement and grafting technique.

Alar and nostril deformity: Malposition or asymmetry of tip cartilage and scarring of vestibular lining may cause either alar or nostril deformity requiring repositioning of tip cartilage and placement of cartilage grafts for correction.

Overresection of upper lateral cartilage: This may cause a pinched cartilaginous dorsum with compromise of nasal valves and airway obstruction. Spreader cartilage grafts between the septum and upper lateral cartilage correct the problem.

RHYTIDECTOMY

Aging is a continuing dynamic process. Noticeable facial aging commences during the third decade and becomes overtly apparent during the fifth decade, when cutaneous and subcutaneous atrophy results in various degrees of facial wrinkling, ptosis, furrowing of the perilabial vertical lines, and changes in the texture of the skin. The extent and degree of the aging process, although chronologic and inexorable, depend on many other nontemporal factors. Heredity, endocrine function, environmental exposure, alcoholism, and smoking all affect the process. With progressive atrophy of the skin, fat, muscle, and bone, gravity leads to sagging of the integuments from areas of firmer attachment (Fig. 14–7).

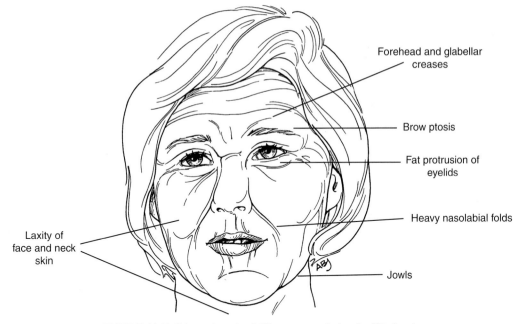

Forehead and glabellar creases

Brow ptosis

Fat protrusion of eyelids

Heavy nasolabial folds

Laxity of face and neck skin

Jowls

FIGURE 14–7. Skin ptosis and wrinkling apparent during the fifth decade.

Atrophy of the skin is reflected microscopically by reduction of elastic fibers and collagen as well as glycosaminoglycan ground substances. Flattening of the dermal-epidermal junction occurs, with reduction in the number of melanocytes and Langerhans cells.

In the individual patient, a thorough medical history and physical examination are essential, and any untoward abnormalities must be thoroughly controlled before the elective cosmetic operation is scheduled.

Local examination of the craniofacial region should document the extent of forehead wrinkles, glabellar vertical creases or corrugations, nasal root wrinkles, forehead-brow ptosis, elasticity, mobility, and caliber of facial skin, symmetry and contour of malar areas and nasolabial folds, and contour, fat deposit, and platysma anatomy of jawline and neck.

Anatomy

Skin and Subcutaneous Layer. Thickness of skin and subcutaneous tissues varies between individuals. Male skin is thicker owing to the beard's hair follicles. Hair patterns in the sideburn and postauricular hairline determine placement of incisions. Elevations of skin flaps must include a thin layer of subcutaneous tissue to preserve the subdermal plexus blood supply to the skin flaps.

Superficial Musculoaponeurotic System (SMAS). This layer runs deep to the subcutaneous tissue and above the parotid capsule. It is continuous with the platysma inferiorly and inserts on the zygoma superiorly, with attachments to the temporoparietal fascia. It becomes attenuated medially, where it blends into the facial muscle investing fascia. Proper handling of this layer is important in the final outcome of a face lift procedure.

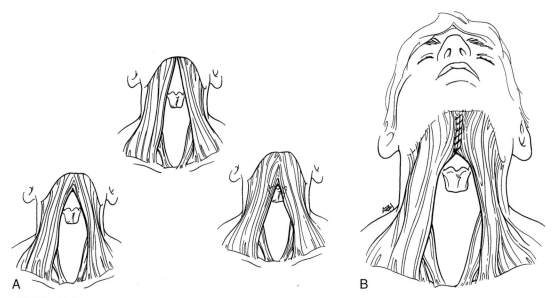

FIGURE 14–8. *A,* The three patterns of platysma insertion on the mandible. *B,* The neck deformity requires approximation of each half of the platysma from the level of the hyoid to the insertion of the mandible.

Platysma. This flat, thin muscle lies between the skin of the neck and the superficial layer of the cervical fascia. Superiorly it attaches to the mandible and overlying skin and becomes contiguous with the SMAS. It extends inferiorly to insert on the skin below the clavicle. The muscle orientation in the midline of the neck is an important factor in the changes that occur with aging. The muscle fibers may decussate from the mandible to the thyroid cartilage, forming a sling mechanism; decussate from the mandible to 2 or 3 cm inferiorly; or not decussate at all, each half inserting separately on the mandible (Fig. 14–8). Minimal decussation leads to more progressive changes, including prominence of submental fat and prominent medial platysmal bands (turkey gobble deformity).

Retaining Ligaments. A series of fascial and fibrous condensations form retaining ligaments that fix skin to the underlying or fascial skeleton. Attenuation of these condensations is at least partially responsible for the changes that occur with aging.

Facial Nerve. The frontal branch of the seventh nerve becomes vulnerable as it crosses the zygomatic arch to run within the temporoparietal fascia to the deep surface of the frontalis muscle. The marginal mandibular branch is also vulnerable in the face lift procedure as it runs along or below the inferior edge of the mandible immediately beneath the platysma muscle. The buccal branches are better protected by the parotid gland, although medially at the anterior border of the masseter muscle they lie immediately beneath the attenuated SMAS.

Anesthesia

Local anesthesia, using lidocaine or bupivicaine with epinephrine for its hemostatic effect, is supplemented by intravenous analgesia. Even if general endotracheal anesthesia is to be used, a local anesthetic agent is administered subcutaneously to permit local hemostasis and a lower plane of general anesthesia.

Technique

Rhytidectomy is directed at the correction or improvement of skin laxity, jowling, heavy nasolabial folds, submental and submandibular fat deposits, and platysma bands.

ELEVATION OF SKIN FLAPS

The patient should be in the supine, semisitting position with the head turned to the side. The planned incisions and the areas to be undermined should be marked on the skin before anesthesia is administered. The incision commences in the temporal scalp 5 cm behind the hairline and 5 cm above the ear. At the ear, it curves forward and then downward in the preauricular crease and is scalloped in front of the ear, then comes under the ear lobe into the postauricular region. The postauricular skin incision lies on the posterior surface of the concha, so that the ear covers the resultant scar, and is continued onto the mastoid area. The incision is extended with a gentle downward curve. Alternatively, if a large amount of neck skin is to be resected, the incision is extended down to and along the hairline, beveling the incision to preserve the hair follicles (Fig. 14–9).

The superficial subcutaneous tissue is then progressively undermined, commencing posteriorly with elevation of the postauricular skin and the skin that lies over the mastoid region. As the posterior scalp flap is elevated, the mastoid fascia, the sternomastoid muscle, and superficial to it the great auricular nerve are identified. The dissection continues and is superficial to the fascia over the muscle and the platysma. The cheek is then undermined anteriorly through the preauricular segment of the incision and continues down to the thyroid cartilage in the neck almost to the midline. The mandibular branch of the facial nerve, which lies deep to the platysma, should not be damaged if dissection is confined to the superficial subcutaneous layer. In the cheek, the undermining continues until the anterior border of the masseter is reached. In the temporal area, the undermining process continues along the plane of the temporal fascia so as to preserve the hair follicles. Anterior to the temporal hairline, however, the dissection may be subcutaneous.

The zygomatic arch region reveals some deep attachments between the superficial fascia and the arch, so dissection should be superficial in this area. The anterior branch of the temporal artery and its veins may be ligated and divided, and hemostasis is assured once the flaps are fully elevated.

ELEVATION OF THE SMAS

The SMAS of the face is continuous with the temporoparietal fascia above and the platysma below and provides the foundation for the overlying skin. The SMAS is connected to the dermis by multiple fibrous septa, and thus lifting and pulling the SMAS pulls the overlying skin to which it remains attached medially.

Usually the SMAS and lateral platysma are elevated and advanced as a single unit. If the flap is elevated to the zygomatic arch and lateral to the anterior border

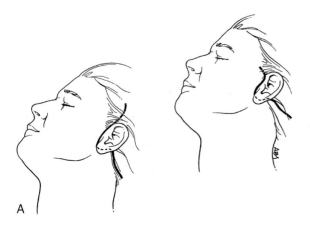

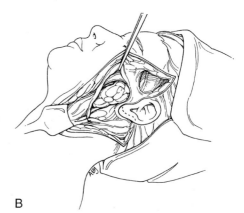

FIGURE 14–9. A, Incisions for a face lift. The anterior incision may extend into the temporal hairline or course beneath the sideburn. The posterior incision may be continued into the hair-bearing posterior scalp or extended down along the hairline. Elevation (B) and plication (C) of the subcutaneous musculoaponeurotic system.

of the masseter, the facial nerve is safe. The flap is plicated to the sternocleidomastoid fascia and parotid capsule, helping to recontour the cheeks, jawline, and neck (Fig. 14–9). The skin flap is pulled upward and backward, and several key anchoring sutures are placed at the posterior angle and at the upper pole of the ear. After redundant skin has been excised, linear closure of the incision is accomplished.

CORRECTION OF THE NECK

Advancement and plication of the skin flaps and SMAS–platysma flaps tighten the skin and significantly improve the cervicofacial angle. Attention must also be directed to the submental and submandibular fat, the lack of platysma decussation, and the platysma bands. Fat is removed by surgical defatting or suction lipectomy. A submental incision exposes the platysma, and hypertrophic bands are directly excised and the platysma plicated in the midline. The plication combined with the SMAS–platysma advancement laterally provides a sling tightening of the neck (Fig. 14–10).

SUBPERIOSTEAL FACE LIFT

Craniofacial techniques have been extended to facial rejuvenation procedures in recent years. Through a coronal and buccal sulcus incision, a subperiosteal

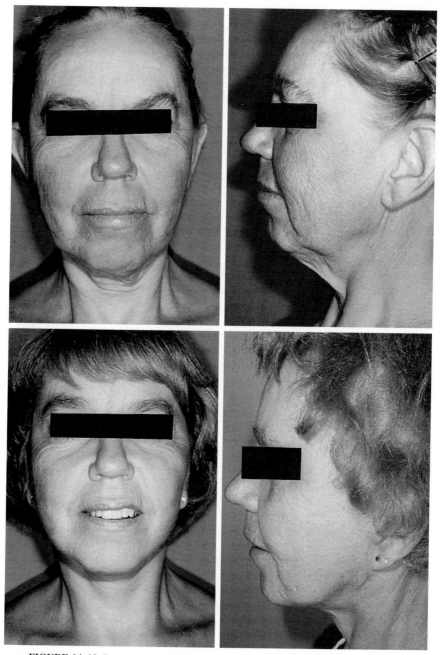

FIGURE 14–10. Preoperative *(top)* and postoperative *(bottom)* photographs of a face lift.

dissection elevates the midfacial soft tissues off the underlying maxilla and zygoma as far medially as the lateral nasal walls. Deep periosteal tacking sutures are used to plicate and suspend the facial soft tissues. Proponents believe that this deeper approach provides a better and longer-lasting correction of cheek jowls, nasolabial folds, and ptosis of the corner of the mouth.

Complications

Hematoma: Hematoma should be prevented by meticulous hemostasis. Firm facial dressings and ice compresses to the face reduce postoperative edema. The incidence of hematoma is twice as high in male as in female patients.

Skin loss: Excessive tension on wound closure, hematoma, and infection may lead to skin slough. Cigarette smoking predisposes to this complication.

Hair loss: Poorly planned incisions, failure to bevel the incisions away from hair follicles, too superficial a dissection plane, and excessive tension on wound closure may lead to significant alopecia.

Nerve injury: The greater auricular nerve is the most vulnerable. Injury results in numbness to the upper lateral neck and lower ear. Symptomatic seventh nerve injury most commonly involves the marginal mandibular branch, with loss or weakness of lip depressor function. Injury to the frontal branch leads to significant ptosis of the ipsilateral brow.

FOREHEAD-BROW LIFT

The forehead-brow lift is indicated for the correction of ptosis of the eyebrows, lateral hooding of the upper eyelids, forehead wrinkles, and glabella frown crease.

The forehead-brow lift may be carried out alone, in combination with a face lift, or in combination with a blepharoplasty. A forehead-brow lift should be done before an upper lid blepharoplasty because it reduces the amount of skin that must be removed in an upper lid blepharoplasty.

Coronal Brow Lift

Local anesthesia is established with lidocaine and epinephrine. A transcoronal incision extends from the superior aspect of the helix across the scalp to the opposite superior helix. If carried out in conjunction with a face lift, incisions are extended to meet with the preauricular face lift incision. The coronal incision runs above and parallel to the anterior hairline. The dissection continues to the periosteum, and a scalp and forehead flap is elevated off underlying periosteum (Fig. 14–11). The periosteum is incised several centimeters above the superior orbital rim, and dissection is continued in a subperiosteal plane to the supraorbital rim and root of the nose. The forehead flap is turned down over the face, and corrugator muscles are identified. If the patient has noticeable glabellar frown lines, the corrugator muscles are resected. If the patient has transverse frown lines, frontalis muscle function is reduced by removing interrupted strips of frontalis muscle, each about 1 cm in width. Care must be taken to avoid injury to the supraorbital nerve

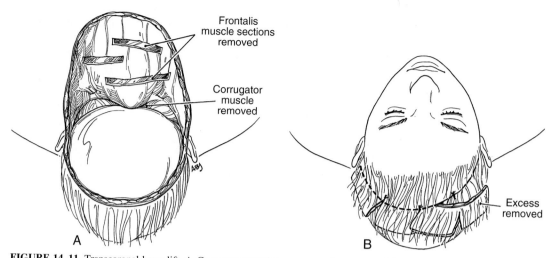

FIGURE 14–11. Transcoronal brow lift. *A,* Corrugator muscles are removed to correct glabella frown lines. Strips of frontalis muscle are removed to minimize forehead wrinkling. *B,* Brows are elevated to desired position with tacking sutures in the scalp, and excess scalp is resected.

centrally and the frontalis branch of the seventh nerve laterally. The forehead-scalp flap is then turned back, and measurements are made to determine the amount of scalp that must be resected in order to elevate the brows to a desired position. After securing several fixation points, the scalp flaps are trimmed accordingly and the wound is closed using polyglycolic acid suture for the galea layer and nylon or polypropylene suture for the skin.

Transcoronal brow lift elevates the anterior hairline. The forehead-brow lift can be done through an anterior hairline incision in patients who already have a high or receding anterior hairline.

Endoscopic Brow Lift

Increasing interest is being directed toward minimally invasive facial rejuvenation. Most of the experience has been with endoscopic brow lift, through limited stab incisions in the scalp. The scalp and forehead are elevated with endoscopic visualization, and corrugator and procerus muscles are resected with specialized instruments. The scalp is allowed to rotate posteriorly, where it is fixed with a lag screw or held in place with a circumferential dressing.

BLEPHAROPLASTY

Eyelid surgery may be carried out as an isolated operation, or it may be done in conjunction with a face lift or other procedures. It may be combined with a supraciliary brow lift for brow ptosis or hooding of the upper eyelid, or with a forehead lift for the wrinkles and glabellar frown of forehead ptosis. The brow lift procedures should be done before the upper lid procedure and the upper lid procedure before a lower lid blepharoplasty.

A preoperative assessment of visual acuity, extraocular muscle mobility, and tear production should be documented, with special note made of keratoconjunctivitis sicca (dry eye syndrome). Any abnormality merits an ophthalmologic opinion.

The Schirmer's test of tear production is done by placing a column of filter paper against the rim of the eyelid near the fornix for 5 minutes. The level of wetness on the filter strip is measured. Patients with dry eye syndrome are not good candidates for blepharoplasty unless they are prepared to use artificial tears and lubrication gel at night.

Patients complain of appearing tired. Lower lids have a baggy or puffy appearance and may be associated with fine wrinkling around the orbits. Upper lids are heavy with skin and have lost a defined supratarsal fold.

Upper Eyelid

Upper eyelid blepharoplasty is directed at removal of redundant eyelid skin and protruding orbital fat (Fig. 14–12). This should produce an upper lid with well-defined pretarsal skin and a supratarsal fold.

After determining the amount of excess skin to be excised from the upper lid, the lines are marked before either local or general anesthesia is administered. The inferior incision is placed 7 to 10 mm above the eyelid margin. The skin marked for excision is incised, dissected, and removed, exposing the underlying orbicularis oris muscle. A narrow strip of muscle is excised along the extent of the skin wound and the muscle edges retracted, exposing the orbital septum. The orbital fat pads are visible behind the septum. There are two fat compartments in the upper lid: The superior oblique muscle separates the medial and central fat compartments. The orbital septum is opened, and fat protruding through the separated septum in response to gentle pressure on the lower lid should be removed. The levator aponeurosis is clearly seen upon removal of the retroseptal fat. Hemostasis is established with electrocautery and the skin closed with a running subcuticular suture.

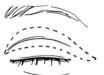

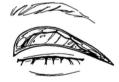

FIGURE 14–12. Elliptical skin excision for upper lid blepharoplasty.

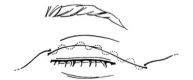

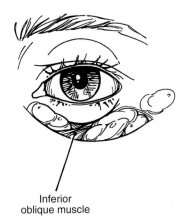

FIGURE 14–13. Fat compartments of the lower lid.

Inferior
oblique muscle

Lower Eyelid

Lower lid blepharoplasty is directed at removal of the bags or puffiness caused by fat protrusion and removal of excess skin. In evaluating the lower lid, it is important to determine lid tone and the risk of lower lid retraction or ectropion following blepharoplasty. Tone may be determined by the speed with which the lower lid returns to a normal position after being pulled down or away from its resting position on the globe.

Transconjunctival Blepharoplasty. This procedure is effective in patients with bags due to fat protrusion but no excess skin. A transconjunctival approach enables removal of fat without visible scar. Care must be taken to avoid injury to the inferior oblique muscle.

Transpalpebral Blepharoplasty. The lower lid is approached through an incision about 2 mm beneath the ciliary margin. The incision extends laterally into a skin crease. Either a skin flap or skin-muscle flap that includes underlying orbicularis oris muscle is elevated. The fat compartments lie beneath the orbital septum. Three fat compartments are found in the lower lid, with the inferior oblique muscle separating the medial and central compartments (Fig. 14–13). The lateral fat compartment is situated under the orbicularis insertion at the lateral canthal area, so the muscle should be pressed at this point to get proper identification of the lateral pocket. After the orbital septum is opened, bulging fat in each of the three compartments is removed and hemostasis established. The skin or skin-muscle flap is draped in a cephalad fashion, and redundant skin with a strip of orbicularis oris is removed (Fig. 14–14). The incision is closed with interrupted suture (Fig. 14–15).

Complications

Postoperative bleeding or hematoma: Re-exploration and evacuation of blood and coagulation of bleeding points are necessary.
Dry eye syndrome: A transitory dry eye syndrome, requiring lubrication with ophthalmic ointments and artificial tears, may occur following blepharoplasty.
Retrobulbar hematoma: A collection of blood behind the globe causes proptosis.

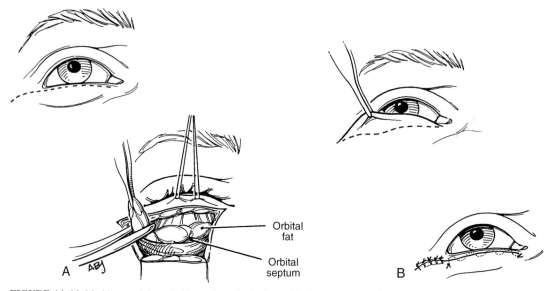

FIGURE 14–14. Markings and fat and skin excision in the lower blepharoplasty operation. *A,* A skin muscle flap is elevated through a subciliary incision. The orbital septum is opened and excess fat removed from the three fat pockets. *B,* Excess skin and a strip of orbicularis oris muscle is removed and the wound is closed.

The incisions must be reopened and any collection of blood evacuated. Ophthalmologic consultation is mandatory.

Upper eyelid ptosis: A true ptosis of the upper lid is indicative of injury to the levator muscle. If ptosis does not improve as the swelling resolves, the eyelid must be re-explored and the levator mechanism repaired.

Ectropion: Excess removal of lower lid skin may result in ectropion. A well-planned and executed procedure, however, may also result in scleral show or frank ectropion if poor lid tone is not recognized preoperatively. This complication can be avoided in eyelids with poor tone by suspension. Prior to closure of the blepharoplasty wound, the orbicularis oris muscle is transposed cephalad and laterally. A superolateral wedge is removed and the muscle sutured to the periosteum of the later orbital wall. This may also be done in conjunction with a tarsal excision at the lateral canthus. The tarsal plate is sutured to the remainder of the lateral canthal tendon, thus providing a lid suspension.

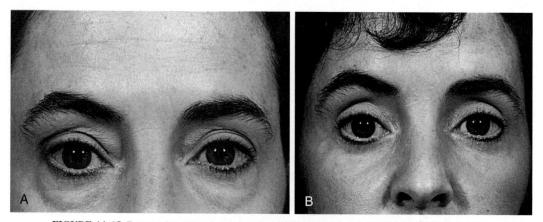

FIGURE 14–15. Preoperative *(A)* and postoperative *(B)* views of an upper and lower lid blepharoplasty.

ANCILLARY AESTHETIC PROCEDURES

MALAR REGION

Augmentation of the malar prominence may be achieved with synthetic implants at the time of rhytidectomy. An intraoral approach is preferred, but implants may also be placed via a subciliary lower lid blepharoplasty incision.

CHIN

Microgenia can be corrected by a chin implant. The ptotic appearance of the chin seen with aging (witch's chin) is corrected by direct excision of redundant submental skin and advancement of a de-epithelialized skin flap from the inferior wound. A chin implant may help the correction.

LIPS

Aging results in a longer upper lip, with loss of vermilion fullness and less exposure of the red vermilion. Loss of visible vermilion is corrected by skin excision above the mucocutaneous junction and advancement of vermilion. Lip fullness may be temporarily achieved by collagen or fat injection.

Liposuction

Liposuction is effective either as an adjunct to rhytidectomy or as an isolated procedure to recontour the submental region. A suction cannula is introduced through a submental stab incision, and redundant fat below the jawline is aspirated (Fig. 14–16). Suction is carried out in a plane between the platysma and overlying skin, leaving a thin layer of subcutaneous tissue attached to the dermis. The cheek fat pads and jowl areas are amenable to liposuction through the face lift incision or intranasal incisions. Poor patient selection or technique results in a sallow or hollowed appearance and the procedure is advisable only in carefully selected circumstances.

Collagen Injection

Bovine collagen has long been available as suture material and as a hemostatic agent. As a major protein component of connective tissue, bovine collagen adapted as a highly purified injectable substance has extended its use to soft tissue augmentation. Administered by injection via a fine-gauge needle, it can be used to correct small contour irregularities and wrinkles and to elevate small depressions to skin level.

Zyderm I, Zyderm II, and Zyplast are all varieties of collagen produced by Collagen Biomedical (Collagen Biomedical, Palo Alto, CA) with varying

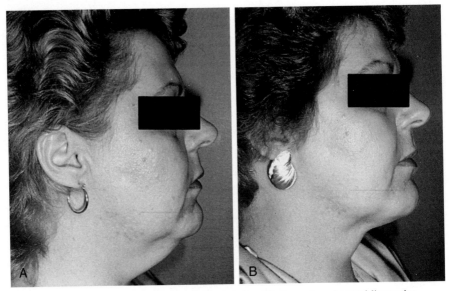

FIGURE 14–16. Preoperative *(A)* and postoperative *(B)* views of a submental liposuction.

concentrations of collagen per milliliter of solvent. Zyplast collagen is more rigid and has to be injected into the deep dermis or superficial lumps develop.

Collagen treatment should not be used in patients with a history of allergies or those who demonstrate a positive skin test to the material. In suitable cases, Zyderm or Zyplast can be used to touch up any residual lines after a face lift procedure, and they may have a place in the treatment of nasolabial and glabellar lines.

Chemical Face Peel

Fine facial wrinkles and superficial keratoses are amenable to correction by the application of some chemicals.

SUPERFICIAL PEELING AGENTS

Trans-retinoic Acid (Retin A). A retinoid or vitamin A compound, this substance is effective in the treatment of fine wrinkles and superficial keratoses. Available in strengths of 0.025, 0.05 and 0.1 per cent, daily topical application shows beneficial effects after 4 to 6 months of treatment.

Alpha-hydroxy Acids. Naturally occurring acids, including glycolic acid and lactic acid, are effective superficial peeling agents. They penetrate into the epidermis only, with minimal effect on dermal collagen.

Jessner's Solution. A mixture of resorcinol, lactic acid, salicylic acid, and ethanol, this solution is an efficient keratolytic agent. It is commonly used to prepare the skin for a deeper peel with trichloroacetic acid.

DEEP PEELING AGENTS

Trichloroacetic Acid. A derivative of acetic acid, this is used clinically in strengths of 10 to 50 per cent. Concentrations of less than 35 per cent produce a superficial peel, whereas deeper peels are achieved with stronger concentrations. Concentrations of 30 per cent or more cause a frosting of the skin within 15 seconds. The frosting subsides within several minutes, leaving the skin erythematous. Increased penetration is also achieved by pretreatment with a course of retin A or immediate preapplication of Jessner's solution.

Phenol. The phenol peel uses a mixture of phenol, liquid soap, croton oil, and water. It results in the deepest and most effective peel. The solution must be applied slowly and carefully to avoid cardiac arrhythmia. Careless application may cause full-thickness skin slough. Many patients experience a permanent hypopigmentation of peeled areas.

Dermabrasion

Dermabrasion, or surgical planing, is effective in correcting fine wrinkles and superficial keratoses as well as contour irregularities caused by acne or traumatic scars. It may be used as an alternative to chemical peel. As the skin is sanded down, wrinkles, pits, and depressed scars become shallower than the surrounding skin. The skin is abraded into the dermis, retaining sufficient dermis to enable re-epithelialization. Results are permanent because the dermis never attains it preabrasion thickness.

Laser Resurfacing

The short pulsed high-energy CO_2 laser is proving effective in facial resurfacing and rejuvenation procedures. The laser removes the skin's keratin layer and induces a tightening effect with minimal thermal injury. Laser resurfacing smooths skin wrinkles and removes superficial lesions. The initial technology used a 3-mm collimated beam, but newer methods treat up to a 2.25 sq cm area with each pulse. The technology is in its infancy and will prove an important adjunct in facial rejuvenation.

HAIR REPLACEMENT

Baldness or alopecia, the result of hair loss, may be frontal, frontoparietal, or frontoparieto-occipital.

Each hair follicle has a life span of its own, but the band of hair around the temporal and occipital region usually survives for the patient's lifetime. Hair transplanted from this area to the area of baldness survives for the rest of the patient's life and continues to grow at the normal rate of 0.5 inch per month as an expression of donor dominance.

The role of cosmetic surgery in providing dynamic hair replacement has become increasingly important in social and economic settings, where the illusion of youthfulness and the significance of an aesthetic appearance are matters of great concern.

Those patients whose total baldness is associated with fine silky hair in the temporo-occipital area are not good candidates for hair transplants and may be best served by a well-constructed hair piece or weave. No matter what technique of hair replacement is used, the planned and proper reconstruction of a new frontal hairline is of paramount importance.

Dynamic hair replacement can be performed surgically by several techniques.

Free Composite Grafts Transplanted as Multiple Punch Grafts or as Strips

Punch Grafts. Using skin biopsy punches, an office or outpatient procedure is performed under local anesthesia. Multiple 4-mm grafts are most commonly obtained from the scalp, as small punches are associated with a higher follicle survival rate and less scarring at both donor and recipient sites. With proper spacing, a total of four sessions may be necessary for placement of several hundred plugs.

A punch graft instrument that is 1 mm smaller is used for the removal of bald plugs from the recipient site, as the donor grafts contract slightly after placing them on a saline sponge and in a sterile container and the recipient sites expand slightly. Any bleeding areas can be controlled by pressure with a cotton applicator soaked in weak epinephrine. The grafts are inserted into the deep recipient sites and covered with nonadherent gauze and a pressure dressing.

Strip Grafts. These consist of long composite segments of hair-bearing skin and subcutaneous tissue 5 to 8 mm wide, harvested from the parieto-occipital area of the scalp for reconstruction of a new frontal hairline. After removal of excess fascia and fatty tissue, the donor area is prepared and incised down through the galea and the strip graft is placed in position, with the hair follicles pointing anteriorly, and sutured with continuous 6-0 polypropylene.

Strip grafts with a running W margin can be harvested using a special instrument, whereas the use of hexahedral or square scalp grafts may produce more hair than a circular graft.

Micrografts. Micrografts are used to establish the final anterior hairline after optimal density has been established by other techniques. Minigrafts of 3 to 4 mm are divided into sections, each containing three to four follicles. These sections are then de-epithelialized, a stab incision is made in the recipient site, and the micrograft is inserted.

Scalp Reduction

Patients with localized occipital baldness are ideal candidates for direct excision and primary closure of the area of alopecia. Midline elliptical excision results in improvement, but rewidening of the scar typically compromises the final outcome. Excellent results may be achieved by a unilateral S-shaped excision along the inner margin of the fringe or a bilateral U-shaped excision along the entire fringe (Fig. 14–17). The wound is allowed to relax over 3 months, and reduction is repeated as necessary until the bald scalp is excised. Hair transplants correct frontal alopecia once scalp reductions are completed.

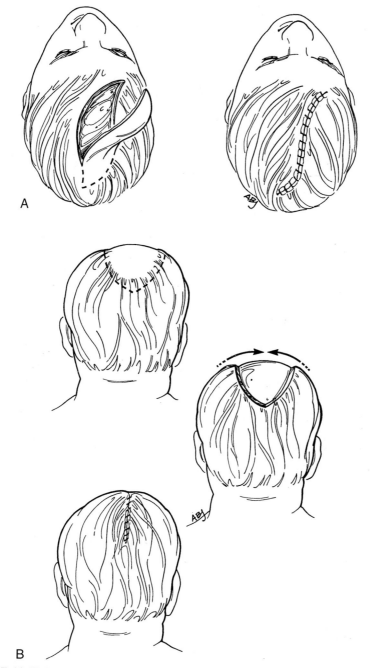

FIGURE 14–17. Patterns of scalp reduction for correction of male pattern baldness. *A*, S-shaped excision. *B*, U-shaped excision.

Scalp Flaps

Local pedicle flaps provide immediate correction of an area of baldness because flaps, unlike grafts, do not temporarily lose their hair. The area of baldness to be corrected is excised and the flap transposed into the defect. The donor site is undermined and closed and the flap inset. Flaps available for correction of baldness include the following:

Temporo-parietal-occipital flap (Juri flap) (Fig. 14–18): A long flap based on branches of the superficial temporal vessels, this is used to reconstruct the entire frontal hairline. Hair must be styled to camouflage the posterior direction of hair growth on the transposed flap.

Lateral scalp flap (Fig. 14–19): A 2.5- to 3-cm-wide flap based anteriorly is raised for a length of 12 to 16 cm and used to reconstruct half the anterior hairline. The second half is reconstructed with a flap from the other side 8 to 12 weeks later.

Temporal vertical flap: A vertical flap based on the parietal scalp extends anterior or posterior to the ear. Its advantage over other flap reconstructions of the anterior hairline is the normal anterior direction of hair growth on the transposed flap.

Occipitoparietal flap: Based on the occipital vessels, this flap corrects high occipital alopecia.

Scalp Expansion

Tissue expanders are placed beneath hair-bearing scalp and inflated over an 8- to 10-week period. Although the density of hair in the expanded scalp is reduced by the stretching that takes place, the increased surface area of hair-bearing tissue more than compensates. The augmented hair-bearing scalp is readily advanced following excision of bald areas. Expansion of traditional flaps also provides wide

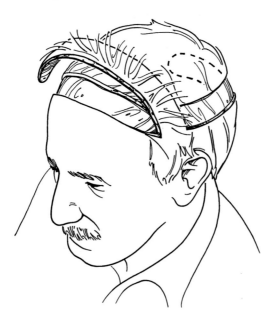

FIGURE 14–18. Temporoparietal scalp flap for correction of male pattern baldness.

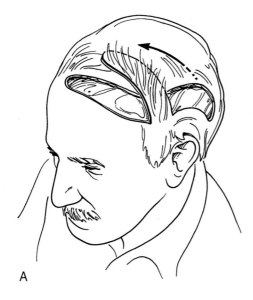

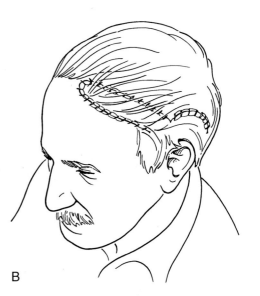

FIGURE 14–19. *A, B,* Lateral scalp flap for correction of male pattern baldness. *C,* The second flap is transferred 8 to 12 weeks later.

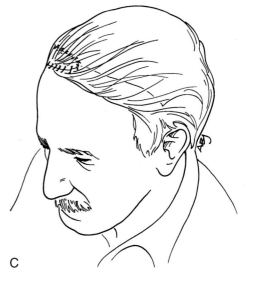

flaps available to resurface larger areas of frontal baldness, with greater ease in closure of the donor defect.

Suggested Reading

Conway H: The surgical face lift–rhytidectomy. Plast Reconstr Surg 45:124, 1970

Daniel RK, Lessard M-L: Rhinoplasty: A graded aesthetic-anatomical approach. Ann Plast Surg 13:436, 1984

Hamra ST: The deep-plane rhytidectomy. Plast Reconstr Surg 86:53, 1990

Juri J, Juri C: Aesthetic aspects of reconstructive scalp surgery. Clin Plast Surg 8:243–254, 1981

Peck GC: Basic primary rhinoplasty. Clin Plast Surg 15:15, 1988

Ramirez OM: The subperiosteal approach for the correction of the deep nasolabial fold and the central third of the face. Clin Plast Surg 22:341, 1995

Sheen JH: Secondary rhinoplasty. Plast Reconstr Surg 56:137, 1975

CHAPTER 15

Breast and Chest Wall: Breast and Developmental Chest Wall Pathology

THE BREAST

Development of the Mammary Gland

During embryonic life, an ectodermal ridge appears on each side of the body and extends from axilla to groin. Normally the whole of this ridge atrophies except for a small portion in each pectoral area from which the mammary glands arise. Failure of disappearance of all of this ridge may result in the development of accessory breasts (polymastia) or accessory nipples (polythelia) along this line. The portion of the mammary ridge that develops into breast enlarges and branches to form slender ductules from which the secreting breast tissue is formed. At puberty, pituitary gonadotrophins foster the ovarian secretion of estrogen and progesterone and stimulate the budding of these ducts with the development of secreting acinar tissue.

Abnormalities of development that may require surgical reconstruction include the following:

1. Ectopic breast tissue
2. Abnormalities of size
   a. Macromastia
   b. Undeveloped or small breasts
   c. Amastia
3. Abnormalities of shape
   a. Tuberous breast deformity
   b. Congenitally inverted nipple

Ectopic Breast Tissue

Accessory breast tissue may develop anywhere along the mammary ridge but is most common in the axilla or inframammary fold. Polythelia or accessory nipple areolar tissue is usually seen below the normal nipples and is corrected by a simple excision. Polymastia or ectopic glandular tissue should be removed for aesthetic reasons and also to avoid breast cancer in these redundant tissues, which can occur just as in normal breasts.

Abnormalities of Size

MACROMASTIA

Breast enlargement may be a consequence either of a normal physiologic state with simple overdevelopment or of an end-organ sensitivity to normal circulating hormones. This latter phenomenon may result in very large breast overgrowth in pubertal and adolescent girls and is termed virginal hypertrophy. When breast size is excessive, it can contribute to progressive musculoskeletal discomfort in the neck and shoulders.

Reduction mammoplasty, originally based on the Biesenberger "inverted T" technique, evolved into the Wise pattern of skin excision used in today's procedures. Strombeck popularized a transverse double pedicle to carry the nipple-areola complex, whereas McKissock transposed the nipple on a vertically oriented dermoglandular bipedicled flap folded on itself. This has since been modified to an inferiorly based pedicle, which enables the safe transfer of a well-vascularized, sensate nipple-areola complex.

Keyhole Pattern (Fig. 15–1). The skin excision for most modern reduction mammoplasty procedures uses the keyhole pattern. Markings are made with the patient in a sitting or standing position. The central breast meridian is established by dropping a line from the midclavicle to the nipple. The inframammary line is marked, the level is measured, and the level is transposed to the anterior surface of the breast and marked on the meridian line. The exact nipple location is established relative to this marking. Usually the nipple location is marked at that position, or about 1 cm lower in heavy pendulous breasts. From the midpoint of the nipple site, two lines are drawn downward, tangential to the areola. A template with a diameter of 3.5 to 4 cm is positioned with its center over the chosen nipple and opened to the spread of these lines. The new areolar window is marked. A distance of 5 cm from the junction of the areolar and diverging line (a and a') is measured and marked (b and b'). From these points lines are drawn medially and laterally to meet the ends of a marking along the inframammary line. This defines the width of the medial and lateral skin flaps and the distance from the lower edge of the areola to the postoperative inframammary line. The identical symmetric lines of markings are then placed on the second breast.

Inferior Pedicle Technique. These markings are usually done with the patient asleep and in a supine position. The inferior pedicle is marked with a base of about 10 cm. The pedicle is de-epithelialized and elevated, leaving the flap attached to the chest wall with a 5-cm-thick base (Fig. 15–2). The medial, lateral, and central flaps of skin and breast tissue are elevated to the prepectoral fascia. All tissue between the inferior pedicle and breast flaps is removed. The breast flaps are draped over the inferior pedicle carrying the nipple-areola complex, and the wounds are sutured with an absorbable dermal stitch and a subcuticular skin stitch.

Free Nipple Graft Technique. Extremely large breasts, requiring resection of 2000 gm or more of breast tissue and an unusually long pedicle, may be

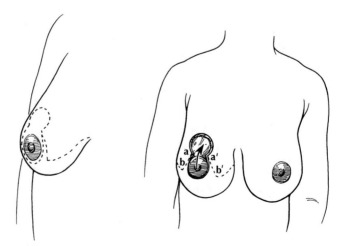

FIGURE 15–1. Markings of the keyhole pattern for breast reduction.

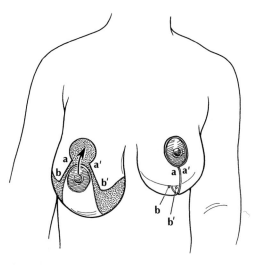

FIGURE 15–2. Inferior pedicle carrying the nipple cephalad in the breast reduction operation.

managed by the free nipple graft technique. The keyhole pattern is marked and breast flaps are elevated without preservation of the nipple-areola complex carrying a pedicle. The nipple-areola tissue is removed from the resected specimen and defatted. The new site for placement of the nipple and areola is de-epithelialized and the nipple-areola complex is replaced as a full-thickness graft.

Complications of reduction mammoplasty include the following:

Infection and hematoma: These may be minimized with meticulous surgical techniques.

Necrosis of skin flaps: This is usually limited to the T junction of the wound closure; it is seen more commonly in heavy smokers. Wounds are managed with dressing changes and allowed to heal secondarily.

Fat necrosis: This is caused by localized areas of ischemia; the breast may develop hard lumps that resolve over several months.

Nipple-areola loss: A small percentage of patients may experience nipple-areola slough, especially if the pedicle carrying the nipple is longer than 30 cm. Care must be taken not to undermine the pedicle and to avoid tension at closure. Irreversible ischemia is managed intraoperatively by removal and defatting of the nipple-areola complex and replacement as a full-thickness skin graft.

Loss of nipple sensation: Nipple sensation may be reduced postoperatively; normal sensation usually returns over several months, although permanent numbness may result from injury to the lateral cutaneous nerves.

HYPOMASTIA

The body image of mature women may be related to the perception of norms pertaining to breast size. Placement of an implant aesthetically augments the breast, although the procedure is currently embroiled in controversy related to the safety of implanting silicone devices. Currently, two types of implantable breast prostheses are available: (1) silicone shell filled with silicone gel, and (2) silicone shell filled with normal saline. The silicone shell may have either a smooth or a textured wall.

At this writing the long-term safety of a silicone gel fill is being debated in the

United States, and gel-filled protheses are not available for cosmetic augmentation mammoplasty. The FDA does allow the use of silicone shell filled with normal saline for cosmetic augmentation. Either device may be used for both acquired and congenital breast deformities.

Capsular contracture is the single greatest obstacle to a successful outcome for augmentation mammoplasty. Capsular contractures result from the periprosthetic scar tissue contracting with sufficient force to distort the implant, and in extreme cases it causes a hard and painful breast. This phenomenon has been reported to occur in 20 per cent of patients undergoing breast implants, although only a small percentage have sufficient capsular contracture to create an aesthetically compromising situation. The cause is not well understood. Whether the textured shells have a lower long-term incidence of capsular contraction than the smooth shell implants is currently being debated.

The procedure may be carried out through one of three incisions (Fig. 15–3): inframammary incision, periareolar incision, and transaxillary incision. Whichever incision is used, the subcutaneous tissues are dissected down to the layer selected for implant placement. The implant may be placed in either the submammary or the subpectoral tissue layer. If the implant is to be placed above the muscle, the dissection is carried out on top of the prepectoral fascia. If a subpectoral pocket is to be used, the pectoralis muscle is elevated at the free margin and the dissection is carried out on top of the rib perichondrium in the lower aspect of the dissection and above the pectoralis minor in the upper portion. The inferior origin of the pectoralis major is taken down, with careful control of the perforating intercostal vessels. The origin must be freed to prevent a restricting band that can displace the implant in a superior or lateral direction.

Whether to place the implant subpectorally or above the pectoralis muscle also remains somewhat controversial. Some believe that placement of the implant below the muscle minimizes the risk of capsular contracture. Others believe that it makes little difference and prefer the subglandular approach because of the ease of dissection under local anesthesia.

Complications of augmentation mammoplasty include the following:

Hematoma

Infection requiring removal of implant. Both of these complications should be preventable by a good technique with meticulous hemostasis. Loss of the implant due to one of these complications is very uncommon.

Capsular contracture: Capsular contracture is classified by grade as defined by Baker:

Grade 1: Breast feels as soft as an unoperated breast.

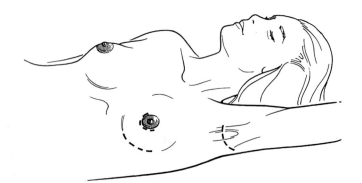

FIGURE 15–3. Incisions used for placement of the implant in breast augmentation.

Grade 2: Mild firmness is detectable but not visible.

Grade 3: Moderate firmness can be easily palpated and some distortion is noted visually.

Grade 4: A hard, painful breast shows marked distortion visually.

Capsular contractures around submammary implants could previously be broken with closed manipulation, but this practice is now discouraged for fear of rupturing the implant. If capsular contraction is symptomatic or distorts the breast, it may require an open approach and surgical freeing of the contracting scar tissue.

Connective tissue disorder: There have been concerns that silicone may stimulate an autoimmune response in some patients. Silicone implants have been implicated in scleroderma and rheumatoid-like illnesses, although no corroborating scientific evidence is available at this time.

Obscuring of mammograms: There does seem to be some risk of obscuring normal gland tissue on mammographic studies of the breast. This raises the possibility of an occult carcinoma being missed, with a delayed diagnosis of breast cancer. The problem is minimized by obtaining a three-view study—craniocaudal, mediolateral, and axillary oblique.

Leak or rupture of the device

AMASTIA AND ATHELIA

Absence of the nipple (athelia) as an isolated deformity is rare, usually being associated with absence of the underlying breast (amastia). If the sternal pectoralis major muscle is absent, the patient has Poland syndrome.

If a patient presents prior to full development of the contralateral breast, a tissue expander is placed and expanded at a rate to maintain symmetry with the developing breast. Once breast growth stabilizes, the expander is removed and replaced with a permanent breast implant. Nipple-areola reconstruction is delayed until reconstruction of the breast mound is completed.

Abnormalities of Shape

TUBEROUS BREAST DEFORMITY

Tuberous breast deformity may be unilateral or bilateral. The breast has a tuberous shape characterized by a constricted base with the appearance of herniation of breast tissue immediately beneath the areola. The breasts are small and asymmetric with a large nipple-areola complex (Fig. 15–4).

Surgery is directed at release of the constricted base, enlargement of size, and reduction of the large areolar circumference

The tuberous breasts are dissected off the underlying pectoralis major fascia, and radial incisions are made through the entire thickness of the breast tissue. This enables the base to expand. An implant is then placed in either a prepectoral or subpectoral pocket. If the patient is a developing adolescent, a tissue expander is inserted, with plans to place the permanent implant once full breast development has occurred. The areola can be reduced at the initial procedure or at a second procedure.

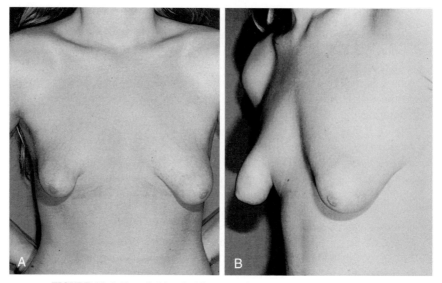

FIGURE 15–4. Frontal *(A)* and oblique *(B)* views of tuberous breast deformity.

INVERTED NIPPLE

The nipple is tethered and inverted by the pull of underlying ducts. There is also a deficiency of fibrous connective tissue bulk beneath the nipple. Correction requires severing of the underlying ducts. The erected nipple's new position may be maintained by circumferential sutures or local flaps of breast tissue to provide bulk below the nipple. A suction cup device applied over the nipple may be effective in everting the nipple without the need for surgical intervention. These devices are available in Europe.

Breast Ptosis

Ptosis of the breast refers to a sagging and hanging of the breast. The degree of ptosis is best defined by the position of the nipple-areola complex and breast relative to the inframammary fold as described by Regnault (Fig. 15–5):

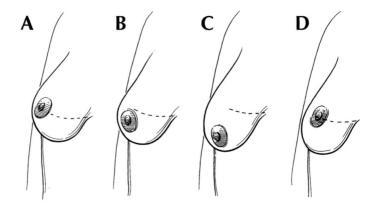

FIGURE 15–5. Degrees of breast ptosis. *A,* Minor. *B,* Moderate. *C,* Severe. *D,* Pseudoptosis.

Minor ptosis: The nipple lies at the level of the inframammary fold.

Moderate ptosis: The nipple lies below the fold but higher than the lower part of the breast.

Severe ptosis: The nipple lies well below the fold, pointing downward.

Pseudoptosis: Also referred to as glandular ptosis; the nipple lies at the level of the fold but the inferior breast quadrants have descended below the level of the inframammary fold.

Mild ptosis of the breast may be corrected by placement of a mammary implant, avoiding the scars inherent in formal mastopexy operations. For moderate and severe ptosis, mastopexy is directed at removal of excess skin, lifting the breast tissue in a cephalad direction, and repositioning the nipple-areola complex above the inframammary fold. Augmentation with an implant may be done in conjunction with mastopexy to increase breast volume if desired. Many procedures have been described to correct breast ptosis, most resulting in a scar around the circumference of the areola and extending into the subareolar breast skin.

Benign Lesions

PREPUBERTAL

Breast masses in children are almost always benign, and biopsy is avoided if possible for fear of creating a disturbance in breast development.

Juvenile thelarche: Prepubertal males and females may develop a firm, 1- to 3-cm nodular mass beneath the nipple-areola complex. The mass may be tender and resolves over a 12- to 24-month period. It is thought to result from hormonal stimulation of a hypersensitive end organ.

Neurofibroma: These lesions may involve the nipple-areola complex, either as solitary lesions or as part of a neurofibromatosis. If a lesion must be excised because of rapid growth, great care must be taken not to resect or injure the underlying breast anlage from which the breast will develop.

Hemangioma: These lesions usually resolve by 6 to 7 years of age and do not require intervention; surgical contouring or scar revision is usually delayed until the breast is fully developed.

Lymphangioma: Lymphangiomata usually do not resolve spontaneously and require surgical management at some time. If the lesion is not troublesome, resection may be delayed until breast development is complete. If earlier intervention is required, partial resection is preferable to complete excision if the breast anlage is involved.

PUBERTAL

Juvenile fibroadenoma: Seen in young women between puberty and 20 years of age, the neoplasm is smooth, lobulated, and encapsulated and may become very large and be confused with virginal hypertrophy. It may occur after the administration of oral contraceptives. Histologic examination reveals a normal, dense, cellular stroma.

Juvenile fibroadenomas are ideally removed through a periareolar incision without injuring normal breast tissue. Large lesions may leave redundant skin, which usually recontours with time. Scar-producing skin excisions should be avoided or dealt with at secondary operations.

Virginal hypertrophy: An end-organ sensitivity to circulating hormone may cause rapid unilateral or bilateral breast growth at puberty or within several years. Stromal hypertrophy may result in significant enlargement with associated social and psychological problems. In these instances, surgery should not be delayed, realizing that breast hypertrophy could recur, requiring repeat intervention. Most patients do well with reduction mammoplasty by the inferior pedicle technique. In rare instances, recurrent virginal hypertrophy may require simple mastectomy with breast and nipple-areola reconstruction.

Gynecomastia: Gynecomastia begins during puberty. The cause is uncertain but is probably due to end-organ receptor sensitivity to circulating hormones. Histologic changes include hypervascularity, fibroblast proliferation, collagen deposition, and connective tissue hyalinization in the breast stroma. The majority of cases are idiopathic, but gynecomastia may be associated with a host of conditions causing hormonal abnormalities, including endocrine-secreting tumors of the testes, adrenal hyperplasia, hypogonadism, Klinefelter syndrome, and liver disease. Use of phenothiazines, digitalis, methyldopa, and spironolactone may cause breast enlargement.

Most cases of gynecomastia resolve spontaneously in 2 to 3 years, but some may persist and require surgery. Once endocrine or drug-induced gynecomastia is excluded, the breast tissue can be removed through a periareolar incision. A core of breast tissue must be left beneath the areola to ensure its blood supply. The margins of the excision are carefully tapered to avoid contour depressions, and suction lipectomy may be helpful in feathering the edges and thinning the chest flap in fatter patients. Redundant skin usually contracts with time, although patients with marked breast enlargement and skin redundancy may require excision of breast skin.

ADULT

Cysts: Breast cysts are common lesions that tend to vary in size with the menstrual cycle. They are epithelium lined, are filled with fluid, and may be single or multiple. They present as a tender or nontender, firm, distinct mass on palpation. Ultrasonography determines if a palpable mass or a lesion noted on mammography is solid or filled with fluid. Large or painful cysts are aspirated. If a residual mass remains after aspiration, bloody aspirate, or abnormal cytology, a breast biopsy must be done.

Fibroadenoma: This is a firm, rubbery lesion most commonly occurring in the second or early in the third decade. It has well-defined, smooth borders on palpation, which differentiates it from carcinoma. It tends to grow slowly and should be managed by excisional biopsy.

Ductal papilloma: These lesions may be solitary or multiple. They present with an abnormal nipple secretion, which is often blood tinged. Occasionally a small nodule is palpable beneath the areola, but in most cases a palpable lesion is not apparent. Palpation of the areola determines from which area the nipple secretion is coming. This area with its ductal system is resected by wedge excision.

Fat necrosis: These lesions are hard and irregular, may have overlying skin dimpling and stippled calcification on mammography, and may or may not be tender. Occasionally there is an antecedent history of trauma, although the majority of patients give no such history. Excisional biopsy is usually necessary to exclude a diagnosis of breast cancer.

Mondor's disease (thrombophlebitis): This presents with tenderness and thrombosis of one or more superficial veins of the breast.

Breast abscess: Infections are most common in lactating breasts within a month or so following delivery. Mastitis is treated conservatively with hot packs and antibiotics. A breast abscess, due either to progression of mastitis or to obstruction of a duct, manifests as a firm, indurated mass with surrounding redness. It is exquisitely tender and is managed by incision and drainage and antibiotics.

Fibrocystic mastopathy: A common affliction of the breast, this process is also referred to as cystic lobular hyperplasia, or fibrocystic disease. It is thought to be a consequence of cyclic changes secondary to circulating ovarian hormones. The incidence increases with reproductive age and manifests with breast lumps and pain. The lumps are usually cystic lesions whose development, regression, and redevelopment relate to the menstrual cycle. There may be an associated clear nipple discharge at times. Large or painful cysts should be aspirated. If the discharge is bloody or if a palpable mass remains after aspiration, excisional biopsy is necessary to exclude carcinoma.

Histologic patterns seen on breast biopsy include glandular hyperplasia; micro- and macro-cyst formation; stromal and periductal fibrosis; sclerosing adenosis—seen in younger women; there is a dense fibrosis with distortion of breast lobules and cellular elements. Sometimes difficult to differentiate from a carcinoma on frozen biopsy section, it is an entirely benign process; and epithelial metaplasia and hyperplasia—epithelial hyperplasia in cyst and duct walls may fill the lumen with a cellular papillary growth.

Fibrocystic mastopathy is a benign disease that does not evolve into breast cancer. A patient with concomitant epithelial hyperplasia with atypia or carcinoma in situ is at increased risk for breast cancer. These patients require close follow-up with physical examination and mammography so that new lesions are identified and biopsied immediately. Patients who have had multiple biopsies, have breasts that are difficult to evaluate by physical examination or mammography, and are excessively anxious about their increased risk of breast cancer may, in carefully selected circumstances, be candidates for subcutaneous or simple mastectomy.

Simple Mastectomy

The entire breast with attached nipple-areola complex is removed using a transverse incision. If the patient so desires, a breast implant or tissue expander is placed submuscularly. The nipple-areola complex may be defatted and replaced as a free graft, or a nipple reconstruction may be accomplished at a later time.

Subcutaneous Mastectomy

Subcutaneous mastectomy is directed at removal of the breast tissue with preservation of the nipple-areola complex. It is ideally done through an inframammary incision but, in large ptotic breasts, may require a keyhole pattern of skin excision so that a pexy of the nipple-areola complex may be accomplished. Preservation of a viable nipple-areola complex requires that a button of breast tissue be left attached to the areola. The breast is reconstructed by placement of a submuscular implant or tissue expander at the time of mastectomy. If a tissue expander is used, a permanent implant is placed at a second procedure following tissue expansion. These patients require continued follow-up by physical examination and mammography because breast tissue remains.

Breast Cancer

Cancer of the breast is the most common malignancy in women living in the United States. The incidence is increasing, and the risk of developing breast cancer is estimated to be about 10 per cent over an 80-year life span. More than 45,000 women die each year, although 5-year survival has improved to about 77 per cent because of earlier detection and better medical management.

A carcinoma of the breast may be noninfiltrative, in which case it is a carcinoma in situ, or infiltrative, termed an invasive tumor.

HISTOLOGIC TYPES OF CANCER

Paget's disease of the nipple: This first becomes apparent as a reddish, weeping lesion involving the nipple. Generally a palpable mass develops beneath the nipple-areola complex if the lesion is allowed to progress.

Ductal carcinoma: Scirrhous adenocarcinoma, the most common type of breast cancer, is infiltrative with pronounced desmoplasia and fibrosis. Diffuse lymphatic spread often occurs within the breast. Papillary carcinoma, a slower growing tumor, metastasizes later to regional nodes than does scirrhous adenocarcinoma. Comedocarcinoma has an obvious intraductal component, and tumor calcification is common. Medullary carcinoma is characterized by infiltration of lymphocytes. This lesion is less invasive, with late lymphatic metastases and a favorable prognosis.

Lobular carcinoma: Less common than ductal carcinoma, this develops in the lobular breast tissues. Histologic diagnosis is based on foci of noninvasive lobular tumor because infiltrative disease has the same pattern as scirrhous adenocarcinoma.

Inflammatory carcinoma: A very aggressive cancer, this is characterized by tumor obstruction of subdermal lymphatics, lymphangitis, and a breast that is red and hot. The prognosis is poor.

Miscellaneous carcinomas: Carcinoma of adnexal origin, mucinous carcinoma, epidermoid carcinoma, and adenoid cystic carcinoma.

Cystosarcoma phylloides: A bulky tumor, cystosarcoma phylloides is a malignant, locally invasive lesion. It rarely metastasizes to regional nodes, although hematogenous spread may occur. Management is by simple mastectomy without the need for axillary node dissection.

DIAGNOSIS

Physical examination: Most commonly involving the upper outer quadrant, a mass may be palpated on self-examination or physical examination. It is difficult to palpate lesions smaller than 1 cm (by which time the lesion has probably been growing for almost 5 years).

Involvement of nipple ducts may cause a bloody discharge or the weepy lesions of Paget's disease. A peau d'orange skin appearance indicates involvement of the subdermal lymphatics.

Mammography: Invaluable in the early detection of breast cancer, characteristic findings include a lesion with irregular borders, stippled calcifications, and greater vascularity of tissues surrounding the lesion. Ultrasonography is useful in determining the solid or cystic nature of a lesion. MR imaging can provide information unavailable with mammography.

Fine-needle aspiration: Fine-needle aspiration distinguishes a cystic lesion from a solid mass, and cytology may be helpful in diagnosis. Biopsy is required before proceeding with definitive management.

Biopsy: Biopsy is necessary for histologic diagnosis of a palpable mass, suspicious lesion on mammography, cyst recurrence following aspiration, and malignant fine-needle aspiration specimen. A palpable mass may be incised for biopsy under local or general anesthesia. A nonpalpable lesion may be localized by wires inserted under mammographic control.

TREATMENT

Intraductal Carcinoma. Intraductal carcinoma may be treated by either wide excision with histologic confirmation of complete excision or simple mastectomy. Patients treated by wide excision require close follow-up owing to the incidence of multifocal in situ disease.

Infiltrating Carcinoma. Invasive carcinoma is treated by either modified radical mastectomy or lumpectomy and radiation. Modified radical mastectomy includes removal of the breast with its nipple and areola, resection of the skin overlying the tumor, and axillary node dissection. The pectoralis major and minor muscles are preserved. The medial and lateral pectoral nerve innervation to these muscles is also carefully preserved to maintain muscle function and bulk.

Lumpectomy and supervoltage radiation are effective treatments provided that the mass is completely excised with histologic confirmation of negative margins. Most advocates of lumpectomy and radiation recommend axillary dissection or node sampling.

Adjuvant chemotherapy is undergoing multiple clinical trials. No widespread consensus has been reached, and recommendations for adjuvant chemotherapy are determined by status relative to menopause, status of axillary nodes, and tumor hormonal receptors. In general, combination chemotherapy is recommended for premenopausal women with positive axillary node(s), regardless of tumor hormone receptors, and for postmenopausal women with positive node and negative hormonal receptors. Tamoxifen is recommended for postmenopausal women with positive nodes and positive hormonal receptors.

Breast Reconstruction After Mastectomy

The trend toward modified radical mastectomy rather than radical mastectomy, as the definitive curative operation for breast cancer, has fostered early or immediate breast reconstruction as part of the aesthetic rehabilitation program for patients.

The introduction of breast implants, tissue expansion, muscle flaps, and microsurgical techniques has provided the essential prerequisites for the early restoration of the patient's chest wall.

TIMING

Breast reconstruction may be initiated or completed either at the time of mastectomy or at a secondary procedure. If a delayed reconstruction is chosen, the patient generally must wait at least 3 months for postoperative swelling and scarring to settle sufficiently.

SURGICAL TECHNIQUES

Tissue Expansion. In the absence of adequate prethoracic soft tissue for the comfortable insertion of an implant, tissue expansion develops enough subcutaneous and subpectoral volume for subsequent placement of a permanent breast implant. When the breast is to be reconstructed with a silicone prosthesis, preexpansion is usually required in patients undergoing immediate reconstruction. A tissue expander is placed submuscularly so that it is covered completely by pectoralis major muscle, origin of rectus abdominus muscle, and origins of the serratus anterior muscle (Fig. 15–6). Following 3 to 4 months of slow, sequential inflations at weekly or biweekly intervals, the tissue expander is replaced with a permanent implant (Fig. 15–7). Tissue expansion is also indicated for secondary reconstructions if soft tissues are inadequate to accommodate the silicone prosthesis.

Breast Implant. Controversy regarding silicone gel is pertinent in the selection of implants for reconstruction. Although gel-filled implants are sanctioned by

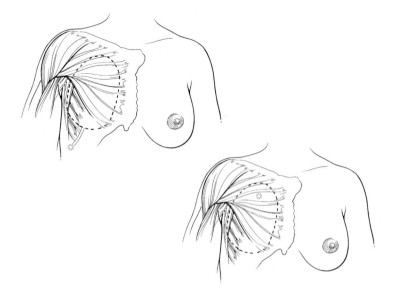

FIGURE 15–6. Placement of the tissue expander for postmastectomy breast reconstruction is completely submuscular. The implant is covered by pectoralis major muscle, origin of rectus abdominis muscle, and origin of serratus anterior muscle.

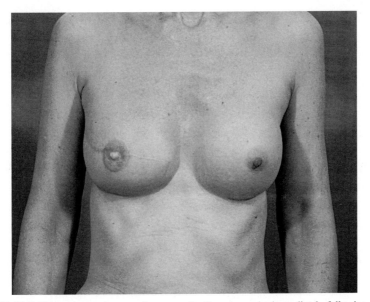

FIGURE 15–7. This patient underwent placement of a tissue expander immediately following mastectomy. She has now had postoperative placement of the permanent implant and nipple reconstruction.

the FDA for reconstructive purposes, a very detailed informed consent must be carried out with the patient in determining whether to proceed with a silicone gel or saline-filled prosthesis. Prostheses are selected according to the size and shape of the contralateral breast. Depending on the contralateral breast and the body habitus, alternatives for implant include the low-profile round, high-profile round, and tear drop–shaped implant. As in the case of augmentation mammoplasty, both smooth-walled and textured implants are available. The size of the implant is selected to provide an aesthetic chest wall contour and symmetry with the contralateral breast.

Musculocutaneous Flaps. The transfer of autogenous tissue as either pedicled or free flaps is an important modality in the reconstruction of ideally shaped and positioned breasts. These procedures are gaining more favor because of the controversy relating to breast implants.

Latissimus Dorsi Musculocutaneous Flap. The latissimus dorsi muscle with a paddle of skin is transferred on the thoracodorsal pedicle to the anterior chest wall (Fig. 15–8). In patients with sufficient subcutaneous tissue, enough soft tissue can be transferred and folded on itself to create an aesthetic breast mound without the need for silicone implant. Generally, however, the latissimus dorsi muscle is used in conjunction with an underlying breast prosthesis.

Transverse Rectus Abdominis Myocutaneous Flap (TRAM Flap). The skin and fat of the lower abdomen may be transferred to the chest wall, providing a mound of autogenous tissue without need for an implant (Fig. 15–9). Although this is an operation of some magnitude, it provides better long-term results than other techniques used in breast reconstruction.

The lower abdominal skin and fat are dissected off the anterior abdominal wall, maintaining attachments to the rectus abdominis muscle. The skin paddle is perfused by perforating vessels from the rectus muscle. The rectus abdominis

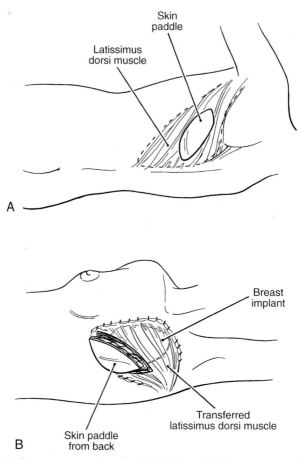

FIGURE 15–8. *A,* Breast reconstruction using the latissimus dorsi myocutaneous flap. *B,* The skin paddle is best placed inferiorly and medially.

muscle is then mobilized on its superior epigastric vascular pedicle and the flap transferred to the chest wall through a subcutaneous tunnel in the upper abdomen and lower chest wall. The skin and fat are sculpted and sutured in place on the chest, creating an aesthetic breast (Fig. 15–10).

A single rectus muscle perfuses the ipsilateral lower abdominal skin and fat and a portion of the contralateral tissues. If the entire lower abdominal tissues are needed for reconstruction of a large breast, both rectus muscles are transferred. Both rectus muscles are also used if the patient has an abdominal scar that limits the amount of skin one muscle can provide.

If a single-pedicled TRAM is used, it is preferable to transfer the contralateral muscle. Bilateral TRAM flaps may be transferred simultaneously, each muscle carrying half the abdominal wall skin and fat for bilateral breast reconstruction. The TRAM flap should not be used in obese patients with a pendulous panniculus or in patients with vascular disease and vasculitis. Risk of tissue loss is significantly higher in diabetics and heavy smokers. The abdominal wall must be carefully repaired after TRAM flap. If a single muscle is transferred, the fascial defect is usually small enough to be reapproximated and closed with sutures. If both muscles are transferred, the fascial defect is reconstructed with polypropylene mesh.

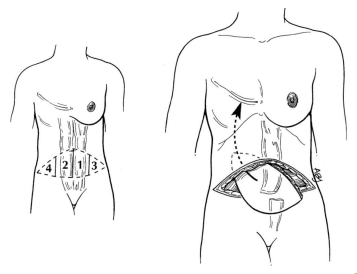

FIGURE 15–9. Outline of tissues used for the transverse rectus abdominis myocutaneous flap breast reconstruction. If the skin and subcutaneous paddle are to be transferred on a single muscle, the paddle is divided into four zones. Zone 4 is not reliable in most patients, and zone 3 must be carefully inspected for adequate vascularity.

Complications of the TRAM flap include the following:

Tissue loss: Partial flap loss is managed by débridement and wound care. Significant or total flap loss is a serious complication and may require secondary reconstruction with a latissimus dorsi flap.

Abdominal wall weakness: This is usually avoided with meticulous surgical technique. Abdominal wall strength below the arcuate line depends on the anterior fascia, a portion of which is taken with the rectus muscle. The fascial defect must be closed without tension using sutures or mesh. If weakness with protrusion of intra-abdominal contents does occur, an abdominal wall plication with mesh reinforcement is necessary.

Free Flap Reconstruction. The free TRAM flap, the gluteus maximus myocutaneous flap, and a lateral thigh free flap have been described for breast reconstruction. In recent years, the free TRAM flap has gained popularity, as it provides an excellent reconstruction and requires less abdominal wall dissection than does the pedicled TRAM. The free TRAM is transferred using microvascular techniques on the inferior epigastric vessels. It is a well-perfused flap, and a single muscle carries both ipsilateral and contralateral skin and fat. Only a small segment of anterior fascia is taken, avoiding the need for mesh reconstruction of the abdominal wall. The epigastric artery and vein are anastomosed to donor vessels in the ipsilateral axilla. Generally, the thoracodorsal or subscapular artery and vein provide the recipient vessels. The internal mammary vessels may also be used as recipient vessels.

Nipple-Areola Reconstruction

The Nipple (Fig. 15–11). Several approaches are available:

Quadripod flap: Four flaps are designed around a central base. The radiating flaps are elevated at the level of the deep dermis. The dermis is incised around the periphery of the base and the quadripod flap teased out of its subcutaneous base. The limbs of the quadripod flap are sutured to themselves. The circular

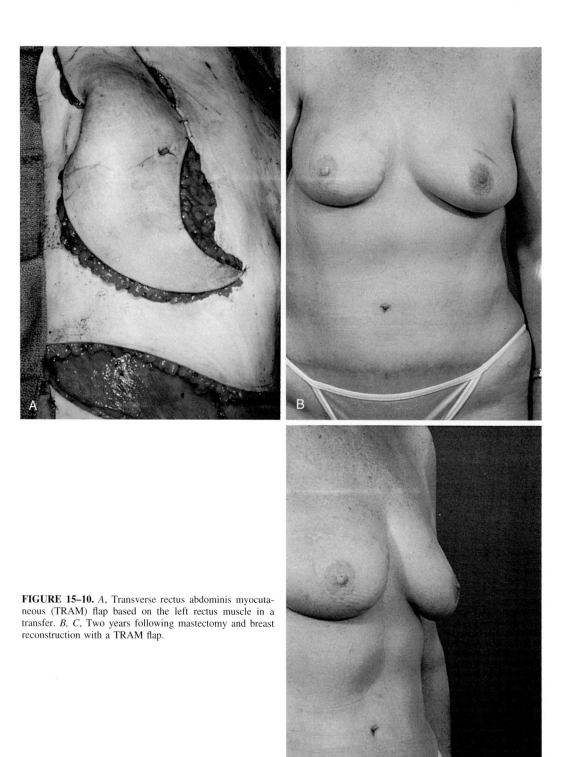

FIGURE 15–10. *A*, Transverse rectus abdominis myocutaneous (TRAM) flap based on the left rectus muscle in a transfer. *B*, *C*, Two years following mastectomy and breast reconstruction with a TRAM flap.

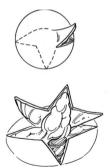
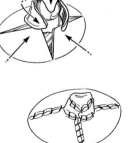
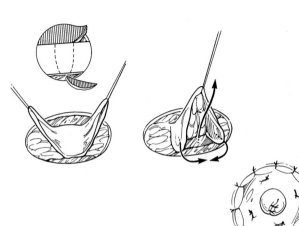
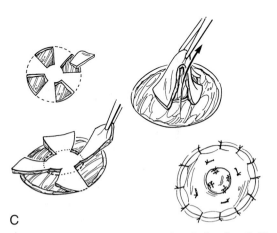

FIGURE 15–11. Techniques for nipple areolar reconstruction. *A*, Star flap. *B*, Skate flap. *C*, Quadri-pod flap.

de-epithelialized area around the neonipple must be grafted to create the areola.

Skate flap: Two wings are elevated on each side of a central base. The wings are elevated at the level of the deep dermis. The dermis at the base of each wing is incised into the subcutaneous tissue and the two wings drawn out at 90 degrees to the surface. The wings are wrapped around their base, and the donor wound is grafted to reconstruct an areola.

Star flap: A star flap is designed as a three-pointed star. The three flaps are elevated deep to the dermis and sutured to themselves to create a nipple. The donor wounds are closed primarily, avoiding the need for an areolar graft. The areola is recreated by tatooing.

Contralateral nipple graft: A composite graft is taken form from the opposite nipple and sutured to a de-epithelialized site on the reconstructed breast. The areola is tatooed.

The Areola. The areola is constructed by harvesting skin from the inner thigh or inner gluteal crease to provide the usual tan color. If dark brown to black areolar tissue is required, the labia minora skin is used. If tattooing of the areola is to be done, skin can be taken from any accessible area or the skin on the mound can be tattooed. Any graft is defatted and a central hole made for the nipple and sutured to the margins of the de-epithelialized mound.

THE CONTRALATERAL BREAST

The objective of reconstruction is to create an aesthetic breast that matches the contralateral breast. This may require an operative procedure on the opposite breast. It is imperative that surgery on the contralateral breast be coordinated with preoperative mammography and oncologic follow-up. It is avoided if it will interfere with or compromise long-term follow-up.

Options include mastopexy, reduction mammoplasty, augmentation, and prophylactic mastectomy and reconstruction.

CONGENITAL MALFORMATIONS OF THE CHEST WALL

EMBRYOLOGY

In the first 2 weeks of embryonic development, the layers of somatopleure develop to overlie the pericardium. The thoracic wall develops as these layers give rise to the skin of the chest and upper abdominal wall. The dorsal mesoderm migrates ventrally, and the substance of the chest wall begins to develop. Ribs start to form in the dorsal mesoderm at about the sixth week and develop ventrally. Paired lower sternal bars fuse and the ribs, which are now developing toward the sternum, begin to form primitive unions with the sternum. These are the future costochondral cartilages.

Pectus Excavatum (Funnel Chest)

This is the most common of the congenital deformities of the sternum, varying in degree from mild to severe. It occurs in one per 300 births and is more common in males. The sternal depression extends from the sternomanubrial junction to the xiphoid and is due to congenital deformation of the costal cartilages, which curve posteriorly, secondarily depressing the sternum. The deformity may present as a broad, shallow depression extending from nipple to nipple or as a very significant sternal depression extending from the xiphoid to the manubrium with little involvement of adjacent ribs.

Although some degree of respiratory compromise may rarely be present, clinical manifestations are usually absent. The cosmetic effect of the deformity is the most significant problem. Patients with severe deformities are noted to have stooped shoulders, kyphoscoliosis, and a protuberant abdomen.

Children with severe or progressive deformities are corrected by subperichondral costal cartilage resection, wedge osteotomy at the sternomanubrial junction, and overcorrection of the sternum. If, however, the patient presents at an age beyond the adolescent growth spurt or as an adult, camouflage of the deformity by placement of a solid silicone implant is simpler and equally, if not more, effective.

A custom-prepared silicone implant is fashioned from mold impressions of the chest wall. Alternatively, an implant can be fashioned using three-dimensional reconstruction of a CT scan. Through a small infrasternal incision a dissection plane is created between the sternal periosteum and overlying tissues. The prosthesis is placed into position, and the edges of the implant are placed beneath the origin of the pectoralis muscle. This provides total filling of the depression, with restoration of a normal chest contour (Fig. 15–12). Female patients often have an associated hypomastia. Augmentation mammoplasty is best delayed until a second procedure because of risk of migration of implants.

Pectus Carinatum

This deformity is characterized by an anterior bulge of the sternum due to malposition of the costal cartilages. Most deformities are actually due to posterior displacement of the costochondral junctions, resulting in an appearance of sternal prominence. A small number of patients, however, do have a true anterior malposition of the sternum relative to normally positioned costochondral junctions. Correction is possible via a sternal or transverse submammary incision. After the sternal origins of each pectoralis major muscle are detached, the deformed ribs and cartilages are resected subperichondrially and the perichondrial beds resected. The pectoral muscles are then reattached to each other and to the sternum and the lower border of the pectoralis muscles. The incision is then closed.

Sternal Clefts

Sternal clefts may be one of three types: They involve the manubrium and gladiolus to the fourth intercostal space; they involve the lower half of the sternum;

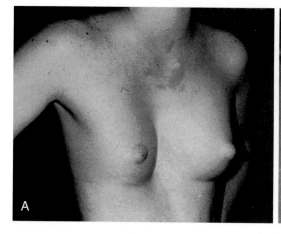

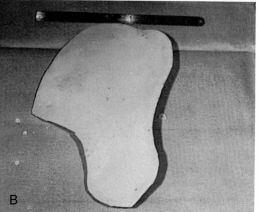

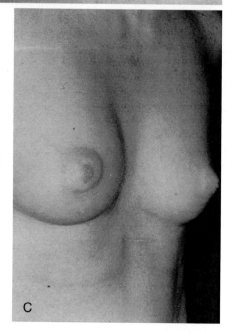

FIGURE 15–12. *A*, Preoperative view of a 16-year-old girl with a pectus excavatum. *B*, A custom silicone implant for correction of the defect. *C*, Five years after operative placement of a custom silicone implant.

and they are complete, often associated with ventral abdominal and diaphragmatic hernia and ectopia cordis.

Treatment is via a midline presternal incision. Superior sternal clefts can often be corrected by excision of associated inferiorly joined bone with chondrotomies and approximation of the sternal bands by encircling sutures. In the more severe varieties of sternal clefts, a prosthetic mesh may be used for its correction.

Poland Syndrome

This syndrome is characterized by absence of the sternal head of the pectoralis major, hypoplasia or aplasia of the breasts, and variable deformities of the thoracic wall, upper extremity, and vertebrae. This syndrome occurs in one of every 25,000 births and is more common on the right side. Specific chest wall deformities include abnormal development of the costal cartilages and abnormalities or absence

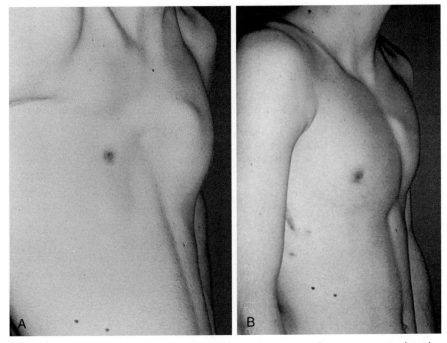

FIGURE 15–13. *A,* 17-year-old male with Poland's syndrome. *B,* Two-year postoperative view following correction of Poland's syndrome chest wall defect with silicone implant and latissimus dorsi muscle flap. (With permission from Marks MW, Argenta LC, Izenberg PH, Mes GB: Management of the chest wall deformity in male patients with Poland's syndrome. Plast Reconstr Surg 87:674–678, 1991.)

of the second, third, and fourth anterior ribs. Associated deficiency of other muscles is often present, including the serratus anterior, latissimus dorsi, deltoid, supraspinatus, and infraspinatus muscles. Other associated anomalies include dextrocardia, pectus excavatum, scoliosis, and winging of the scapula. Associated upper extremity deformities are most frequently associated with brachysyndactyly, although significant hypoplasia and aplasia have been described.

Correction of the deformity is directed at reconstruction of the chest wall and breast reconstruction in women. Chest wall reconstruction is directed either at repositioning of the deformed ribs in the most severe cases or at correction of the contour deformity by insertion of a preformed, custom-built silicone implant. The repositioned ribs or implant is then covered with a latissimus dorsi muscle flap, if available. The latissimus dorsi muscle is adequate to correct very mild defects but, once it atrophies, is too thin to correct moderate or severe deformities. When transferring the latissimus dorsi muscle, it is important to detach its insertion and transfer it anteriorly to the humerus, thereby reconstructing the anterior axillary fold (Fig. 15–13). The breast is reconstructed by expansion of the chest wall soft tissues and secondary placement of a permanent implant. If associated athelia is present, a nipple-areola reconstruction is done at a later date.

Suggested Reading

Argenta LC, Vander Kolk CA, Friedman RJ, Marks MW: Refinements in reconstruction of congenital breast deformities. Plast Reconstr Surg 76:73–80, 1985
Baker JL Jr: Classification of spherical contractures. Augmentation mammoplasty. *In* Owsley JQ Jr,

Peterson RA (eds): Symposium on Aesthetic Surgery of the Breast. St. Louis, CV Mosby, 1978, pp 256–263

Biggs TM, Yarish RS: Augmentation mammoplasty: A comparative analysis. Plast Reconstr Surg 85:368, 1990

Courtiss E, Goldwyn RM: Reduction mammoplasty by the inferior pedicle technique. Plast Reconstr Surg 59:500, 1977

Elliott LF, Hartrampf CR Jr: Breast reconstruction: Progress in the past decade. World J Surg 14:763, 1990

Gibney J: The long-term results of tissue expansion for breast reconstruction. Clin Plast Surg 14:509, 1987

Hartrampf CR, Scheflan M, Black PW: Breast reconstruction with a transverse abdominal island flap. Plast Reconstr Surg 69:216, 1982

Letterman G, Schurter M: The surgical correction of gynecomastia. Am Surg 35:322, 1969

Marks MW, Argenta LC, Lee DC: Silicone implant correction of pectus excavatum: Indications and refinement in technique. Plast Reconstr Surg 74:52, 1984

McKissock PK: Reduction mammoplasty with a vertical dermal flap. Plast Reconstr Surg 49:245, 1972

Ravitch MM: Atypical deformities of the chest wall: Absence and deformities of the ribs and costal cartilages. Surgery 59:438, 1966

Regnault P: Breast ptosis. Clin Plast Surg 3:193, 1976

CHAPTER 16

Trunk and Lower Extremity

ACQUIRED CHEST WALL DEFECTS

The aim of chest wall reconstruction is to cover vital structures, achieve an air-tight closure of the pleural cavity, re-establish chest wall stability, and provide a stable and aesthetic wound closure. The flaps commonly used for reconstruction of the chest wall are the rectus abdominis, lattisimus dorsi, pectoralis major and serratus anterior muscle flaps, and omentum.

Reconstruction may be indicated for the following conditions:

Resection of a Chest Wall Malignancy

Latissimus dorsi or rectus abdominis myocutaneous flaps provide adequate tissue for most of these defects. A wide lateral wall defect that includes loss of four or more ribs and lateral wall defects associated with loss of the sternum may require skeletal stabilization with prosthetic material. Polypropylene mesh is the material of choice (Fig. 16–1).

Post–Median Sternotomy Infection

Acute infection of a median sternotomy wound or chronic infection due to sternal osteomyelitis may necessitate aggressive débridement of the sternum and adjacent rib cartilages. The pectoralis major muscles cover the superior two thirds of the defect. They may be transposed on the thoracoacromial vessels or based medially on the perforating branches of the anterior intercostal vessels as turnover flaps.

The rectus abdominis muscle pedicled on the superior epigastric artery provides an ideal flap that often covers the entire sternum to the level of the sternal notch. The rectus abdominis is not used if the internal mammary artery, which becomes the superior epigastric artery, has been used in a coronary artery bypass. If neither rectus is available, the omentum can be used for coverage of the lower portion of the wound. The skin overlying the lateral chest walls can be undermined and approximated over the muscle flaps or the flaps can be skin grafted.

Empyema

Infection of the pleural cavity following pneumonectomy carries significant morbidity. It may be associated with a bronchopleural fistula. Management is initially directed at drainage of infected pleural fluid with a chest tube or preferably an Eloesser procedure. One or two lateral rib segments are removed, and the pleura is sewn to the wound's skin edges. Dressing changes are continued for several weeks until the pleural cavity is clean and granulating. At a second operation the pleural space is eliminated by transfer of local muscle flaps, and the skin is closed.

The latissimus dorsi muscle is the flap of choice but is usually not available owing to transection at the initial thoracotomy. Patients at high risk for bronchopleural fistula or empyema preferably have had a muscle-sparing incision at initial thoracotomy. The pectoralis major and serratus anterior muscles are used

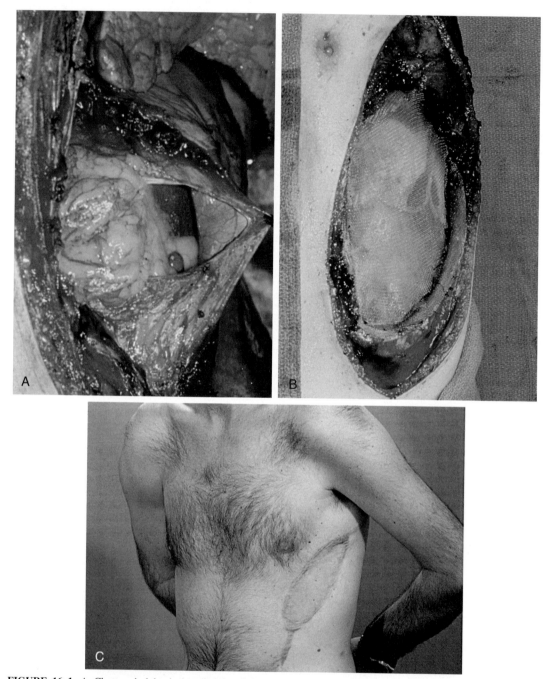

FIGURE 16–1. *A,* Chest and abdominal wall defect following excision of a sarcoma. *B,* The diaphragm and chest wall integrity has been reconstructed with polypropylene mesh. *C,* The mesh has been covered with a latissimus dorsi muscle, with reapproximation of wound edges and a split-thickness skin graft to the remaining defect.

when the latissimus dorsi cannot be transferred. An anterior segment of the second and third ribs is removed for transfer of the pectoralis muscle. The rectus abdominis muscle, pectoralis minor, and omentum also reach into the pleural cavity if needed.

Radiation Wounds

As radiation techniques improve, this complication is becoming rarer. The chest wall must be radically débrided, removing all ischemic, infected, and necrotic tissue. Often the pleura is stuck to the chest wall and must also be removed. Prosthetic materials should not be used in these chronically infected wounds. Usually the soft tissues are sufficiently fibrotic that musculocutaneous flap closure suffices in re-establishing skeletal stability. The latissimus dorsi musculocutaneous flap is the preferred method of reconstruction. The rectus abdominis muscle with either a vertical or transverse skin paddle (TRAM) can also be used.

BACK

Spina Bifida

Spina bifida results from the failure of fusion of the neural groove. It is the most common central nervous system congenital anomaly, occurring in about 1 of every 1000 live births in the United States.

SPINA BIFIDA OCCULTA

One or several spinous processes are hypoplastic or aplastic without involvement of underlying neural tissues. Patients who present with overlying skin lesions such as lipoma, hemangioma, patch of hair, or dermal sinus may have tethering of the spinal cord. Failure to correct a tethered cord can result in a progressive neurologic injury. Any patient with these skin lesions overlying the spinal column requires evaluation by MR imaging and neurosurgical assessment.

SPINA BIFIDA CYSTICA

The dorsal defect involves underlying meninges or meninges and nerve tissue.

Meningocele. Aplasia of the dorsal aspect of one or several vertebrae is present, along with herniation of meninges. The meningeal sac is usually filled with cerebrospinal fluid. Because neural elements are not involved, the patient is neurologically intact. The deformity generally involves the lumbosacral area but may occur anywhere along the length of the spinal column.

Meningomyelocele. This dorsal defect involves meninges and neural tissues. Most commonly occurring in the thoracolumbar area, it may also occur in other parts of the spinal cord. An associated posterior displacement of the medulla and

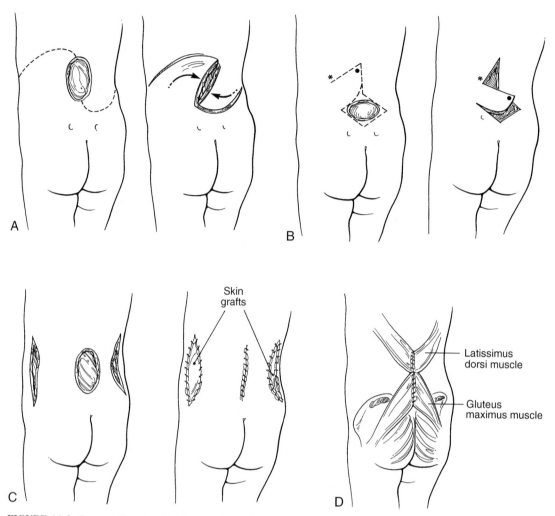

FIGURE 16–2. Common flaps for skin closure of a myelomeningocele include *(A)* rotation lumbosacral flap, *(B)* rhomboid transposition flap, *(C)* bipedicle fasciocutaneous flap with skin graft to the lateral relaxing incisions, and *(D)* bilateral muscle flaps.

pons (Arnold-Chiari malformation) is present. Depending on the level of involvement and degree of spinal cord dysplasia, the neurologic symptoms vary from weakness to complete absence of sensation and motor function below the level of the defect.

Closure. Defects are generally closed within the first day of life. The herniated cord is reduced and the meninges are closed in layers, with careful closure of overlying deep fascia and skin. Patients with significant skin defects require closure with a local flap. Multiple flaps have been described, including rotation lumbosacral flaps, rhomboid transposition flaps, bipedicled skin or fasciocutaneous flaps, and bilateral musculocutaneous flaps (Fig. 16–2).

Acquired Defects

Defects due to trauma, tumor resection, débridement of soft tissue infection, and radiation injury may require coverage with local skin flap, fasciocutaneous flap, or muscle flap. The trapezius muscle is useful for upper back defects. The latissimus dorsi muscle, based proximally on the thoracodorsal vessels or distally as a reverse lattisimus dorsi flap on perforating vessels from the ninth, tenth, and eleventh posterior intercostal vessels, are useful flaps.

ABDOMINAL WALL DEFORMITIES

The cephalic, caudal, right lateral, and left lateral folds develop to form the abdominal wall. The intestinal tract develops exterior to the abdominal cavity between the fifth and tenth weeks and then slowly returns to the abdominal cavity. The umbilical ring contracts as the abdominal wall forms.

Gastroschisis

Failure of differentiation of the lateral abdominal wall results in a full-thickness defect on the right side adjacent to the umbilical cord. The abdominal viscera herniate through this defect, and an associated malrotation of the bowel is usually present.

Omphalocele

Failure of the midgut to return to the abdominal cavity presents as a large umbilical defect, with abdominal viscera external to the abdominal wall covered only by amniotic membrane.

Correction of gastroschisis and omphalocele is similar and is determined by the size of the defect and amount of extraabdominal viscera. Small defects may be closed primarily by direct approximation of fascia and overlying skin. Large defects may be closed in two stages, with the skin closure being accomplished in the early hours of life after appropriate resuscitation. The rectus muscles and fascia are re-approximated at a later date once the abdominal cavity is sufficiently developed to return the viscera to their normal position.

Large defects may require correction by placement of a prosthetic cover over the exposed viscera and suturing the material to the edges of the defect. The dome of the silo is sequentially clamped over a 1- to 2-week period, reducing the size of the silo. This in turn pushes the viscera into the abdominal cavity, which is progressively stretched by the newly returned viscera. Once the viscera have been completely reduced into the abdominal cavity, the abdominal wall fascia and skin are operatively approximated.

Prune-Belly Syndrome

Failure of the abdominal muscles to develop results in a wrinkled appearance to the abdominal skin. There may be concomitant urologic anomalies. Correction is by wide dissection and approximation of the hypoplastic muscles and resection of excess skin.

Reconstruction of Acquired Abdominal Wall Defects

An optimal abdominal wall closure requires approximation of the posterior and anterior abdominal fasciae and approximation of skin and subcutaneous tissue. If adequate fascia is not available, abdominal wall integrity and strength are achieved by suturing prosthetic mesh to the edges of the fascial defect (Fig. 16–3). Skin may be closed over the mesh, or granulation tissue may be allowed to develop through the mesh and the wound secondarily skin grafted. There are situations, however, in which mesh should not be used. These include patients with intra-abdominal or local soft tissue infection and patients with bowel fistulae. Patients may also have their mesh removed because of chronic drainage or splitting of the mesh.

The rectus abdominis muscles provide an ideal source of soft tissue for reconstruction of a fascial layer in these patients. The muscles may be transferred on either their inferior or their superior pedicle or turned over as a bipedicled turnover flap and sutured to each other in the midline. If added strength is needed, mesh may be sewn over the rectus flaps by plication to the external oblique fascia.

Lower abdominal wall defects may be reconstructed by transfer of distant flaps from the leg. Either the rectus femoris muscle, with overlying fascia and skin if needed, or a tensor fascia lata flap may be transposed to cover a large portion of the lower abdominal wall.

LOWER EXTREMITY

Trauma

Management of an acute injury to the lower extremity requires control of bleeding, stabilization of fractures, restoration of arterial inflow, and repair of soft tissues.

Significant injury may lead to a compartment syndrome, whereas fractures may be complicated by nonunion or osteomyelitis. Deficiency of soft tissues in the pretibial area and foot may require sophisticated reconstructive techniques.

COMPARTMENT SYNDROME

The lower leg has four compartments: anterior, lateral, superficial posterior, and deep posterior compartments. Diagnosis of compartment syndrome is determined by the presence of pain on stretching of involved compartment muscles, weakness of involved muscles, loss of sensation in the distribution of involved nerves, and swelling. Pulses may be present, and loss of pulse is not necessary to make the diagnosis. Compartment pressure should not rise above 35 to 40 mm Hg.

Compartment syndrome requires fasciotomy and decompression of all four muscle compartments.

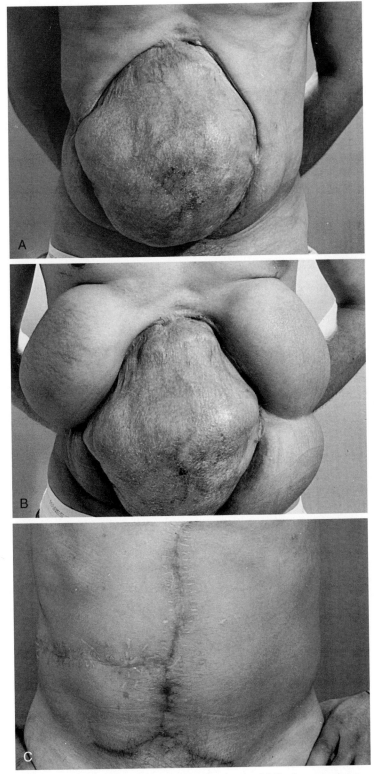

FIGURE 16–3. *A,* A 25-year-old patient with skin graft on bowel following a gunshot wound to the abdomen. *B,* Three 700 ml expanders were inflated over 10 weeks. *C,* Patient underwent transposition of the rectus muscles to obtain abdominal wall closure. This was reinforced with a layer of mesh and a primary skin closure obtained with the expanded abdominal wall subskin.

OPEN FRACTURES

Open tibial fractures are classified by the type of bone injury and the extent of overlying soft tissue injury. These injuries mandate irrigation and débridement and stabilization of bones. Preferred treatment is open reduction and internal fixation with compression plates and screws or intramedullary rod fixation and simple wound closure. Injuries with a bone gap or significant soft tissue defect are stabilized with external pin fixation. The soft tissue defect is reconstructed by flap transfer and the bone gap secondary grafted with iliac bone. Gaps in excess of 8 cm are best managed with a vascularized bone graft. The adjacent fibula can be pedicled or the contralateral fibula transferred as a free vascularized graft. Alternatively, the traumatic gap is closed by distraction osteogenesis.

Distraction Osteogenesis. A corticotomy is fashioned above or below the fracture and a specialized external fixator applied. The fixator stabilizes the two segments and allows distraction parallel to the bone axis by the turn of a screw. One week after corticotomy, distraction is initiated at a rate of 1 mm/day. The bone segment adjacent to the fracture is transported through the fracture gap until it docks. Fracture healing may then take place.

Soft Tissue Defects. The femur is well padded by muscle and soft tissue so that problems most commonly occur below the knee. Soft tissue deficiency is often associated with open tibial fractures and foot and ankle injury. Large defects require flap closure and depend on the level of injury (Fig. 16–4).

Upper Third of Lower Leg. The medial and lateral heads of the gastrocnemius muscle may be transferred on the appropriate sural artery to resurface the upper third and the knee. The medial head of the gastrocnemius has a longer muscle belly and is used preferentially.

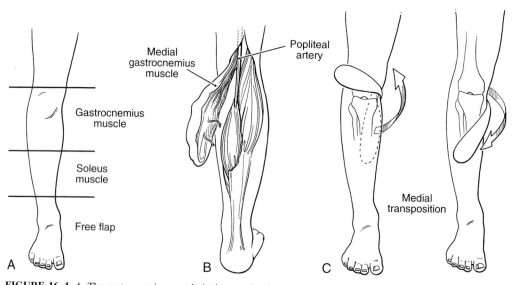

FIGURE 16–4. *A,* The gastrocnemius muscle is the muscle of choice for coverage of defects involving the knee and proximal one third of the lower leg. The soleus muscle provides coverage for the middle one third of the lower leg. Soft tissue defects involving the lower one third of the leg often require free flap coverage if a local flap is not available. *B,* The gastrocnemius muscle is elevated on the sural artery and vein. *C,* The arc of rotation of the medial gastrocnemius muscle on the sural vessels provides coverage to the knee and upper one third of the lower leg.

Middle Third of Lower Leg. The soleus muscle is transferred on segmental perforating vessels from the posterior tibial and peroneal vessels.

Lower Third of Lower Leg. Lower third defects represent difficult reconstructive problems owing to the lack of tissue for local muscle flaps. Large defects require coverage by a free flap, whereas smaller defects may be amenable to local fasciocutaneous flaps.

Ankle and Foot. Flaps described for coverage include the dorsalis pedis, lateral calcaneal, flexor digitorum brevis, and abductor hallucis flaps. These injuries provide difficult problems, often requiring distal flap transfer such as a cross-leg flap or free tissue transfer.

Osteomyelitis

Open fractures complicated by infection require aggressive débridement of infected and nonviable bone, bacterial culture, and specific systemic antibiotics. Internal fixation materials must be removed and an external fixator applied if stabilization is needed. Once the wound is surgically clean, it is covered with well-vascularized soft tissue. Bone gaps are secondarily grafted.

Chronic Ulceration

Venous Insufficiency. Incompetence of the valvular mechanism leads to progressive venous insufficiency and venous stasis. The skin develops a stasis dermatitis with hyperpigmentation secondary to hemosiderin deposition. Ulcers typically develop in the lower leg, most commonly over the medial or lateral malleoli.

Conservative management with bed rest and leg elevation is often successful. A compression dressing impregnated with zinc oxide, glycerin, and gelatin (Unna boot) may be effective. A necrotic ulcer requires débridement with wet-to-dry saline solution dressing changes or surgical débridement. The clean ulcer may be dressed with a skin substitute such as cultured keratinocytes and the dressing changed every 3 to 5 days.

If conservative methods are unsuccessful, the ulcer must be excised, underlying perforating veins ligated, and the wound skin grafted.

Arterial Insufficiency. Ulcers due to inadequate arterial flow are typically small lesions with a punched-out appearance. They may be associated with other signs and symptoms of extremity ischemia such as claudication, rest pain, shiny and hairless skin, and absence of palpable pulses.

Noninvasive Doppler flow studies or duplex scanning is helpful in determining the likelihood of healing with local wound care. If flow is inadequate, the patient requires arteriography and appropriate revascularization procedures. Large ulcers with exposed tendon or bone or those on the plantar surface of the foot may require concomitant or secondary flap reconstruction.

Diabetic Ulcers. Diabetes mellitus may result in polyneuropathy with anesthesia of distal extremities, advanced atherosclerosis with ischemia of distal extremities, and compromised healing of wounds with soft tissue infection, deep space abscesses, and osteomyelitis. Each of these may cause a nonhealing ulcer, and the cause must be determined. Necrotic tissues are aggressively débrided and invasive infections treated with culture-specific antibiotics. Arterial insufficiency is dealt with appropriately. Small or superficial wounds may be amenable to a skin graft, but ulcers typically involve the heel or plantar surface.

Failure to respond to conservative wound care often requires limb salvage by free tissue transfer. Patients with neurotrophic feet should be fitted with orthotic shoes, as ulceration is likely to recur.

Vasculitis. Collagen-vascular diseases may result in necrotizing vasculitis with skin ulceration. Ulcers are treated by local wound care methods, including dressing changes, débridement, cultured homograft, and, if necessary, excision and skin grafting. Occasionally recalcitant ulcers lead to exposure of tendon, bone, or joint, requiring local or free tissue transfer.

Lymphedema

Abnormalities of lymphatic drainage cause a build-up of lymph fluid in the interstitial spaces and swelling of the involved extremity. Primary lymphedema results from congenital maldevelopment of the lymphatics, whereas secondary lymphedema is due to an acquired obstruction of lymphatic drainage.

PRIMARY LYMPHEDEMA

Lymphedema praecox: Comprising 80 per cent of cases, it appears during childhood or adolescence (Fig. 16–5).
Lymphedema tarda: Occurs later, usually in patients older than 35.
Milroy disease: Familial primary lymphedema.

The skin has a brawny, scaly appearance with nonpitting edema of the tissues. The patient often has recurrent bouts of cellulitis.

Extremities are treated conservatively with compression garments. Severe bouts of swelling are treated with pneumatic pressure devices, elevation, and antibiotics for associated infections. Surgery is reserved for patients with progressive or uncontrolled lymphedema.

Lymphatic drainage beneath the deep fascia is better than that above, and excision is directed at skin and subcutaneous tissues.

Charles procedure: Skin and subcutaneous tissues are excised and split-thickness grafts applied to the deep fascia or muscle.
Staged excision: Skin flaps are elevated and underlying subcutaneous tissues resected in staged serial excisions. This is the more popular approach owing to the better cosmetic results.

SECONDARY LYMPHEDEMA

Obstruction of lymphatic channels may be due to direct extension of a tumor, lymphatic metastases, lymphadenectomy, or radiation-induced fibrosis. In tropical

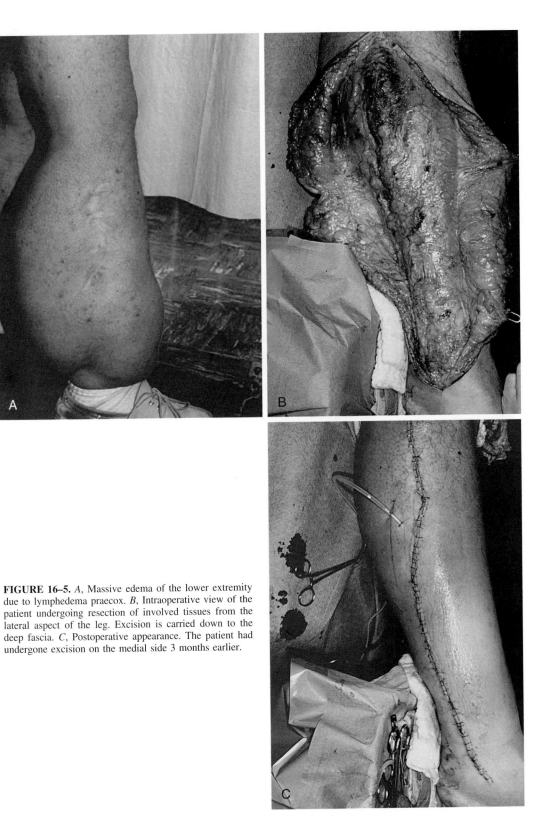

FIGURE 16–5. *A*, Massive edema of the lower extremity due to lymphedema praecox. *B*, Intraoperative view of the patient undergoing resection of involved tissues from the lateral aspect of the leg. Excision is carried down to the deep fascia. *C*, Postoperative appearance. The patient had undergone excision on the medial side 3 months earlier.

regions, infection with the filaria parasite may lead to dramatic cases of lymphedema of the groin and lower extremity.

THE PRESSURE SORE

Pressure, or decubitus, ulceration of the skin is a common condition characterized by the development of a pressure sore over bony prominences when a patient sits or lies in the same recumbent position for several hours without pressure relief. The compression of the tissues over a bony point causes local ischemia that, if uncorrected, progresses to the development of the pressure sore. Because muscle and fat are more vulnerable to pressure than skin, these sites undergo primary extensive necrosis so that by the time skin ulceration occurs, the margins of the ulcer are found to be widely undermined, with a large mass of deep necrotic tissue and a relatively small skin ulcer.

The development of a secondary infection may spread to adjacent structures such as bones and joints. Culture biopsy is necessary to identify a quantitative degree of infection. The number of organisms per gram of tissue attests to the presence of infection, usually represented by a mix of gram-positive and gram-negative bacteria—aerobic and anaerobic.

Pressure sores develop in about 3 per cent of patients in acute care hospitals and about 40 to 50 per cent of patients in chronic care facilities. In paraplegic patients, the absence of sensation allows pressure sores to reach a large size.

Etiology

A neurogenic trophic factor due to central nervous system injury was proposed by Charcot but never proved.

Pressure on a local area of soft tissue for a prolonged period results in ischemia and mechanical injury. It is believed that the pressure must exceed 32 mm Hg, which is the arterial capillary blood pressure.

Shear forces tend to increase the amount of pressure applied to the skin, as well as cause direct injury to muscle-perforating vessels to the skin.

Predisposing local factors include compromised innervation, loss of sensation, soft tissue ischemia and fibrosis, and soiling with stool or urine.

Malnutrition and anemia, so common in debilitated individuals, may be contributory factors. They also impair healing once ulceration has occurred.

Prevention

Turning of the patient or change of position every 2 hours, either actively or passively, is essential to prevent the development of pressure sores, as it avoids continued localized pressure over bony points. Thus, good nursing care and availability of air-fluidized beds, which reduce shearing forces, as well as padding of the heels, are important.

Amelioration of malnutrition, hypoproteinemia, and anemia must be attended to.

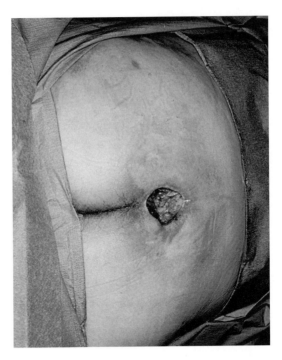

FIGURE 16–6. A grade IV decubitus ulcer with necrosis of tissue down to the sacrum.

Treatment

Once infection is diagnosed, identification of the specific organisms is necessary. *Bacteroides fragilis, Staphylococcus aureus, Proteus mirabilis, Pseudomonas aeruginosa*, and *Escherichia coli* are the usual contaminants.

Early wound débridement, frequent changes of moist saline dressings, or bacteriostatic dressing solutions may prevent progression of infection. Systemic antibiotics may control associated cellulitis or systemic infection but cannot reach the ischemic necrotic ulcer or granulation tissue.

Pressure sores are graded according to depth of involvement.

Grade I: Partial skin thickness into the dermis
Grade II: Full-thickness skin to subcutaneous tissue
Grade III: Through subcutaneous tissue into muscle
Grade IV: Through all layers of soft tissue to bone or into joint (Fig. 16–6)

Surgical Management

Surgery is an integral part of pressure sore management. The timing of surgical treatment is important because the systemic sepsis due to pocketing of infection may require urgent operation to remove sloughs, drain the wound, and improve the patient's general status.

Where possible, closure should be deferred until the sore is in a healing phase with a clean granulating surface.

With urinary infection controlled in the paraplegic, good nutrition, a normal hemoglobin, and good local antiseptic dressings, some ulcers heal or the granulating surface is amenable to free skin grafts to foster healing. As the graft becomes adherent to underlying tissues, it ultimately breaks down, requiring more definitive surgical treatment as a final stage in the rehabilitation of the patient.

INDICATIONS FOR FLAP COVERAGE

1. Thin unstable scar over prominent bony protuberance
2. Abnormal bursa under scar
3. Chronic pyoarthrosis
4. Failure of sore to heal
5. Progression of decubitus ulcer

PRINCIPLES OF OPERATIVE MANAGEMENT

1. Excision of the ulcerous tissue in a well-prepared patient
2. Removal of the underlying bony prominence
3. Removal of all infected bone and heterotopic bone
4. Postoperative wound care: Hemovac suction of the wound; air-fluidized bed.

PRINCIPLES OF FLAP CLOSURE

Flaps are designed to achieve tension-free closure of both recipient and donor sites, obliteration of dead space, padding over bony prominences, and suture lines that do not lie over pressure points.

CLOSURE OF SPECIFIC ULCERS

When designing a flap, one must remember that the patient may develop future ulcers at other sites. Ideally a flap does not compromise adjacent territories that can provide flaps for other wounds. Flaps described for closure of pressure sores include skin flaps, musculocutaneous flaps, and fasciocutaneous flaps. The following are the most common transfers:

Sacrum (Fig. 16–7)
Skin flaps
   Gluteal rotation flap
   Transverse lumbosacral flap
   Thoracolumbar flap
Musculocutaneous flap
   Gluteus maximus rotation flap
   Gluteus maximus island flap
   Gluteus maximus VY advancement flap

Ischium (Fig. 16–8)
Skin flaps
   Gluteal rotation flap
   Posterior thigh VY advancement flap

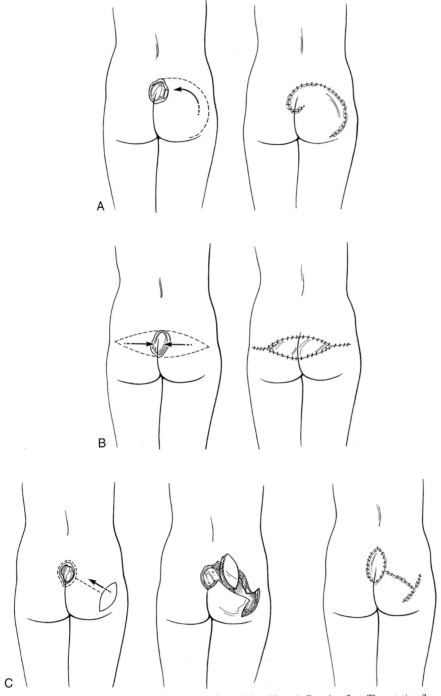

FIGURE 16–7. Common flaps used for closure of sacral decubitus. *A,* Rotation flap: The rotation flap may include the skin and subcutaneous tissue or may be a myocutaneous flap by including the underlying gluteus maximus muscle. *B,* Closure of a large sacral ulcer with bilateral V-Y gluteus maximus musculocutaneous flaps. *C,* The gluteus maximus myocutaneous island flap may be based on either the superior or inferior gluteal vessels.

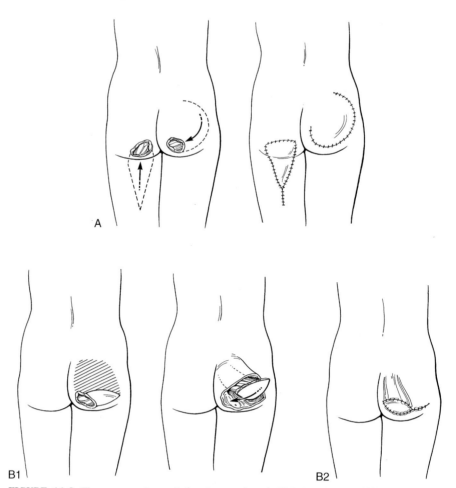

FIGURE 16–8. Flaps commonly used for closure of an ischial decubitus: *A,* V-Y advancement myocutaneous flap including the hamstring muscles to close the left ischial sore. A rotation flap is demonstrated closing the right ischial sore. The rotation flap may include skin and subcutaneous tissue or include the underlying gluteus maximus muscle as a rotation myocutaneous flap. *B,* Gluteus maximus island myocutaneous flap based on the inferior gluteal vessels for closure of an ischial pressure sore.

Musculocutaneous flaps
  Gluteus maximus rotation flap
  Gluteus maximus island flap
  Hamstring VY advancement flap
  Gracilis flap
Fasciocutaneous flaps
  Gluteal thigh flap

Trochanter (Fig. 16–9)
Musculocutaneous flaps
  Tensor fascia iata flap
Muscle flaps
  Vastus lateralis muscle flap
Fasciocutaneous flaps
  Gluteal thigh flap

POSTOPERATIVE MANAGEMENT

Air-fluidized bed
No sitting or direct pressure on the operative site for 3 to 6 weeks

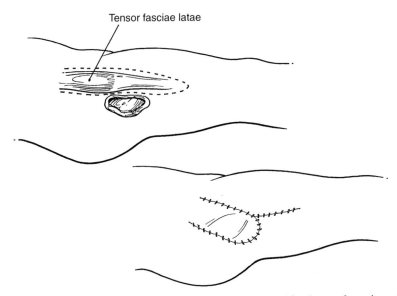

Tensor fasciae latae

FIGURE 16–9. The tensor fascia lata flap provides the simplest method for closure of a trochanteric ulcer.

Gradual remobilization at 3 to 6 weeks, with sitting time slowly increased over a 2- to 3-week period

RECURRENT WOUND BREAKDOWN

Closure of pressure sores is one of the most difficult and frustrating of all reconstructive endeavors. Recurrent breakdown is unfortunately all too common, resulting from (1) inadequate débridement of devitalized tissue or infected bone, (2) failure to eliminate wound dead space and achieve a tension-free closure, and (3) poor hygiene, nutrition, and care once the patient is discharged.

HIP DISARTICULATION

Recurrent wound breakdown leads to multiple operative procedures and eventual exhaustion of available donor sites for closure. These patients, in addition to those with recalcitrant hip joint infection and persistent femoral osteomyelitis, require hip disarticulation. An anterior thigh flap is fashioned to achieve closure of the disarticulation wound. A long flap may be preserved to resurface wounds of the sacrum.

BODY CONTOURING

Abdomen

Abdominoplasty and abdominal dermolipectomy are procedures aimed at the correction of abdominal wall contour. The most common candidates are women after several pregnancies, patients who have undergone significant weight loss, and patients with an excessive abdominal panniculus. In evaluating patients for abdominoplasty, four factors must be considered: (1) amount of redundant abdominal skin, (2) amount of subcutaneous fat, (3) abdominal wall protrusion due to a laxity of fascia and diastasis of underlying rectus muscles, and (4) pattern of scars from previous abdominal operations.

ABDOMINOPLASTY

The ideal feminine abdominal wall is flat, with a narrow waist and hour-glass shape of the torso. Abdominoplasty is an aesthetic procedure designed to achieve optimal abdominal wall contour, with careful attention to placement of scars.

Markings for skin excisions are made with the patient standing. The intent of the procedure is to create a scar that is low on the abdominal wall so as to easily be covered by underwear or bathing suits.

The two most common incisions are the W-shaped incision extending across the pubis and into the suprainguinal area and a low abdominal incision lying in an established crease or fold (Fig. 16–10). The incision is continued down to the anterior abdominal wall and the flap of fat and skin elevated to above the costochondral margins laterally and the xiphoid centrally. The patient is then placed in a flexed position, and the abdominal flap is pulled down and marked as to where it may safely be resected. The aim is to resect the tissues of the hypochondrium from the umbilicus down.

The umbilicus is dissected free on its stalk and is later transposed into an incision on the abdominal flap that has been positioned inferiorly. The diastasis of the rectus muscles is then repaired by plication of the anterior rectus fascia with nonabsorbable sutures. The patient is placed in a flexed position, the abdominal flap is pulled downward, and the wound is closed in two layers using absorbable dermal sutures and a subcuticular continuous suture in the skin. The position of the umbilicus is carefully measured and marked, and an opening is made in the abdominal wall.

The area is defatted and the umbilicus pulled through on its stalk. Polyglycolic acid sutures between the anterior fascia and umbilicus are placed to create an aesthetic umbilical dimple. The umbilicus is sutured in position, and drains are placed to avoid collection of blood and serum. A light pressure dressing is applied (Fig. 16–11).

ABDOMINAL DERMOLIPECTOMY

Abdominal dermolipectomy is reserved for patients with significant abdominal wall adipose tissue and patients with a large hanging panniculus. The procedure is directed at simple excision of redundant skin and fat with primary closure. Tissues may be resected through a transverse elliptical excision, with closure resulting in a horizontal scar along the lower abdomen or a fleur-de-lis pattern with a resection of skin and fat in both horizontal and vertical directions. (Fig. 16–12).

The fleur-de-lis pattern provides a better abdominal contour because not only is the panniculus resected but advancement of tissues from lateral to medial improves the waist line. This approach results in both a lower abdominal transverse scar and vertical midline scar extending to the xiphoid. With either approach only

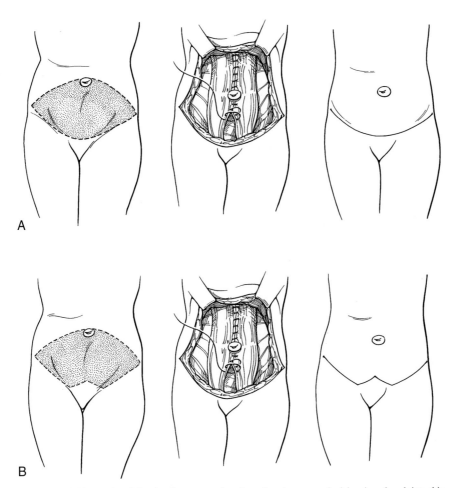

FIGURE 16–10. *A*, The abdominoplasty operation through a transverse incision in a low-lying skin crease. Plication of the rectus muscles to correct any diastasis is an important part of the abdominoplasty procedure. *B*, The W pattern for abdominoplasty.

enough tissue is resected to enable a tension-free closure because undermining of fat abdominal wall tissues is best avoided.

Patients with excessive fat and skin extending around to the back may be corrected with a belt lipectomy. This procedure is also effective in patients who have had a significant weight loss, with loose hanging skin encircling the torso.

MINI-ABDOMINOPLASTY

Patients with mild to moderate deformity involving the lower abdomen may be candidates for mini-abdominoplasty. The procedure is carried out through a low abdominal incision, which does not have to be extended as far laterally as in the standard abdominoplasty. The abdominal wall soft tissues are dissected off the anterior abdominal wall as far superiorly as the umbilicus, which is not freed from its native position.

Abdominal wall laxity due to diastasis recti and attenuation of anterior abdominal wall fascia results in more protrusion of the lower abdominal wall because of the weakness of the posterior fascia below the arcuate line. Plication

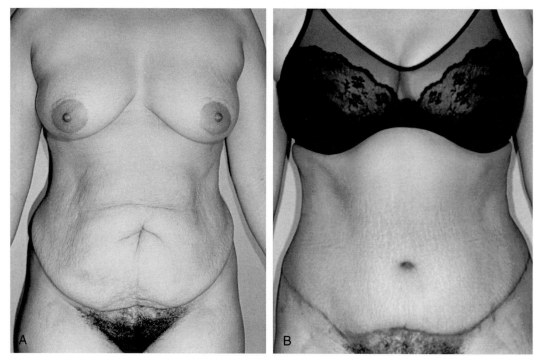

FIGURE 16–11. *A*, Preoperative photograph of a patient who has had multiple pregnancies. *B*, Three months after operative abdominoplasty and correction of the diastasis recti.

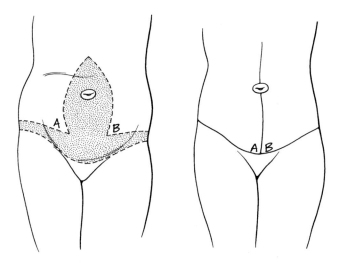

FIGURE 16–12. The fleur-de-lis dermolipectomy.

of the anterior fascia in the lower part of the abdomen can be achieved with the mini-abdominoplasty and provides adequate recontouring in a significant number of patients. If excess fatty tissue is present in the upper part of the abdomen, this may be addressed with suction lipectomy concomitantly with mini-abdominoplasty.

Complications

Hematoma and Seroma. These complications are minimized with careful hemostasis, avoiding injury to the superficial inguinal nodes during the lower part of the dissection, and placement of suction drains. Hematomas should be surgically evacuated, thereby avoiding secondary infection. Persistent seroma following removal of drainage tubes may require periodic needle aspiration and compression dressings.

Skin Slough. Skin sloughs most commonly occur in the midline. An eschar develops and, if small, may be treated conservatively with Silvadene or dressing changes and allowed to heal secondarily. In rare instances a large slough may extend from the incision to the umbilicus, requiring débridement and skin graft. Unacceptable scars may be dealt with at a later date by excision and primary closure. This results in a vertical scar extending from the suprapubic area toward the umbilicus.

A higher incidence of skin slough occurs in patients who are heavy smokers, and patients should therefore be encouraged to stop smoking in the perioperative period. Skin slough is also more likely to occur in patients with previous abdominal incisions. Abdominoplasty in patients with existing abdominal scars must be carefully planned relative to those scars.

Pulmonary Embolus. Abdominoplasty and abdominal dermolipectomy carry a very slight but real risk of pulmonary embolus. Pneumatic stockings should be used intraoperatively and ambulation initiated on the first postoperative day.

Thigh Dermolipectomy

Excess skin and fat may be removed from the thighs and hips by a semicircular or circular thigh reduction (Fig. 16–13). Redundant tissues in the medial thigh require resection of tissues through a vertical incision. These procedures result in significant scarring in the hip, thigh, and infragluteal regions. A thigh lift may also be accomplished by resection of skin and fat from the bikini line. Tissues are undermined toward the thigh to obtain a lift of the flank, thigh, and buttock with a superficial fascial suspension. These procedures are reserved for patients with significant skin redundancy because most of the deformities can be adequately corrected by suction lipectomy.

Brachioplasty

Patients with excessive arm skin that hangs as a bat-wing deformity or patients with excessive skin and adipose tissue may be corrected by direct excision of tissues through an elliptical excision extending from the medial epicondyle to the

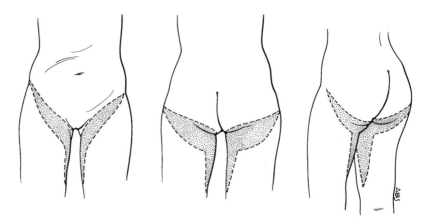

FIGURE 16–13. Circumferential markings for a thigh reduction.

axilla. This results in a visible scar, and care must be taken to avoid axillary contracture and injury to cutaneous nerves.

Suction Lipectomy

The areas where localized accumulations of fat engender flabbiness include the abdomen and flanks, the medial aspect of the thigh, the upper part of the thigh, the gluteal areas, the trochanteric region with or without semicircular adiposity, and Barraques-Simon disorder, characterized by congenital, firm adiposity of the lower part of the body with a normal lean upper body.

There are two layers of fat in the lower extremity and trunk. The superficial layer is composed of dense fat surrounded by fibrous septi, and the deep layer is composed of a much less dense fatty tissue surrounded by less well-defined fibrous septi.

Patients with well-defined and localized fat deposits in the trochanteric, gluteal, and thigh areas are ideally managed by suction lipectomy. The skin tone must be carefully evaluated, as the skin must redrape over suctioned areas. A patient with significant excess skin or compromised skin elasticity is not a candidate for suction lipectomy but can be managed by surgical excision.

Patients with localized fat accumulation with good skin tone are well suited for suction lipectomy. Proper patient selection and the avoidance of this modality in patients with generalized obesity ensure a successful outcome for suction lipectomy.

The procedure may be done under general, spinal or epidural, or local anesthesia, depending on the size of the area to be suctioned. Suction lipectomy causes significant fluid shifts, and patients must have fluid and electrolytes adequately replaced intraoperatively and immediately postoperatively. As a general rule, 30 to 33 per cent of the aspirate is blood if epinephrine has not been infiltrated preoperatively, and patients undergoing large aspirations (greater than 2500 ml) should provide autologous blood preoperatively.

The effective instrument is a blunt cannula. The larger and shorter cannulas remove more fat than smaller or longer ones. Cannulas with multiple holes remove more fat than those with a single hole. Tubing connects the cannula to a vacuum source that produces a pressure of 1 atmosphere. The vacuum pressure extracts the fat into glass collecting containers. Patients must be marked while standing.

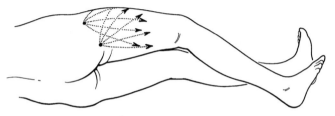

FIGURE 16–14. Cross-tunneling technique for suction lipectomy.

Small stab incisions are placed in hidden creases such as the infrainguinal, gluteal, pubic, periumbilical, and medial popliteal creases. Incisions need be no longer than 0.5 cm, providing enough room to insert the instrument. Once the cannula is inserted into the subcutaneous tissue layer, the vacuum is turned on and multiple tunnels are created by propelling the instrument backward and forward. Multiple tunnels are created in a fan fashion. It is best that any given area be treated from incisions placed in several areas so that a cross-tunneling effect is created (Fig. 16–14).

The amount of fat aspirated is quite subjective and is determined by pinching the aspirated skin and removing fat until the area has been thinned to the desired degree. It is imperative that the area not be oversuctioned, or dimpling and depression result. Postoperatively the patient is placed in a compression garment to be worn continuously for the first several weeks. Depending on the amount of fat suctioned and the quality of skin tone, patients may have to wear the compression garment for up to 6 weeks (Figs. 16–15 and 16–16).

TUMESCENT TECHNIQUE

The tumescent technique has become popular in recent years. The area to be suctioned is infiltrated with 1 liter of saline containing 500 mg lidocaine and 1 mg epinephrine. The engorged tissues are easier to suction, and blood loss is minimal

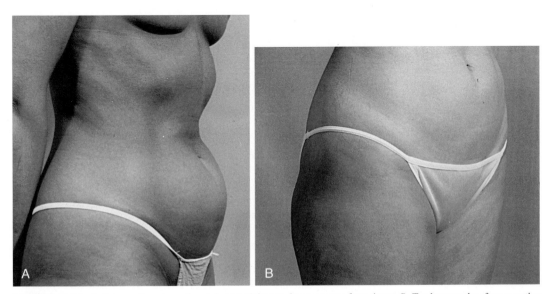

FIGURE 16–15. *A,* Preoperative view of protuberant abdomen due to excess fatty tissue. *B,* Twelve months after operative liposuction of abdominal fat.

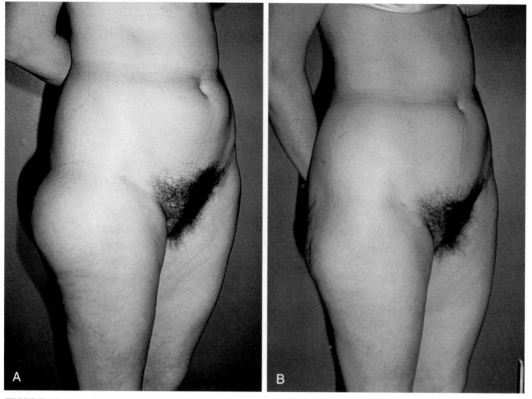

FIGURE 16–16. *A*, Preoperative view of excess fat in the trochanteric distribution. *B*, One year after operative liposuction of the trochanteric regions.

owing to the epinephrine-induced vasoconstriction. This technique enables suction with a finer cannula.

Suggested Reading

Byrd HS, Spicer TE, Cierny G III: Management of open tibial fractures. Plast Reconstr Surg 76:719, 1985

Daniel RK, Faibisoff B: Muscle coverage of pressure points: The role of myocutaneous flaps. Ann Plast Surg 8:446, 1982

Ilizarov GA: Clinical application of the tension-stress effect for limb lengthening. Clin Orthop 250:8, 1990

Illouz Y-G: Body contouring by lipolysis: A 5-year experience with over 3000 cases. Plast Reconstr Surg 75:591, 1983

McGraw JB, Penix JO, Baker JW: Repair of major defects of the chest wall and spine with the latissimus dorsi myocutaneous flap. Plast Reconstr Surg 62:197, 1978

Nahai F, Rand RP, et al: Primary treatment of the infected median sternotomy wound with muscle flaps: A review of 211 consecutive cases. Plast Reconstr Surg 84:433, 1989

Pitanguy I: Aesthetic plastic surgery of the upper and lower limbs. Aesthet Plast Surg 4:363, 1980

Ramirez OM, Ramasastry SS, Granick MS, et al: A new surgical approach to closure of large lumbosacral meningomyelocele defects. Plast Reconstr Surg 80:799, 1987

Regnault P: Abdominoplasty by the W technique. Plast Reconstr Surg 55:265, 1975

CHAPTER 17

Genitourinary System

DEVELOPMENT OF THE UROGENITAL SYSTEM

The development of the urinary tract is related to three distinct sets of excretory apparatus: the pronephros, the mesonephros, and the metanephros.

The pronephros disappears after a brief existence, leaving no trace. The mesonephros and wolffian body consist of several minute tubules embedded in mesoderm which drain directly into the body cavity by developing a long excretory channel within the substance of the wolffian body, which connects its various segments as far as the cloaca.

The wolffian duct provides an important basis for the development of the urinary tract. The definitive kidney has a double origin, being derived from the wolffian duct and the metanephros, which is a mass of tissue at the distal end of the wolffian body. A small bud from the wolffian duct provides the beginning of the primitive ureter, which increases in length in a cephalad direction. By undergoing canalization, it thereby forms the ureter, renal pelvis, calyces, and collecting tubules of the kidney.

The metanephros appears and covers the growing end of the ureter by a nephrogenic cap of tissue. Each unit of kidney is accordingly composed of two elements: metanephric, which produces urine, and mesonephric, which excretes the urine. The two components fuse to provide a continuous unit.

In early development, the kidney lies at the level of the second sacral vertebra in close contact with its fellow but soon migrates in a cephalad direction. At first, the hilum of the kidney is directed anteriorly so that the ureter and vessels enter on this aspect, but during its ascent the kidney rotates so that the hilum assumes its adult position, directed medially. Malrotation may occur so that the hilum is directed laterally.

Congenital malformations of kidney and ureter include the following:

Total agenesis of one kidney. In addition to absence of ureter and kidney, the corresponding half of the bladder trigone is deformed and is so visualized at cystoscopic examination.

Supernumerary ureter or kidney.

Faulty insertion of the ureter due to error in partition of the cloaca. The ureter may open into the male prostatic urethra or into the female vagina, resulting in urinary incontinence.

Failure of renal ascent, remaining in the retrorectal position.

Fusion of kidneys. As a result of crossed ectopia, one kidney may cross over to the opposite side so that both kidneys are fused and are situated on one side of the body.

Horseshoe kidney develops if each kidney lies on its correct side, but they are connected across the front of the aorta by an isthmus of renal parenchyma or fibrous tissue.

Miscellaneous anomalies include congenital stricture of the ureter, congenital hydronephrosis, and polycystic disease of the kidneys.

The Cloaca

The development of the lower urinary tract, the genitalia, and the infraumbilical part of the abdominal wall depends on the normal maturation of the cloaca. The cloaca is a common chamber, with a dilated hindgut dorsally, which extends ventrally into the allantois and caudally into the tailgut.

The wolffian ducts enter the chamber laterally, establishing communication with the urinary tract, while the development of a longitudinal urorectal septum separates the rectum from the urinary bladder. The development of a solid perineal body heralds the creation of a dorsal anal outlet and a ventral urogenital sinus.

The anterior cloacal wall fuses with the ventral abdominal ectoderm, representing the cloacal membrane, and extends over a large segment of the ventral abdominal wall.

By the sixth week of intrauterine life the urinary bladder has developed. At this time, in the female, the müllerian ducts differentiate into uterus and vagina. It is easy to envisage how maldevelopment in this area may give rise to a rectovesical fistula in the male and a rectovaginal fistula in the female.

Exstrophy of the bladder represents a defect in cloacal maturation which affects the anterior abdominal wall and anterior wall of the bladder. Thus, the inside of the bladder is exposed on the abdominal wall without an anterior covering.

The Urethra

The male urethra commences as a genital tubercle that appears at the cranial end of the cloacal membrane and lengthens to form the phallus, which becomes grooved.

Defects in development may result in the following:

Epispadias: The roof of the urethra is incomplete and is usually associated with urinary incontinence. It may occur concomitantly with exstrophy of the bladder.
Hypospadias: Failure in complete formation of the urethra, its orifice terminating on the ventral surface of the penis, either at the level of the scrotum, along the shaft of the penis, or at the glans.
Congenital valves at the vesicourethral junction may cause difficulties in bladder evacuation, with back-pressure changes in the bladder, ureters, and kidneys.

The female urethra is only about 4 centimeters long, lies upon the anterior wall of the vagina, and, after piercing both layers of the urogenital diaphragm, terminates at the external orifice between the labia minora 1 inch beneath the clitoris.

The Genital Tubercle

The genital tubercle is a conical prominence that appears during the sixth week of intrauterine life between the umbilical cord and the tail. On its caudal slope is a median groove between two lateral folds. The genital tubercle elongates to form the phallus, with an expanded end that becomes the glans. If the embryo is a male, this structure represents the primordium of the penis. In the female it becomes the clitoris.

Rupture of the urogenital membrane creates a surface sinus. Genital folds develop on each side of the urogenital sinus and unite over the sinus. Hypospadias results from failure of fusion of these folds. In the female these folds become the labia minora.

A second pair of lateral folds, the genital swellings, develop and fuse in the male to form the scrotum. In the female they become the labia majora.

Fusion of the distal segments of the müllerian ducts leads to formation of the uterus and vagina, which are at first solid but later become canalized.

Normal development of the uterus and failure of canalization of the vagina result in menstrual blood accumulating above the obstruction, the uterus and proximal vagina distending as hematocolpos and hematometra. Further accumulation of blood in the fallopian tubes results in hematosalpinx.

Whereas the fused portions of the müllerian ducts form the uterus and vagina, the unfused portions form the fallopian tubes. Failure of proximal fusion causes the development of a bicornuate uterus, or one half may remain as a rudimentary horn. Failure of distal fusion results in a persistent vaginal septum or vaginal atresia. Portions of the wolffian duct may persist, in the female, as tubular remnants, providing the ducts of Gartner, which may develop into cystic lesions within the broad ligament or in the lateral wall of the cervix or vagina.

The ovaries develop from the germinal ridge on the anterior surface of the mesonephros, which represents the primitive undifferentiated gonads. During the 12th week, they descend to the pelvic brim on the posterior surface of the broad ligament. The round ligament attaches the ovary to the uterus and prevents gonadal descent to the labia majora.

The testes in the male develop from the germinal ridge in close proximity to the wolffian body and its efferent tubules. Persistent rudiments of the wolffian tubules result in the formation of the appendix epididymis and the paradidymis or organ of Giraldes.

At the lower pole of the testis is the gubernaculum testis, a fibromuscular band that extends inferiorly to the lower part of the anterior abdominal wall. During the 12th week of fetal life, the gubernaculum guides testicular descent to the future internal inguinal ring. At this time the processus vaginalis, an evaginated process of peritoneum, descends to the scrotum, and the testis, guided by the gubernaculum, traverses the inguinal canal to reach the scrotum at the ninth month, at which time the peritoneal communication of the processus vaginalis becomes obliterated. Persistence of the processus vaginalis provides the basis of a congenital inguinal hernia, hydrocele of the testis, or hydrocele of the cord.

Anomalous descent of the testis may produce one of the following:

Cryptorchism: The testis is retained in the abdominal retroperitoneal locale.

Undescended testes: There is an arrest in descent within the inguinal canal.

Ectopic testis: The testis descends beyond the external inguinal ring and instead of migrating to the scrotum, migrates along gubernacular fibers to either the front of the symphysis pubis, the thigh, or the perineum.

Retractile testis: The cremasteric action causes retraction of the gonad out of the scrotum. The testis can, however, be held in the scrotum manually. Children with retractile testis do not require surgical intervention, whereas those with the other conditions do.

HYPOSPADIAS

With an incidence of 1 per 300 live male births, this congenital penile deformity is characterized by the urethral meatus being located on the ventral surface of the penis, proximal to its normal position at the tip of the glans. The condition is probably mediated by the intrauterine cessation of androgen production, with incomplete masculinization of the external genitalia.

Associated with hypospadias may be varying degrees of cryptorchism and associated abnormalities of the urinary tract defined by intravenous pyelography. If voiding difficulty occurs, the possibility of vesicourethral valves suggests the need for cystoscopy and cystourethrography.

The classification of hypospadias is best defined by the site of the urethral meatus: perineal, scrotal, penoscrotal, penile, or glans.

Anatomy of Hypospadias

The prepuce at the flattened glans is incomplete, with absence of the ventral surface, creating the illusion of an unduly long, hooded dorsal preputial component. The perineal, scrotal, and penoscrotal varieties of hypospadias are associated with a bifid scrotum and a deep groove of hairless skin between the two sacks.

Although hypospadias may occur without chordee, chordee is an almost invariable companion of hypospadias. The skin on the ventral penile surface distal to the meatus is very thin. The normal dartos fascia, Buck's fascia, and corpus spongiosum are absent and replaced by a fan-shaped band of dense fibrous tissue, named chordee, which causes the penis to curve ventrally.

Chordee is usually absent in the glanular form of hypospadias, which may be simply managed by circumcision and, if necessary, meatotomy. Occasionally chordee is present without hypospadias, justifying excision of the chordee without need for a urethroplasty.

Surgical Repair of Hypospadias

Repair of hypospadias should, ideally, be completed before the child commences school and may be initiated by one and a half to two years of age.

The principles of repair consist of release of the penile curvature due to chordee and urethroplasty to bring the meatus to the tip of the glans.

Based on the surgical report by Duplay, Denis Browne popularized the two-stage repair. After release of chordee as a first stage, urethroplasty was deferred for 6 months. At the second stage a perineal urethrotomy deviated the urinary flow, and a buried strip of skin was used to form a new urethral tube. Incisions on the ventral penile surface extended from the meatus to the glans. The median skin strip would become the new dorsal urethral layer. The lateral skin was undermined and approximated in the midline over a catheter to create the new ventral urethral roof. Any undue tension was relieved by a dorsal relaxing incision. Through-and-through wire sutures through the lateral skin folds were secured by beads and metal stops to relieve tension on the skin edges, which were approximated by interrupted sutures.

Scrotal and perineal hypospadias can be corrected by creating a tube of scrotal skin to advance the meatus to the penile shaft and then at another stage to reconstruct the penile urethra.

One-Stage Repair

The procedure designed by Horton and Devine has the merit of completion at one operative sitting but requires meticulous attention to detail. It consists of resection of chordee, its completion being tested by induction of an erection. The urethroplasty is done by reconstructing the urethra with a full-thickness tubed skin graft obtained from the dorsal foreskin hood. The grafted tube is sutured to the spatulated natural urethral meatus and brought through a tunnel in the glans. The new urethra is then covered with flaps of dorsal skin.

Complications After Hypospadias Repair

Fistula: Prolonged diversion of the urinary stream may permit healing of the fistula. If the fistula persists, a delay of 6 months is recommended before it is repaired.

Meatal stenosis or urethral stricture requires appropriate treatment by either dilation or urethroplastic correction.

EPISPADIAS

In the male, epispadias may vary from the glanular form with a groove on the dorsum of the glans to a complete dorsal cleft involving the entire penile urethra with associated exstrophy of the bladder and diastasis of the symphysis pubis.

The female with epispadias presents with a bifid clitoris and widely spaced labia minora. The urethra opens between or above the two halves of the clitoris.

Examination of the male penis demonstrates the urethral opening on the dorsum, beyond which is a gutter lined by mucosa. The corpora cavernosa are separated, and the prepuce is deficient dorsally with excessive skin ventrally. There is associated dorsal curvature of the penis.

Incontinence is almost invariably present, except in the mildest forms of the abnormality, owing to insufficient or absent development of the sphincteric musculature. Fortunately, the condition is rare, with an incidence of 1 in 30,000 births.

Management has two objectives.

Control of Incontinence. Operative repair of the sphincter mechanism should be attempted. The bladder neck is approached via an incision through the separated symphysis, and the channel is opened. After uncrossing the bladder neck, the lumen is narrowed and any tissue containing muscle fibers is carefully incorporated in the suture. Urinary diversion via a suprapubic cystotomy is carried out until bladder neck healing has occurred.

Failure to establish functional control of incontinence requires the construction of an ileal loop with ureteric transplantation.

Repair of Epispadias. Closure of the dorsal cleft is designed to obtain control of the urinary stream, provide sexual function, and achieve normal appearance. A one-stage repair, which is the mirror-image of hypospadias repair, attains these objectives.

The chordee-like fibrotic dorsal tissue is excised and the urethroplasty carried out by using a tubed fine full-thickness skin graft from the ventral preputial skin. The tube is anastomosed to the urethra, and the separated corpora are approximated over the constructed urethra. Lateral penile and preputial tissue is used for skin coverage, with the new meatal opening brought to its normal position through a tunnel in the glans. Urinary diversion is provided to protect the repair.

EXSTROPHY OF THE BLADDER

This serious abnormality, with absence of the anterior bladder wall, eversion of the mucosa, separation of the symphysis pubis, and urinary incontinence, may cause death from ascending urinary infection or bladder carcinoma.

There are two divergent therapeutic philosophies in the management of these patients, many of whom have other urogenital malformations as well as associated congenital abnormalities such as cleft palate, cleft lip, and anorectal atresia. (1) Reconstruction of bladder with closure of the anterior abdominal wall using the mobilized, rotated rectus abdominis muscles as well as mesh or fascial grafts. Bilateral ilial osteotomies are essential for closure of both the bladder and the abdominal wall, as they allow the symphysis pubis to be approximated. Skin flaps are required to close the external layers of the defect. The epispadias repair is carried out at the same time, with bladder neck reconstruction. (2) Cystectomy with urinary diversion: Because bladder cancer may develop in patients with reconstructed bladders and because bladder reconstructive procedures may be associated with much morbidity and many complications, an alternate approach is to perform early cystectomy, repair of the anterior abdominal wall, and urinary diversion by ileal loop with transplantation of ureters or ureterosigmoidoscopy.

INJURIES TO THE MALE GENITALIA

Contusion injuries of the genitalia usually respond to conservative management until edema resolves. The development of a hematoma requires its evacuation, and urinary diversion or placement of a transurethral catheter may be indicated until healing occurs in a urethral injury. Urinary extravasation indicates the need for cystourethrography and appropriate urologic repair.

Fracture of Penis. Trauma to an erect penis may tear the tunica albuginea and the corpus cavernosum. Evacuation of the hematoma, control of bleeding, and repair of the disrupted fascia and corpus restore the normal penile alignment and prevent its continued angulation.

Avulsion Injuries of Penis and Scrotum. Tissue loss may result from entrapment in moving machinery or as a result of Fournier gangrene of the scrotum.

Residual scrotal skin can be used to cover the penile shaft. Early skin grafting after débridement is preferred with hairless skin harvested from the buttocks. Total loss of scrotal skin can be treated by burying the testes and spermatic cords in superficial pouches within the skin of the upper thighs.

Loss of Penis. Reattachment of a partially or totally amputated penis is practically feasible using microsurgical techniques, with repair of two dorsal veins, the dorsal arteries, and two dorsal nerves. The reapproximation of one or both corpora cavernosa and urethral anastomosis and reapproximation of the tunica albuginea, penile septum, and Buck's fascia should restore penile stability before the skin is sutured.

Indurative Cavernositis. Fibrosis of the tunica albuginea results in pain and curvature of the erect penis. Also known as Peyronie disease, it may be due to a chronic inflammatory process unassociated with trauma. Although spontaneous remission may occur, progression of the process requires surgical relief.

Total excision of the fibrosed tunica albuginea is complemented by placement of a dermal graft to cover the erectile tissues of the corpora cavernosa. This restores normal erection without painful curvature of the penis.

RECONSTRUCTION OF PENIS

Loss of the penis from trauma, thermal or electrical burns, or sex change surgery provide the main indications for phalloplasty. Among the many techniques that have been described, a composite of two procedures has been given pride of place:

The Radial Forearm Flap. The procedure is performed in one stage using a large forearm flap to construct the penis and neourethra. The vascularized structure requires the anastomosis of the radial artery and its veins to the inferior epigastric, pudendal, or femoral vessels. The anastomosis of the cutaneous nerves of forearm in the flap to the internal pudendal nerve provides sensitivity to the part. The glabrous nature of the skin prevents the development of calculi or hair balls in the neourethra. A costal cartilage graft or silicone prosthesis provides stiffening (Fig. 17–1).

An Abdominal Tube Pedicle Flap. The tube flap developed in the lower abdomen is used as an inside-out flap that is covered by a skin graft, adds bulk, and provides a second channel for placement of the stiffener.

PENILE IMPLANTS FOR IMPOTENCE

Loss of erectile-ejaculatory competence has many possible causes: neurogenic, endocrine, vascular, and psychogenic. Once an organic cause for the problem has been established, consideration should be given to the beneficial role of a penile implant.

Types of implant include the following:

Simple rod: Currently a silicone rod can be placed, under local anesthesia, through a dorsal penile incision, within the tunica albuginea between the corpora cavernosa. It does not produce a full erection but permits intercourse. It is useful in the elderly patient.

Solid double rods create a permanent erection. A Small-Carnon device is implanted

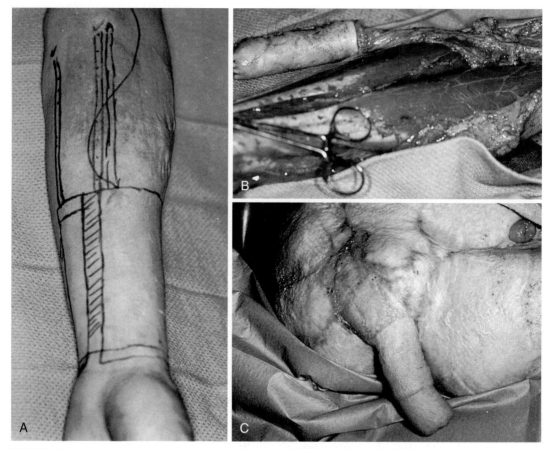

FIGURE 17–1. *A*, Design of the radial forearm flap for reconstruction of the penis. The shaded area will be de-epithelialized and that portion of the flap tubed on itself to create the new urethra. *B*, The flap has been tubed around a catheter to reconstruct the urethra and the flap then folded to create the body of the penis. *C*, Six months after operative reconstruction of the penis.

into each corpus through the crura, using a perineal approach. The procedure may be appropriate in the young patient.

Inflatable prosthesis: The prosthesis consists of a single or double inflatable cylinder placed in the corpora cavernosa. A scrotal pump that can inflate and deflate the cylinders and a fluid reservoir are placed in the prevesical space. The many potential mechanical problems associated with the inflatable prosthesis need to be kept in mind.

SEX IDENTIFICATION

The differences between male and female, based on essential sexual and gender characteristics, are usually easy to enumerate and recognize. Anomalies of genitourinary embryologic development may, at times, create difficulties in correlating sex and gender.

Gender

The transmission of genetic matter is mediated by chromosomes, which are paired collections of DNA found in cell nuclei. The normal chromosomal complement of the human species comprises 22 paired autosomes and 2 sex chromosomes. The essential gender difference is represented by a chromosomal XX pattern in the female and XY in the male. The female ovum carries two X chromosomes, and the spermatozoon harbor an X chromosome and a smaller Y chromosome. An XX combination at fertilization determines female development and XY male development.

Chromatin cell staining can further determine the gender of an individual, as the nuclear chromatin in the female cell contains the Barr body, an area of deep staining which is absent in the male.

Sex

The specific sex of the newborn baby is customarily based on examination of the external genitalia. The proper differentiation of the male secondary sexual characteristics requires the response to stimulation. If inadequate, the resultant hypospadias, small penis, and undescended testicles may suggest that the baby is female. Contrarily, a female child with congenital adrenocortical hyperplasia may present with features of virilism and, although chromatin positive, the hirsutism, large clitoris, and ambiguous external genitalia may, at first sight, be thought to be male.

The diagnosis of intersexuality and definition of pseudohermaphroditism and hermaphroditism may require diligent physical, psychological, chromosomal, and endocrinologic study with gonadal biopsy before a final correlation of gender and sex can be made.

Based on the final diagnosis, early surgical correction may require feminization with construction of a vagina. The desire for masculinization requires phalloplasty and endocrinologic manipulation.

RECONSTRUCTION OF THE VAGINA

Failure of vaginal development may result in the following:

Simple aplasia of the vagina and uterus, although ovaries are present and confirmed by gonadal biopsy.

Atresia of the distal vagina, although proximal vagina and uterus are present and ovaries are normal. This is usually the result of congenital adrenogenital hyperplasia.

There is a short distal vagina but the proximal vagina and uterus are absent. The gonads, either intra-abdominal or inguinal, are testes, proven at biopsy. The syndrome is one of testicular feminization.

Genital deficiencies: Attributable to rare chromosomal aberrations, Klinefelter syndrome, Turner syndrome, and other forms of genitourinary intersexuality.

In addition, patients who have an overwhelming desire to be of the opposite sex—that is, express trans-sexual urges—may, after due and careful consideration, be candidates for emasculation and vaginal construction.

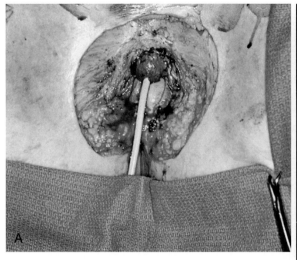

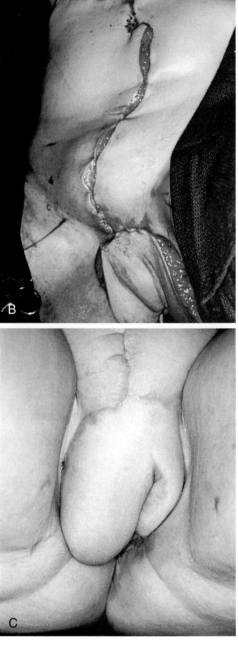

FIGURE 17–2. *A,* The patient has undergone vulvectomy and resection of the vagina and distal portion of the urethra for invasive vulvar carcinoma. *B,* A transverse rectus abdominis myocutaneous flap has been elevated on the inferior deep epigastric vessels and transposed to the perineum. *C,* The flap has been used to reconstruct the vulva, vagina, and distal urethra.

Vaginal Agenesis. Under general anesthesia, with the patient in the lithotomy position, a bladder catheter is placed and a pack placed in the rectum for its later identification. An inverted V-shaped incision is made in the perineum extending from 2 cm behind the urethral meatus to 2 cm in front of the rectum. The labia minora and majora are sutured together and retracted and the fourchette is divided. Blunt dissection is initiated, and a cavity is created between bladder and rectum which is able to accommodate an acrylic mold of suitable size and shape. The mold is covered with a thin tubed skin graft taken from the thigh or buttock and inserted into the cavity. The perineal wound is then repaired in layers. After 6 months the mold can be removed, the patient having been taught how to change it.

Acquired Perineal Defects. Patients requiring vaginal reconstruction after resection for cancer are best managed with flap transfer. A groin flap and medial thigh flaps may be used, but patients are best managed with myocutaneous flap transfer. These flaps adequately eliminate dead space, reconstruct the pelvic floor, and provide skin for vaginal reconstruction. Bilateral gracilis flaps or the inferiorly based rectus abdominis flap with a transverse skin paddle is ideally suited to reconstruct perineal defects following pelvic exenteration (Fig. 17–2).

Suggested Reading

Chang T-S, Hwang W-Y: Forearm flap in one-stage reconstruction of the penis. Plast Reconstr Surg 74:251, 1984

Hendren WH, Donahoe PK: Correction of congenital abnormalities of the vagina and perineum. J Pediatr Surg 15:751, 1980

Tobin GR, Day TG: Vaginal and pelvic reconstruction with distally based rectus abdominis myocutaneous flaps. Plast Reconstr Surg 81:62, 1988

Vorstman B, Horton CE, Devine CJ Jr: Current hypospadias techniques. Ann Plast Surg 18:164, 1987

CHAPTER 18

The Hand and Upper Limb

The structural and functional complexities of the hand, the number of clinical conditions affecting it, and its capacity for function and fine movement emphasize the importance of the surgeon's role in planning reconstructive operations on the hand.

The functional elements of the hand may be divided into four categories of specialization:

The thumb and its metacarpal: The evolution of a highly specialized opposable thumb, with a large central element, distinguishes the human hand from that of other species. Five intrinsic and four extrinsic muscles are specifically involved in controlling thumb activity and position.

The index finger: This finger is capable of independent action, within the range of motion allowed by its joints and ligaments, by virtue of three intrinsic and four extrinsic muscles.

The middle (long), ring, and little finger: With the fourth and fifth metacarpals, these fingers collaborate as a single unit in grasping objects for fine manipulation by thumb and index finger or in concert with the other units in a powerful grasp.

The fixed hand unit: Comprising the distal row of carpal bones and the second and third metacarpals, this unit creates a fixed transverse arch of carpal bones and a fixed longitudinal arch by the anatomic convexity of the metacarpals.

THE WRIST

Surgical Anatomy of the Radiocarpal or Wrist Joint

This joint exists between the lower end of the radius and the articular disc proximally and the first row of carpal bones distally, represented by the scaphoid, lunate, and triquetral bones, firmly held together by their ligaments, presenting a continuous articular surface. The joint capsules are weak anteriorly and posteriorly but strong laterally, where they are reinforced by ligamentous consolidation representing radial collateral and ulnar collateral ligaments. The former is attached to the styloid process of the radius proximally and to the lateral side of the scaphoid distally. The latter is attached to the ulnar styloid proximally and to the medial side of the pisiform distally.

At the radiocarpal joint or wrist joint proper, flexion is possible to about 70 degrees and extension to about 60 degrees with the forearm. A great part of this movement occurs at the midcarpal joint. Lateral movement is less extensive, abduction representing movement to the radial side and adduction movement to the ulnar side (Fig. 18–1).

Carpal Bone Injuries

SCAPHOID FRACTURES

These result from falls on the hyperextended outstretched hand, which, if not adequately immobilized, may result in non-union.

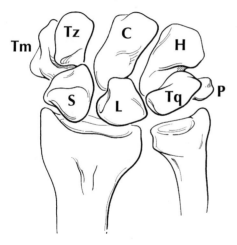

FIGURE 18–1. The carpal bones form three vertical columns. The scaphoid (S), trapezium (Tm), and trapezoid (Tz) form the radial (stabilizing) column, the lunate (L) and capitate (C) form the central (flexion-extension) column, and the hamate (H), triquetrum (Tq), and pisiform (P) form the ulnar (rotation) column. The carpal bones also form a distinct distal row, including the trapezium, trapezoid, capitate, and hamate, and a proximal row, including the scaphoid, lunate, triquetrum, and pisiform.

The *tuberosity of the scaphoid* may rarely suffer fracture, but the fracture is usually stable and undisplaced and heals after 8 to 10 weeks of immobilization.

Fracture through the *waist of the scaphoid* is the most common form of fracture. It is often the result of a trans-scaphoid–perilunate dislocation that has spontaneously reduced. Severe associated ligamentous damage usually occurs. The condition should be suspected if pain, swelling, and tenderness are present over the scaphoid in the anatomic snuffbox, associated with limitation of movement.

Radiologic examination of the area should be taken with several views to visualize the fracture, which may not always be apparent. Plaster immobilization should be instituted and repeat radiologic examination several weeks later may reveal the fracture line. Failure to immobilize the joint leads to non-union and subsequent development of osteoarthritis of the wrist joint.

Fracture of the *proximal pole of the scaphoid* may be associated with its avascular necrosis and subsequent arthritis. Treatment of scaphoid fractures requires adequate immobilization until union occurs. Open reduction and internal fixation are necessary for persistent displacement, carpal instability, scaphoid fracture associated with carpal dislocation, and non-union after adequate immobilization.

DISLOCATION OF THE LUNATE

A fall on the hyperextended wrist may cause anterior dislocation of the lunate, trans-scaphoid perilunate dislocation, and perilunate dislocation with scaphoid rotation.

Displacement of the lunate anteriorly may cause compression of the median nerve where it is confined by the transverse carpal ligament, resulting in paresthesia of the palmar surface of the index and middle fingers.

Diagnosis requires multiple radiographic views of the wrist, with the lateral views providing the significant position of the lunate.

Treatment with manipulative reduction, under general anesthesia, is usually successful if achieved early. With anterior dislocation of the lunate, the carpus must be manipulated posteriorly so that the lunate is reduced on the articular surface of the radius, and with traction applied to the hand the carpus is replaced upon the lunate. Prolonged immobilization of the wrist for 8 to 10 weeks provides time for healing of the ligamentous disruption. If there is delay in diagnosis, manipulative treatment may be unsuccessful, and open reduction of the dislocated lunate, if it still retains a blood supply, is required via a dorsal or volar approach.

TRANS-STYLOID RADIOCARPAL DISLOCATION

Stability of the joint, after manipulative reduction, may be achieved only by internal fixation of the radial styloid process. If the articular surfaces of the joint have been seriously damaged and radiocarpal ankylosis does not develop, then fusion of the joint becomes necessary.

THE HAND

SURFACE ANATOMY

With the wrist flexed, the scaphoid and lunate bones may be felt as dorsal prominences adjacent to the curved line, which creates the radial articulation. Similarly, the capitate bone may be felt, as well as its articulation with the base of the third metacarpal bone. The dorsal surfaces of the metacarpal bones are covered by the extensor tendons but can be palpated, and the prominences of the knuckles are formed by the expanded heads of the metacarpal bones (Fig. 18–2).

With the metacarpophalangeal joints flexed, the joint line may be felt dorsally about 0.5 inch distal to the prominence of the knuckle, and, similarly, the proximal interphalangeal joint may be felt 0.25 inch distal to the prominence formed by the head of the first phalanx with the joint flexed. On the palmar surface of the hand, the metacarpophalangeal joint lies midway between the webs of the fingers and the more distal of two transverse palmar creases.

The palm of the hand forms a concavity lying between two elevations: the thenar eminence, which is the lateral eminence formed by the short muscles of

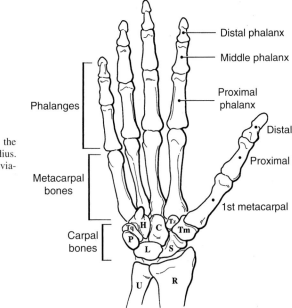

FIGURE 18–2. The bones of the hand and wrist. (U) ulna, (R) radius. See Figure 18–1 for other abbreviations.

the thumb, and the hypothenar eminence, formed by the short muscles of the little finger.

The position of the superficial palmar arch may be marked on the surface by a line extending from the lateral side of the pisiform bone, curving laterally across the middle third of the palm in a line with the outstretched thumb. The deep palmar arch lies upon the metacarpal bones about 1.25 cm nearer the wrist than the superficial arch.

THE SKIN AND SUPERFICIAL FASCIA

The skin on the dorsum of the hand is thick and freely movable, whereas on the palm it is densely adherent to the palmar aponeurosis, being devoid of hair follicles.

The superficial fascia is extremely dense and is traversed by numerous fibrous septa, which closely unite the skin to the underlying palmar fascia. As a result, in infections of the hand and fingers, inflammatory edema becomes more apparent on the dorsum even if the basic inflammatory focus is in the palm of the hand.

Over the tips of the fingers, the superficial fascia is known as the pulp and is closely connected by fibrous septa to the periosteum or the terminal phalanx.

A pulp space infection, called a felon, may result in the development of a great amount of local tension, with avascular destruction of the tip of the terminal phalanx, but the base of that phalanx, which receives blood supply from the vessel running with the flexor digitorum profundus, usually remains unaffected. Thus, early incision and evacuation of pus are essential.

THE FLEXOR RETINACULUM

This is a strong band of deep fascia, also known as the transverse carpal ligament, which binds down the flexor tendons of the fingers at the wrist. It is attached medially to the pisiform and the hook of the hamate bones and laterally to the tuberosity of the scaphoid and the ridge of the trapezium.

Proximally, it is continuous with the deep fascia of the forearm, and distally it merges with the palmar aponeurosis. The palmaris longus tendon and ulnar vessels and nerve lie superficial to it.

THE PALMAR APONEUROSIS

This is a strong layer of deep fascia in the palm which has its apex at the wrist but expands toward the fingers, covering nearly the whole palm of the hand. Proximally the aponeurosis receives the tendon of the palmaris longus and is connected to the flexor retinaculum.

Distally, it divides into four processes that continue as the fibrous flexor sheaths of the fingers. Each fibrous flexor sheath terminates just beyond the insertion of the flexor digitorum profundus, where it blends with the periosteum of the terminal phalanx.

From the margins of the palmar aponeurosis, two lateral fascial layers, which are rather thin and weak, spread out to cover the muscles of the thenar and hypothenar eminences, respectively.

The palmaris brevis is a small, flat muscle about 3 to 4 cm wide which arises from the palmar aponeurosis, its fibers being directed transversely to their insertion into the skin at the medial border of the hand. The muscle covers the ulnar vessels and nerve, receiving its innervation from the ulnar nerve. It wrinkles the skin on the ulnar side of the palm.

Dupuytren contracture is a disease of the palmar aponeurosis and its digital prolongation. It is due to the progressive conversion of the palmar fascia into fibrous tissue. It involves the longitudinal layers of the fascia, including the pretendinous bands, natatory ligaments, spiral bands, and Grayson ligaments. The cause is unknown, although constitutional predisposition may induce a familial incidence. It usually appears after the age of 40 years, being more common in males than females. It may be bilateral in 50 per cent of cases.

The condition commences as a firm nodule at the base of the ring finger and spreads on the ulnar side of the hand into the ring and little fingers. Rarely, all the fingers become affected, or it may affect the thumb first. The fibrotic process progresses slowly, with early involvement of the overlying skin. Nodules gradually coalesce until the skin is bound down to the fascia over a wide area. The fingers undergo contracture, with the joints ultimately becoming rigid with disuse. Treatment should be instituted when flexion of the metacarpophalangeal joint commences and not delayed until the deformity becomes well established.

Although massage and passive stretching may permit elderly patients to maintain reasonable function without operation, surgical amelioration provides the only definitive treatment. Surgical options include the following:

Fasciotomy: This provides simple division of a contracting band without the removal of any tissue. The procedure is appropriate only for an elderly individual with a limited life span, as it releases the metacarpophalangeal deformity for only a limited period of time.

Regional fasciectomy: The procedure is aimed at excision of the identifiable elements of the contracting tissue from each flexed joint as well as the palm. Through a longitudinal incision, the deformity is corrected by the removal of the pathologic tissue from the midpalm to the crease line beyond the last flexed joint.

Extensive fasciectomy: Through a zig-zag palmar incision, skin flaps are raised and the palmar aponeurosis is excised, with total digital clearance to remedy the interphalangeal deformities. The latter clearance requires additional longitudinal incisions over the affected digits.

Dermofasciectomy: In patients with recurrence of deformity or a strong diathesis with skin infiltration, excision of the area with a free graft replacement may be indicated.

Ectopic pads or Dupuytren tissue may develop over the dorsum of the interphalangeal and metacarpophalangeal joints. These may require excision of the knuckle pads with placement of a split-thickness skin graft.

Flexor Surface

Along each finger the flexor tendons are retained in place against the phalanges by a fibrous flexor sheath. Opposite the center of the proximal and middle phalanges the sheath is strengthened by a fibrous band, but opposite the joint it consists of a thin layer.

Under cover of the flexor retinaculum at the wrist, the flexor tendons of the fingers are surrounded by a common synovial sheath that projects proximally into the forearm for about 2.5 cm and distally into the palm of the hand as far as the level of the distal border of the outstretched thumb.

The synovial sheath sends a prolongation into the fibrous flexor sheath of the little finger. A separate synovial sheath belonging to the tendon of the flexor pollicis longus is also in continuity from wrist to thumb. The synovial sheaths of the index, middle, and ring fingers are separated from those at the wrist, commencing opposite the heads of the metacarpal bones. The *common palmar bursa* is the name given to the common synovial sheath extending from the forearm down to the palm.

The swelling, due to distention of the bursa, is constricted in its middle by the transverse carpal ligament, resulting in fluctuation from above to below that structure.

INFECTIONS OF THE PALM

Most tendon sheath infections of the palm are the result of spread from the fingers as a suppurative tenosynovitis (Fig. 18–3).

The palmar bursa: Spread to the palmar bursa usually occurs by extension of infection along the tendon sheath of the little finger, although direct infection from the palm via a breach of its integuments is possible.

The radial bursa: This represents extension of infection along the tendon sheath of the flexor pollicis longus to the palmar portion of the sheath, which is defined as the radial bursa.

The treatment of these infections includes antibiotic therapy and incision of the appropriate tendon sheath with evacuation of the pus.

The spread of hand infection may extend beyond the confines of the synovial membrane sheaths and invade the cellular tissue of the palm deep to the flexor tendons. Two spaces exist in this area.

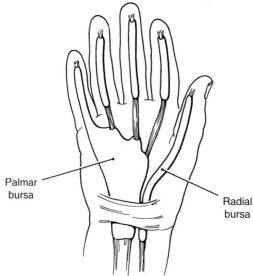

FIGURE 18–3. The palmar and radial bursae of the hand.

Palmar bursa

Radial bursa

The midpalmar space of Kanavel lies deep to the flexor tendons, their synovial sheaths, and the lumbrical muscles of the three medial fingers. It is bounded on the ulnar side by the fifth metacarpal bone, and on the radial side it is separated from the adjacent thenar space by a thin septum attached to the palmar aspect of the third metacarpal bone. The space extends up into the forearm for about 2.5 cm and is situated in front of the pronator quadratus muscle, as the space of Parona, terminating distally in three diverticula that extend along the lumbrical muscles.

Purulent infection in this space points along the tendons of the lumbrical muscles to the interdigital web, where incisions for draining the midpalmar space are made.

The thenar space is bounded in front by the thenar muscles and the thinner portion of the palmar fascia, whereas its floor is composed of the adductor pollicis and part of the first dorsal interosseous muscle. On its radial side it is bounded by the first metacarpal bone, and on its ulnar side it is separated from the midpalmar space by the fibrous septum.

The space is best drained by an incision along the dorsal surface and radial side of the shaft of the second metacarpal bone; a dissector is then passed into the thenar space.

FLEXOR TENDON INJURY

Changing concepts in the surgical repair of tendon injuries have led to a preference for primary tendon repair over delayed repair, subject to the following conditions:

The procedure is performed under ideal conditions by a trained hand surgeon.

The advantages of primary tendon repair include early restoration of the tendon to its normal length, reduction in the period of disability, and reduced incidence of joint stiffness.

Where the operating conditions are less than ideal or there is lack of expertise in the field, delayed primary flexor tendon repair best serves the patient's interest.

Because tendon repair requires an appreciation of pulley anatomy and tendon vascular supply, it is convenient to categorize flexor tendon injuries into their various anatomic zones (Fig. 18–4).

Zone I extends from the insertion of the superficial flexor on the middle phalanx to the insertion of the flexor digitorum profundus on the distal phalanx.

Zone II is often defined as the "critical zone" or "no-man's land." It is the area where the sublimis and profundus tendons run together in the flexor sheath. It commences at the A1 pulley in the palm and reaches the insertion of the sublimis tendon at the base of the second phalanx.

Zone III represents the palm or lumbrical muscle area.

Zone IV is the carpal tunnel.

Zone V is proximal to the carpal tunnel.

Zone I Tendon Repair. The profundus insertion may be avulsed from the insertion by forced extension with the digit flexed. Early repair prevents hyperextension of the distal phalanx and restores distal interphalangeal flexion. Delayed primary repair can be done equally successfully.

Reinsertion of the profundus tendon can be done by advancing the tendon, if

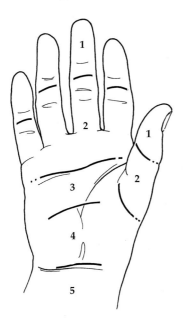

FIGURE 18–4. The flexor tendon zones.

the laceration is within proximity of the insertion. Advancement of a greater distance causes flexion contracture of the joint. The reinsertion can be done by raising a distal osteoperiosteal flap. The proximal tendon stump is passed through the pulley and maintained in position by a stainless steel suture that transfixes the distal phalanx and emerges through the nail, where it is tied over a buttress for removal 5 weeks later. Reinforcing fine sutures are placed between the distal tendon stump and the tendon.

Clean transaction of the tendon in Zone I is repaired by direct tendon anastomosis, as in Zone II repair.

Zone II Tendon Repair. The juxtaposition of the superficial and deep tendons in a narrow fibro-osseous canal led, in the past, to the recommendation that primary treatment involve only skin suture. At a later date, restoration of active flexion was mediated by tendon grafting.

It is currently recommended that, in sharp tendon lacerations, primary repair be directed to both tendons because it provides better functional results. If, however, the tendons are badly contused or mutilated, only the profundus tendon should be repaired, the distal stump of sublimis being left undisturbed so as not to compromise the vincular blood supply to the profundus tendon.

The tendons can be approached via a midaxial or a zig-zag incision. In elevating the tendon sheath, the essential pulley system should be preserved.

The retracted tendon ends are retrieved and approximated by flexing all the appropriate joints and carefully trimmed and sutured by either the modified Bunnell or the Kessler technique without tension (Fig. 18–5). The margins of the tendon juncture are then approximated by a continuous fine suture. The tendon sheath is repaired, thereby covering the tendon and preventing adhesion formation.

After dressings are applied to the wound, a dorsal plaster cast is applied from forearm to fingertips with the wrist in moderate flexion. The metacarpophalangeal and interphalangeal joints are flexed, and rubber bands may be attached to the fingernails by transfixion sutures and to the dressings at the wrist. This permits dynamic finger extension against resistance. Alternatively, early passive range of motion without rubber band tension is initiated postoperatively.

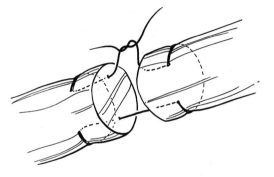

FIGURE 18–5. The modified Kessler repair is one of several popular techniques for the repair of a flexor tendon.

If multiple structures are injured in Zone II, each structure should be repaired primarily; fractures should be stabilized with Kirschner wires; and digital vessels and nerves are repaired as the final maneuver, using the operating microscope.

Zone III Tendon Repair. Primary repair begins with bony fixation and interosseous muscle repair. Both superficial and deep flexor tendons are repaired, followed by vessel and nerve repair.

Zone IV Tendon Repair. Lacerations in the carpal tunnel area may suffer associated ulnar and median nerve and arterial injuries. If possible, primary repair of all the structures in the area is accomplished.

Zone V Tendon Repair. All structures are repaired in standard fashion.

The Flexor Tendon Pulley System. A study of the flexor retinaculum in the fingers defines five annular (A) and three circular (C) pulleys that are important biomechanically in keeping each tendon applied to the phalanges and thereby promote efficient digital motion (Fig. 18–6).

The five annular pulleys are sturdy and are located as follows:

A1 is situated over the metacarpophalangeal joint.
A2 is a long pulley covering the tendon over the proximal half of the first phalanx.

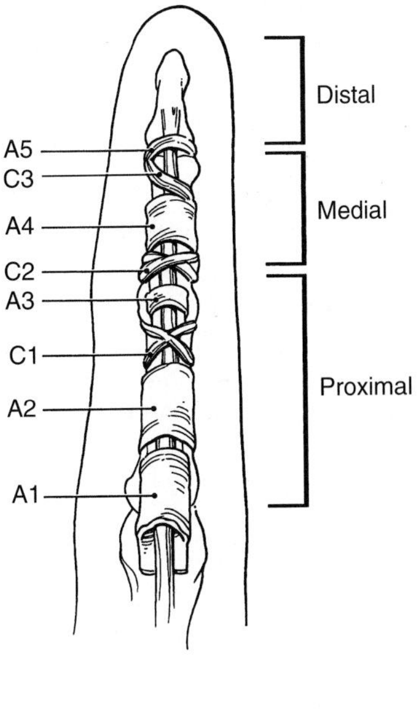

FIGURE 18–6. The pulley mechanism of the finger flexor tendons. There are five annular pulleys and three cruciate pulleys.

A3 is located over the proximal interphalangeal joint.
A4 is over the middle of the middle phalanx.
A5 is over the base of the distal phalanx.

The three thin, pliable cruciate pulleys provide flexibility to the tendon sheaths while retaining their integrity.

C1 is located between A2 and A3.
C2 is located between A3 and A4.
C3 is located between A4 and A5.

Because normal flexor tendon function requires the presence of a pulley system, injury or surgical disruption of the system impairs function. At a minimum, the A2 and A4 pulleys are needed. Pulley reconstruction can be accomplished by using a strip of tendon which is tunneled through fibro-osseous holes created on either side of the volar phalangeal surface so as to roof over the flexor tendons.

A strip of the palmaris longus or extensor digiti minimi tendon provides a sturdy replacement of the pulley and is sutured in place at the time of tenolysis.

Flexor Tendon Grafting. At the present time primary repair or delayed primary repair is recommended as the main objective in the management of flexor tendon injuries. If such repair, within its digital sheath, is not possible because of mutilation of the tendon, then tendon grafting becomes necessary. Success in tendon grafting requires an uninfected wound with good skeletal alignment and a full range of passive joint motion.

Donor tendons that may be harvested for grafting include the palmaris longus, the plantaris, a slip of the extensor digiti minimi, and the extensor digitorum longus tendons to the second, third, or fourth toes.

Surgical exposure of the site to be grafted is gained by a midaxial or zig-zag volar incision. Dissection around the digital sheath should be minimal. All tendon junctures must clear the sheath, with sutures placed at the distal phalanx and proximally in the palm or forearm through a separate incision.

At the completion of the grafting procedure the grafted finger should be in slight flexion, but it should be capable of extension when the wrist is fully flexed.

Staged Tendon Grafting. If a severely damaged digit is extensively scarred and contracted, the excision of scar tissue, release of contractures, and reconstruction of the pulley system should be performed as a first stage. At this time a Silastic rod of appropriate size is inserted as a space maintainer. A new sheath forms around the rod and provides a gliding bed for the tendon graft when it is placed. The Silastic rod is inserted beneath the pulleys and is sutured distally to the stump of the profundus tendon. The proximal end can be left unattached in the palm or forearm.

The second stage is delayed for 3 months, by which time tissue reaction has subsided and joint mobility has been restored. Only the proximal and distal areas where tendon suture will be accomplished need to be exposed. The rod is removed and replaced with the tendon graft.

The Thumb Flexor. The flexor pollicis longus, after its origin from the anterior surface of the radius and interosseous membrane, becomes tendinous at the wrist and continues under cover of the flexor retinaculum, where it enters its fibrous flexor sheath and is inserted into the base of the distal phalanx of the thumb.

Most injuries to the tendon occur at the interphalangeal crease, where primary repair can usually be performed. At the time of tendon suture, its sheath is resected widely to 1 cm beyond the excursion area of the thickened tendon at the site of its suture. More proximal injuries, whether in the region of the metacarpal pulley or in the area of the thenar eminence, may be amenable to primary or delayed primary tendon suture. If the lesion is in the vicinity of the A1 pulley, the latter should be excised widely.

Stenosing Digital Tenosynovitis. Also known as trigger finger, this condition is due to a focal narrowing of the flexor sheath, generally at the A1 pulley, resulting in a caliber discrepancy between the tendon and its sheath. There is a progressive inflammation and swelling around the tendon, impairing tendon excursion. Eventually, the tendon cannot glide through the pulley and it locks in flexion. A congenital trigger thumb may occur in young children. The underlying pathologic basis of the condition in adults may be caused by trauma, granulomatous inflammation, or rheumatoid disease.

Although anti-inflammatory agents or cortisone injection may be helpful in the early stage, once the trigger state develops, surgical relief is required.

Under regional or local block anesthesia with tourniquet hemostatic control, the pathologic area is approached by a longitudinal or oblique incision on the distal palm. The superficial and deep flexor tendons and sheaths are exposed and the A1 pulley is divided.

Extensor Tendons

The subcutaneous course of the extensor tendons over the dorsum of the wrist, hand, and fingers makes them very vulnerable to injury.

The forearm extensor muscles are arranged in a superficial and a deep layer. The superficial layer consists of seven muscles placed in the following order, from radial to ulnar side: brachioradialis, extensor carpi radialis longus, extensor carpi radialis brevis, extensor digitorum communis, extensor digiti minimi, extensor carpi ulnaris, and anconeus, which is continuous with the fibers of the triceps muscle. The extensor tendons to the wrist and digits pass through one of six compartments (Fig. 18–7).

The deep layer on the back of the forearm consists of five muscles innervated by the posterior interosseous nerve: the supinator, the abductor pollicis longus, the extensor pollicis brevis, the extensor pollicis longus, and the extensor indicis proprius.

THE EXTENSOR EXPANSION

The extensor digitorum communis has its origins from the common extensor tendon of the lateral epicondyle and from the adjacent fascia. In the distal part of the forearm, the muscle ends in four tendons, which pass through the fourth compartment of the extensor retinaculum in company with the extensor indicis proprius, to be inserted at the base of the proximal phalanges of the fingers. The muscle is supplied by the posterior interosseous branch of the radial nerve and is the main extensor of the metacarpophalangeal joints of the fingers.

On the dorsum of the proximal phalanx, each tendon forms an extensor expansion, which receives the tendons of insertion of the lumbrical and interosseous muscles, whose functions include flexion of the metacarpophalangeal joints and extension of the interphalangeal joints.

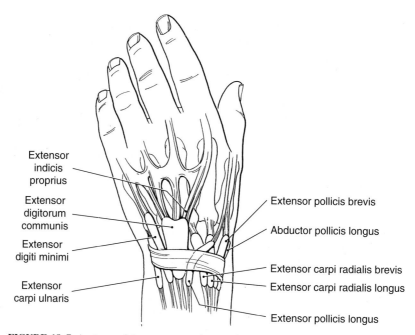

Extensor
indicis
proprius

Extensor
digitorum
communis

Extensor
digiti minimi

Extensor
carpi ulnaris

Extensor pollicis brevis

Abductor pollicis longus

Extensor carpi radialis brevis

Extensor carpi radialis longus

Extensor pollicis longus

FIGURE 18–7. Anatomy of the extensor tendons as they pass through their respective tunnels.

At the lower end of the proximal phalanx, the expansion divides into three parts—a central segment that is fixed to the base of the middle phalanx and the two lateral segments, which re-unite and continue to be inserted into the base of the distal phalanx. As a result, injury to an extensor tendon may not demonstrate an immediate deficit, becoming apparent only after a lapse of some days as intact components of the extensor system begin to weaken.

Tenosynovitis. Excessive use of wrist and fingers may induce tenosynovitis, which may require splint immobilization of the wrist joint.

De Quervain Disease. A stenosing tenosynovitis may involve the sheaths over the abductor pollicis longus and the extensor pollicis brevis as they lie over the distal radius. It is more common in women and is due to overuse syndromes. It is characterized by severe pain on flexion and adduction of the thumb, especially if the hand is pronated and flexed (Finklestein sign).

Tenderness, crepitus, and a vague fullness over the area are present. Radiologic examination excludes any bone or joint abnormality, although calcific tendinitis may, on occasion, be noted. Injection of steroid solution and splinting the wrist and thumb may provide some relief in mild and moderate cases.

Excision of the thickened sheath is performed via a skin incision overlying the fibro-osseous canal in which the tendons are situated. Great care is taken to avoid injury to the superficial sensory branch of the radial nerve.

Rupture of Extensor Pollicis Longus Tendon. An old Colles fracture of the lower radius or the presence of rheumatoid arthritis may cause excessive friction of this tendon as it lies over the wrist joint, with rupture of the tendon. Loss of extension of the interphalangeal joint of the thumb requires suture repair of the tendon. If primary repair is not possible, the extensor indicis proprius may be transferred to the extensor pollicis longus.

Mallet Finger. This deformity results from injury, either open or closed, to an extensor tendon distal to the proximal interphalangeal joint. The patient is totally or partially unable to extend the distal interphalangeal joint, with flexion at the joint due to continuous and uncompensated action of the long flexor. An open transection of the tendon should be treated by immediate primary tendon repair and splinting of the finger for about 6 weeks.

Closed mallet deformity is due to avulsion of the extensor tendon from its insertion by a sudden forced flexion of the distal phalanx. There may be an associated intraarticular fracture of the dorsal lip of the distal phalanx, which may require surgical exploration with fixation of the reduced fracture with a Kirschner wire. A closed mallet deformity without fracture is splinted with the distal interphalangeal joint in slight hyperextension for a period of 6 to 8 weeks.

Boutonniere Deformity. This deformity is represented by flexion of the proximal interphalangeal joint and hyperextension of the distal interphalangeal joint. It results from untreated disruption of the central slip of the extensor tendon at the level of the proximal interphalangeal joint (Fig. 18–8).

With the disruption of the central slip, the two lateral bands become displaced volarly, aggravating the deforming flexion force on the proximal interphalangeal joint and increasing the hyperextension on the distal interphalangeal joint. If neglected, ligamentous contraction creates a fixed deformity, so that passive extension of the proximal joint and flexion of the distal joint are lost.

If the cause is an open injury, primary suture repair is carried out immediately and the finger splinted for about 6 weeks with the proximal interphalangeal joint extended. Closed injuries are customarily treated by appropriate splinting, having been caused by avulsion of the central extensor slip by forced flexion of the joint. If there is an associated avulsion fracture, then Kirschner wire fixation, after operative reduction, is indicated.

In a long-standing chronic deformity, capsulectomy and release of the joint ligaments become necessary, followed by transfer of one or both lateral bands to the central slip.

General Injuries. Injury at the metacarpophalangeal joint level results in inability to fully extend the proximal phalanx. If the underlying joint capsule has been penetrated, it should be repaired, the continuity of the extensor mechanism restored by suture, and the finger splinted.

Tendon injury over the dorsum of the hand should be repaired as soon as it is diagnosed and the part splinted for 6 to 8 weeks. Extensor tendon injury in the

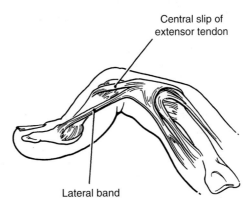

FIGURE 18–8. The boutonniere deformity is characterized by flexion of the proximal interphalangeal joint with extension of the distal interphalangeal joint.

Central slip of extensor tendon

Lateral band

forearm may involve the tendon or the musculotendinous junction. Repair of tendons should be complemented by preservation or repair of the extensor retinaculum to prevent bow-stringing of the repaired tendons.

Repair of the musculotendinous compartment in the forearm should be done as soon as possible, before shortening of the contracting muscle belly occurs. The fascia over this area should be closed separately, thereby creating a satisfactory soft tissue bed so that the repaired musculotendinous unit can glide smoothly.

Soft Tissue Lacerations

Simple lacerations of the hand and digits, uncomplicated by involvement of any other structures, are treated by débridement of wound edges, irrigation of the wound, and careful suture. In general, if associated structures are involved, the pattern of management is débridement of the wound, osseous stabilization, restoration of vascular flow, and tendon repair.

Fingertip Injuries

The nature of the reconstructive response depends upon the amount of tissue lost. Whereas amputations through the level of the distal interphalangeal joint require microvascular replantation, lesser degrees of soft tissue loss or even loss of a small amount of distal phalanx may be treated by replacement of the block of composite tissue that suffered the amputation.

Local flaps may be used to cover a digital tip defect with exposed bone (Fig. 18–9):

Hueston flap is a local axial flap with an intact neurovascular bundle. It provides good coverage for the exposed tip, whereas a full-thickness graft is used to cover the donor site at the base of the digit.

Kutler lateral advancement flap is created by inverted triangular flaps that are raised on either side of the affected fingertip. After the flaps are undermined and mobilized, they are sutured to the distal part of the nail bed.

Atasoy-Kleinert volar advancement flap is a single triangular flap raised from the volar fingertip tissue and sufficiently mobilized to permit its advancement. After the bony phalanx is contoured and the nail trimmed, the flap is sutured to the nail bed over the defect.

Moberg volar advancement flap is formed by bilateral lateral digital incisions that mobilize a neurovascular pedicled volar flap. The flap can be advanced to cover the tip defect.

Littler island transfer flap can be raised from a digit and transposed via a subcutaneous tunnel to cover a defect of the thumb.

Holevich flap can be raised as a radially innervated flap from the dorsum of the index finger to cover a thumb defect. The residual donor defect is covered by a split-thickness skin graft.

Noninnervated regional flaps include the laterally based cross-finger flap, with transposition of a dorsal flap from an adjacent digit to a volar defect. The donor area is covered by a skin graft. Similarly, a distally based cross-finger flap of the adjacent digit can be used to cover a fingertip defect.

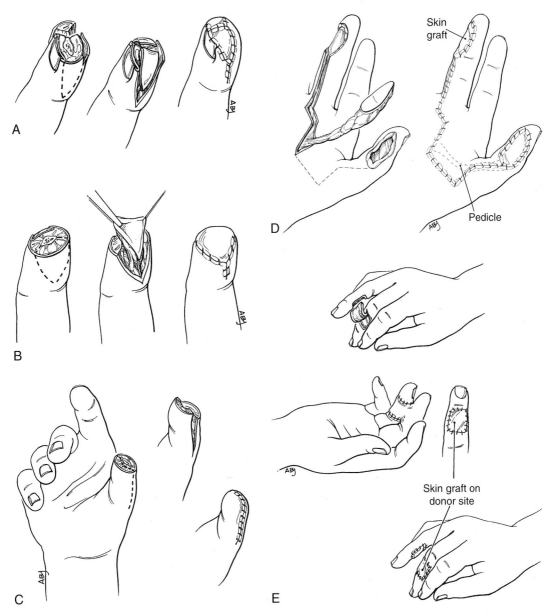

FIGURE 18–9. Local flaps for closure of fingertip injury. *A,* Kutler lateral advancement flap. *B,* Atasoy-Kleinert volar advancement flap. *C,* Moberg volar advancement flap. *D,* Littler island flap. *E,* Cross-finger flap.

A distally based thenar flap can be raised on the thenar eminence and the index or middle fingertip apposed to it for coverage. Flexion contracture of the proximal interphalangeal joint in the elderly limits this procedure to younger patients.

Coverage of hand defects can be accomplished by the use of a reversed radial forearm flap or ulnar forearm flap; use of distant pedicle flaps: anterior chest wall flaps, abdominal flaps, or groin flap; and use of free flaps: radial and ulnar forearm flaps, lateral arm flap based on the posterior radial collateral branch of the profunda brachii artery, or temporoparietal fascia free flap based on the superficial temporal vessels.

The Thumb

The thumb represents 40 per cent of the hand function, so its loss creates a serious disability, with loss of the hand for fine movement requiring a pinch grip. Retention of even a small part of the thumb becomes important as long as it can be covered with stable skin of normal sensation.

If half the proximal phalanx is retained, reconstruction is not needed, but the presence of adherent scar at the end of the stump may be replaced by a flap from the dorsal surface of the first interosseous space.

The levels of thumb amputation require different repair strategies:

Subtotal amputation at the metacarpophalangeal level, proximal or just distal to the joint, with preservation of the commissure and intrinsic musculature.

Replantation: If possible, amputation should be treated by replantation using microsurgical techniques. The amputated member should be kept at 4°C if transportation to a distant center is contemplated, permitting the procedure to be accomplished hours after injury.

Phalangization: The length of the residual stump can be improved by deepening the first web. The interosseous space is opened up and the cleft maintained by placement of a free skin graft. If the area is not unduly scarred, a four-flap Z-plasty may be used, and the adductor pollicis insertion may be transposed from the base of the residual phalanx to the metacarpal to increase the length of the proximal phalanx.

Amputation with loss of the commissure, basal joint, and intrinsic musculature. Total absence of the thumb may be congenital or traumatic. Among the techniques available for thumb reconstruction are osteoplastic lengthening and pollicization.

Osteoplastic lengthening can provide thumb length by use of a bone graft from rib or iliac crest covered by a tube pedicle graft harvested from the groin.

Pollicization provides a well-functioning thumb with near-normal mobility and sensation.

Pollicization of the index finger is done using a broad-based volar flap. The neurovascular bundle to the index finger is conserved, whereas that to the middle finger is ligated. The fascia and transverse metacarpal ligament are divided through their proximal end, and the finger is freed by division of the digit through its proximal phalanx. After removal of the proximal phalanx and metacarpal of the index finger, the index finger is fixed to the stump of the thumb metacarpal by an intramedullary bone graft and one or two Kirschner wires. If the transposed index extensor tendons are slack, a shortening procedure is necessary. The skin flap is closed. Use of the index finger is especially indicated if it also suffered injury during the thumb trauma.

Pollicization of the ring finger, in the presence of an intact index finger, may be preferable, although the thumb function and the aesthetic appearance are inferior to those provided by the index finger transposition. After ring finger pollicization, its extensor tendon needs to be divided and sutured to the proximal end of the extensor pollicis longus or to its own proximal end.

Transplantation of a toe with its tendons, nerves, and vascular supply using microsurgical techniques (Fig. 18–10).

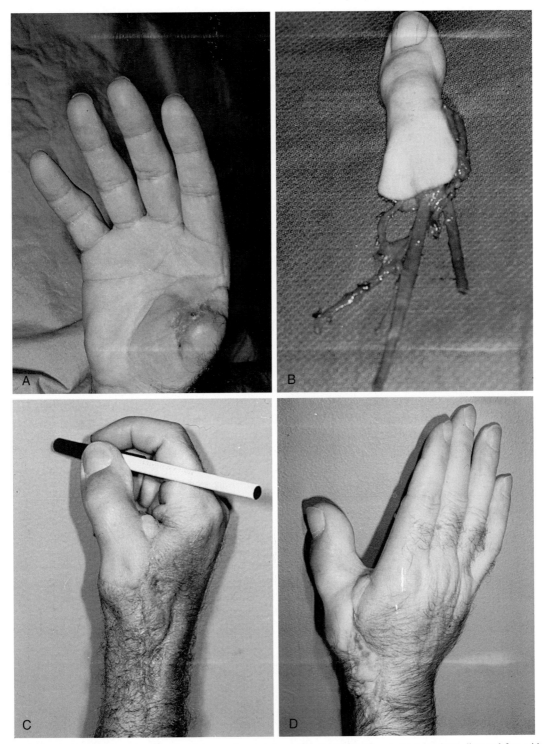

FIGURE 18–10. *A*, Patient after electrical injury and amputation of his thumb. *B*, The great toe has been dissected free with its tendons and neurovascular bundles. *C*, Six months after toe-to-thumb transfer. *D*, By 1 year patient has return of flexion and extension and sensation.

Joints of the Digits

In each metacarpophalangeal joint, the round head of the metacarpal bone is received into the concave facet at the base of the proximal phalanx. The palmar ligament is a strong band that is firmly fixed to the phalanx but loosely to the metacarpal bones, so as not to interfere with free flexion. The palmar ligaments of the metacarpophalangeal joints of the four fingers are bound together by a strong band called the deep transverse ligament. At the sides of each metacarpophalangeal joint are thickenings in the articular capsule called the collateral ligaments. On the dorsum of the joint, the articular capsule is replaced by the extensor expansion. The movements that occur at these joints are those of flexion, extension, abduction, and adduction.

Similarly, in the interphalangeal joints, the heads of the proximal and middle phalanges are marked by articular surfaces with double facets, whereas the middle and distal phalanges present corresponding double concavities for the articulations. The ligaments are arranged in a plan similar to that of the metacarpophalangeal joint, but the movements at these joints are of only two kinds—flexion and extension.

Sprains and dislocations, which are ligamentous injuries of hand joints, vary in their degree of severity, depending on the final degree of joint instability. This in turn depends on the extent of the disruption of surrounding ligaments and the joint capsule.

The metacarpophalangeal joint of the thumb is the most prone to subluxation or dislocation in response to violent hyperextension injury, whereby the phalanx is forced backward onto the dorsum of the metacarpal bone. In addition to the disruption of the volar ligamentous and capsular structures at the base of the first metacarpal, the tendon of the flexor pollicis longus becomes displaced to the ulnar side of the metacarpal head. The ensuing tension then flexes the terminal phalanx.

Although a simple dislocation is readily reduced by appropriate manipulation, manipulative reduction may not be possible in a more complex situation, or the trauma of manipulation may create a more complex state. As the volar plate is disrupted, it comes to lie on the dorsum of the metacarpal head, which in turn is forced onto the palm. Open reduction becomes necessary. Any prolonged residual instability may require continued immobilization or operative repair of torn collateral ligaments.

Interphalangeal dislocations may be dorsal, palmar, or lateral. Dorsal displacement of the middle phalanx is the most common form, with varying degrees of volar plate and collateral ligamentous disruption. Manipulative reduction is invariably possible, with restoration of a stable joint.

Metacarpal and Phalangeal Fracture

Patients with hand injuries should undergo radiologic examination with appropriate views to demonstrate the presence or absence of fractures. Similar views are necessary for sprains and dislocations to demonstrate the corresponding deformity and to identify associated avulsion fractures.

In children, radiologic examination of the normal hand should also be carried out so that comparative identification of epiphyses can be made. Epiphyseal fractures are categorized by the Salter-Harris classification (Fig. 18–11).

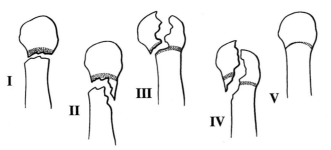

FIGURE 18–11. The Salter-Harris classification of epiphyseal fractures. Type II is the most common fracture. Types I, II, and III have a favorable prognosis. Type IV has an intermediate prognosis, whereas the compression type V injury has a poor prognosis.

Fractures of the Thumb. Fractures of the first metacarpal and its two phalanges are usually due to a direct blow with the fist clenched. Proper treatment includes reduction of the fracture, immobilization until stability of the bone is restored, followed by remobilization to prevent finger stiffness. Fracture of the first metacarpal may be extra-articular, with a transverse fracture through the shaft, or intra-articular.

Intra-articular Fractures

Bennett Fracture. As a result of direct violence, the fracture at the base of the first metacarpal is associated with disruption of the joint surfaces. The small fractured segment is fixed by its ligamentous attachments to the trapezium. Reduction under anesthesia is achieved by application of traction with the thumb abducted while pressure is directed at the base of the metacarpal so that the main mass of the metacarpal shaft is replaced on the fixed smaller fragment. With reduction achieved, a Kirschner wire is placed subcutaneously through the metacarpal shaft and into the carpus. A plaster cast is then applied to incorporate forearm, wrist, and thumb for 6 weeks.

If there is failure in its reduction, the fracture should be treated by open reduction and fixation by two Kirschner wires. One traverses the metacarpal shaft and the carpus, and the second wire traverses the metacarpal shaft and the medial fragment. A plaster cast is then applied.

Inadequate reduction of a Bennett fracture results in the accelerated development of osteoarthritic changes in the joint.

Rolando Fracture. This comminuted intra-articular fracture of the first metacarpal base is best treated by immobilization of the forearm, wrist, and thumb, with the thumb in abduction or by maintenance of traction by placing a Kirschner wire through the proximal phalanx and incorporating a rubber band outrigger in the thumb spica cast for 6 weeks.

FRACTURE OF METACARPALS

Metacarpal Neck. The fourth and fifth metacarpal necks often sustain fracture after a blow with the closed fist. The dorsal angulation deformity can usually be reduced by closed manipulation. If reduction is not stable, it requires a percutaneously placed intramedullary pin to maintain reduction. After 3 weeks of splint immobilization, the pin is removed.

Metacarpal Shaft. Fractures may be spiral, transverse, or oblique and are readily reduced by closed manipulation. Dorsal angulation must be rectified during reduction. Percutaneous passage of a Kirschner wire for 3 weeks maintains the reduction during plaster cast immobilization if the reduction is unstable.

Shaft fractures of the border, little, and index finger metacarpals often require percutaneous K-wire fixation or open reduction and internal fixation with plates and screws.

PHALANGEAL FRACTURES

Undisplaced fractures can be treated by taping the affected finger to an adjacent finger. Any angulation is treated by manipulative reduction. Unstable reductions require percutaneous K-wire fixation or open reduction and fixation. Immobilization should not exceed 3 to 4 weeks, or active motion will be compromised.

Intra-articular fractures may require open reduction and Kirschner pin stabilization.

Nerves of the Hand

MEDIAN NERVE

The nerve enters the forearm at the antecubital fossa and, passing between the two heads of the pronator teres, descends toward the wrist between the superficial flexor muscles anteriorly and the flexor digitorum profundus posteriorly. As it approaches the wrist, the nerve becomes more superficial, lying between the tendons of the palmaris longus and flexor carpi radialis, and enters the hand deep to the transverse carpal ligament.

The muscular branches of the nerve are given off a short distance below the elbow and are distributed to the pronator teres, flexor carpi radialis, palmaris longus, and flexor digitorum sublimis. The anterior interosseous branch also arises below the elbow and passes down the forearm, with its companion artery, to supply the flexor pollicis longus, the radial portion of the flexor digitorum profundus, and the pronator quadratus.

The palmar cutaneous branch is given off above the transverse carpal ligament and descends in front of it, to be distributed to the skin over the thenar eminence of the radial side of the palm. The median nerve has five palmar digital nerve branches, the first two belonging to the thumb on each side and the third directed to the radial side of the index finger, which provides a branch to the first lumbrical muscle. The fourth furnishes a nerve to the second lumbrical muscle before dividing to supply the contiguous sides of the index and middle fingers. The fifth branch divides into two branches, which are distributed to the opposite sides of the middle and ring fingers.

Thus, the palmar digital nerves of the median nerve provide sensory innervation to the lateral three and a half fingers as well as motor fibers to the first two lumbrical muscles. The remaining one and a half fingers are subserved by the ulnar nerve, which also provides motor branches to the remaining lumbrical and interosseous muscles.

Clinical effects of this arrangement of nerves are as follows: High median nerve lesions result in loss of pronation and radial deviation of the hand, loss of flexion of the radial three digits, loss of opposition of the thumb, and loss of palmar sensation of the radial three and a half fingers. Low median nerve lesions result in loss of thumb opposition and loss of palmar sensation of the radial three and a half fingers.

ULNAR NERVE

Entering the forearm in the groove behind the medial humeral epicondyle, the ulnar nerve passes between the two heads of the flexor carpi ulnaris to lie on the deep surface of that muscle. It passes distally as far as the wrist, where it crosses the superficial surface of the transverse carpal ligament to reach the hypothenar eminence. In addition to muscular branches to the flexor carpi ulnaris and the ulnar portion of the flexor digitorum profundus, the ulnar nerve gives off two sensory branches in the forearm—the palmar and dorsal cutaneous nerves.

The palmar branch descends in front of the lower part of the ulnar artery to supply the tissues over the hypothenar eminence. The dorsal branch arises from the ulnar nerve about 7 cm above the wrist and reaches the dorsum of the forearm by passing backward between the shaft of the ulna and the tendon of the flexor carpi ulnaris, supplying the dorsum of the ulnar side of the wrist and hand, the dorsum of the little finger, and the dorsum of the ulnar side of the ring finger.

When the ulnar nerve reaches the flexor retinaculum, it divides into superficial and deep terminal branches. The superficial terminal branch provides branches to the palmaris brevis muscle as well as to the skin of the ulnar margin of the hand and ends by dividing into the palmar digital nerves for the supply of both sides of the little finger and half the ring finger.

The deep terminal branch accompanies the deep branch of the ulnar artery and the deep palmar arch as far as the muscles of the thumb, where it ends in branches to the two parts of the adductor pollicis. Near its origin, the nerve provides branches to the short muscles of the little finger, and in the palm it supplies all the palmar and dorsal interosseous muscles and the medial two lumbrical muscles, as well as the adductor pollicis and deep head of the flexor pollicis brevis.

Clinical effects are as follows: High ulnar nerve lesions result in loss of ulnar deviation of the wrist on flexion, loss of flexion at the metacarpophalangeal joints and extension at the interphalangeal joints of the little and ring fingers, loss of finger abduction and adduction, and instability of thumb pinch. There is loss of sensation of the ulnar one and a half digits and the dorsoulnar aspect of the palm.

For low ulnar nerve lesions, apart from retention of ulnar deviation at the wrist, all other functional losses are as for high nerve lesions. Paralysis of the medial lumbrical and the interosseous muscles results in extension at the metacarpophalangeal joints by the antagonistic muscles and flexion at the interphalangeal joints by the long flexor, producing the so-called clawhand (main en griffe), as well as sensory loss of the ulnar one and a half fingers.

RADIAL NERVE

The radial nerve is the largest terminal branch of the posterior cord of the brachial plexus. The brachial plexus reaches the musculospiral groove of the humerus and emerges by piercing the lateral intermuscular septum of the arm midway between the deltoid tubercle and lateral epicondyle of the humerus.

On the anterior part of the arm, the radial nerve comes to lie between the brachialis and brachioradialis muscles, terminating opposite the lateral condyle by dividing into its terminal branches—the superficial radial nerve and the posterior interosseous nerve.

The radial nerve provides muscular branches to the triceps, anconeus, brachioradialis, and extensor carpi radialis longus as well as twigs to the brachialis muscle.

The lower cutaneous nerve of the forearm arises near the distal end of the groove to supply a strip of skin on the posterior surface of the forearm from the elbow to the wrist.

The superficial radial nerve, which is the smaller of the two terminal branches, is entirely sensory and traverses the forearm on the lateral side of the radial artery to supply the dorsum of the hand and wrist on the radial side and the dorsum of the thumb, index, middle, and radial side of the ring fingers, ending in digital branches.

The posterior interosseous nerve, which supplies the extensor muscles of the forearm, is the larger of the two terminal branches and is given off opposite the lateral condyle of the humerus entering the supinator muscle, within whose substance it winds around the lateral side of the radius. Here the nerve is vulnerable to injury in fractures of the neck of the radius or in operative intervention in this area.

On emerging from the distal border of the muscle, the nerve passes down the back of the forearm between the superficial and deep extensor muscles and then upon the interosseous membrane as far as the dorsum of the wrist. Its branches supply the supinator and extensor carpi radialis as well as the extensor carpi ulnaris, extensor digitorum, extensor digiti minimi, extensor indicis proprius, abductor pollicis longus, extensor pollicis longus, and extensor pollicis brevis.

Clinical features of this nerve are as follows: Injury to the nerve below the origin of the posterior brachiocutaneous nerve results in minimal sensory loss confined to a small area over the dorsum of the hand. Wrist drop is the main motor feature of radial nerve paralysis. Extension of the interphalangeal joints remains intact by virtue of lumbrical and interosseous activity. Injury to the proximal part of the radial nerve also paralyzes the triceps and anconeus muscles. Suture of the divided radial nerve is more often successful than is repair of any other upper limb nerves, in view of its predominant motor function.

The Short Muscles of the Hand

The Thenar Eminence. This consists of three short muscles of the thumb: the abductor pollicis, the flexor pollicis brevis, and the opponens pollicis. The former two are inserted into the radial side of the first phalanx of the thumb, whereas the latter is inserted into the radial border of the metacarpal bone of the thumb, all three being supplied by the median nerve. The deep head of the flexor pollicis brevis is innervated by the deep branch of the ulnar nerve.

The Adductor Pollicis. This muscle lies deeply in the palm and consists of two heads: The oblique head arises from the palmar surface of the carpal bones and from the base of the second and third metacarpals, and the transverse head

arises from the shaft of the third metacarpal. These two parts join into one tendon, which is inserted into the ulnar side of the base of the proximal phalanx of the thumb. This deep, short muscle of the thumb receives its nerve supply from the ulnar nerve, and it acts to draw the thumb toward the center of the palm.

The Hypothenar Eminence. This is composed of the abductor digiti minimi, the flexor digiti minimi, and the opponens digiti minimi, all being supplied by the ulnar nerve.

The Lumbrical Muscles. These four short muscles arise from the tendons of the flexor digitorum profundus in the palm of the hand. The two lateral ones are attached on the radial side of a single tendon, whereas the other two are each connected with two tendons. They are, accordingly, numbered from one to four from the thumb side. The small tendons of the lumbricals are directed to the radial side of the finger to be inserted into the extensor expansion of the proximal phalanx.

The first and second lumbricals are supplied by the median nerve, the third and fourth by the deep branch of the ulnar nerve. The lumbricals assist in flexing the metacarpophalangeal joints and in extending the interphalangeal joints.

The Interosseous Muscles

There are four dorsal and three palmar interosseous muscles that arise from metacarpal bones and are situated in the intermetacarpal spaces. Their tendons are inserted into the dorsal extensor expansion.

The dorsal interossei abduct the fingers from the middle line of the middle finger, whereas the palmar interossei adduct the fingers toward the same line. Acting together, the interossei flex the metacarpophalangeal joints and extend the interphalangeal joints of the fingers in unison with the lumbricals. All the interossei are innervated by the deep branch of the ulnar nerve.

NERVE COMPRESSION SYNDROMES

Carpal Tunnel Syndrome

This condition, also known as median neuritis, is due to compression of the median nerve by the transverse carpal ligament at the wrist.

Underlying causes of the condition include tenosynovitis of the digital flexors, which may be associated with diffuse adhesions of the perineural and peritendinous tissues. Rheumatoid proliferation of the flexor synovia is often noted. The syndrome may be associated with trigger finger and olecranon bursitis. Occupational trauma may be a factor in its causation. The condition often complicates a Colles fracture of the radius. Other associated causes include pregnancy and the abnormal presence of lumbrical or flexor digitorum sublimis muscle bellies within the tunnel. The condition may affect both hands.

Numbness of the thumb, index, middle, and ring fingers, as well as nocturnal burning pain and weakness and clumsiness on using the hand, represents the main clinical symptom.

Physical examination should exclude neuropathic problems in the neck and thoracic outlet. Thenar atrophy, as well as motor and sensory impairment in the course of the median nerve in the hand, is a hallmark of the median nerve entrapment condition. It is noteworthy that normal sensation is present in the proximal palm as the palmar cutaneous branch of the median nerve passes above the transverse carpal ligament.

The Tinel sign is positive. Percussion over the median nerve causes tingling in the tips of the middle and index fingers and less often in the thumb and ring fingers.

The Phalen wrist flexion test is positive. Acute flexion of the wrist intensifies the numbness and paresthesia, with immediate relief when the wrist is returned to its neutral position.

The tourniquet test—inflation of a blood pressure cuff above venous pressure—may precipitate discomfort and pain as well as loss of sensation in the median nerve distribution.

Nerve conduction study confirms delay in nerve transit time below the level of median nerve entrapment.

Treatment is initially conservative management with a wrist splint and antiinflammatories. Injection of triamcinolone or methylprednisone acetate into the carpal tunnel may be effective in mild cases. If the patient does not respond to conscientious effort at conservative management, surgical release is indicated.

Operative management is straightforward. Using a tourniquet for hemostasis, release of the transverse carpal ligament is carried out. Because the flexor retinaculum lies distal to the volar wrist crease, the incision commences at the transverse palmar crease and skirts the hypothenar eminence to the wrist crease. The proximal incision lies ulnar to the midaxis of the ring finger to avoid injury to the palmar cutaneous branch of the median nerve.

Once the fibers of the transverse carpal ligament are identified, a dissector is passed along its deep surface and its entire width is divided. The nerve is identified and well exposed because it might need freeing from any surrounding adhesions or encasement.

The skin only is sutured, a padded dressing is applied, and the wrist is splinted for 10 days.

Ulnar Tunnel Syndrome

The ulnar nerve may be compressed in Guyon canal, which is bounded by the pisiform and pisohamate ligament medially and the hook of the hamate radially. Less common than ulnar nerve compression at the elbow, it is characterized by pain and paresthesia in the ulnar half of the ring finger and little finger, with weakness and atrophy of the intrinsic muscles of the hand.

The most common cause of the ulnar tunnel syndrome is pressure by a ganglion, anomalous muscles, and repetitive trauma.

Operative management is carried out through an incision made along the radial side of the flexor carpi ulnaris. The fibers of the volar carpal ligament are divided, and the ulnar nerve and vessels are retracted medially. A compressive ganglion may be noted and should be removed.

Upper Limb Entrapment Neuropathies

Nerve entrapment may occur in other upper extremity locations:

Pronator teres syndrome: The median nerve is compressed by the lacertus fibrosus, pronator teres, or the arch of origin of the flexor digitorum sublimis. The anterior interosseous branch of the median nerve may be entrapped in the forearm.

Cubital tunnel syndrome: The ulnar nerve is compressed between ulnar and humeral origins of the flexor carpi ulnaris by bony spurs or as the result of pericondylar trauma.

Radial tunnel syndrome: The radial nerve is most commonly compressed in the radial tunnel between the radial head and supinator. It is compressed at one of four points by fibrous bands at the tunnel entrance, the radial recurrent vessels to the brachioradialis and extensor carpi radialis longus muscles, the tendinous margin of the extensor carpi radialis brevis, or, most commonly, at the arcade of Frohse, which is a ligamentous band lying over the deep radial nerve as it enters the supinator. The superficial branch of the radial nerve may be compressed at the wrist.

Thoracic outlet syndrome: The lower trunks of the brachial plexus (C8, T1) may be compressed as they pass between the medial and anterior scalene muscles, producing pain and paresthesia in the nerve root distribution.

TENDON TRANSFER FOR MUSCLE PARALYSIS

Muscle paralysis, whatever its cause, provides scope for tendon transfer in order to restore certain lost functions. Certain prerequisites are essential before consideration can be given to specific tendon transfers:

1. The joint that is to be mobilized must be supple and capable of a full range of passive mobility.

2. Direction of action produces the best function when it is a straight line between the origin of the muscle and the newly acquired point of insertion. Although insertion directly into bone provides the best results, transfer of the active tendon to the tendon of the paralyzed muscle is equally effective.

3. The transposed musculotendinous unit must retain its nerve and vascular supply in order to retain its structural and functional integrity.

4. The musculotendinous unit to be transposed should be capable of sufficient excursion that the required function can be satisfied, and the unit should be capable at least of contracting against gravity and resistance.

The regional transposition of musculotendinous units can restore functional use of the elbow, wrist, digits, and thumb. Techniques have also been developed to restore intrinsic digital balance in the correction of clawing of the fingers.

The Elbow

RESTORATION OF FLEXION

1. Flexor origin transfer: The common flexor origin is detached from the medial epicondyle and adjacent septa and is transposed to the junction of the middle and lower thirds of the humeral shaft.

2. The common origin of the brachioradialis and extensor carpi radialis is detached from the lateral epicondyle and is similarly transposed to the lateral aspect of the humeral shaft.

3. Segmental pectoral transposition: The lower one-third segment of the pectoral sternocostal origin is detached and elevated. The muscular strip is brought through a tunnel in the anterior compartment of the upper arm and is attached to the biceps tendon with the elbow at 70 degrees flexion. The elbow is immobilized in this position for a month, and then graduated extension is commenced.

4. Transfer of triceps: The triceps is detached from its olecranon insertion and transposed medially across the antecubital fossa to reach the neck of the radius, where it is attached to the biceps tendon or through drill holes into the neck of the radius with the elbow at 70 degrees flexion.

RESTORATION OF EXTENSION

1. Transposition of the posterior third of the deltoid, after freeing it from its tendon of insertion, to the triceps tendon

2. Transposition of the biceps tendon into the triceps

The Wrist

In wrist drop due to radial nerve injury, restoration of wrist extension can be achieved by transfer of the pronator teres to the extensor carpi radialis brevis, transfer of the flexor carpi ulnaris to the extensor digitorum communis, and transfer of the palmaris longus to the extensor pollicis. Working in concert, the three transfers restore wrist extension, and the power of wrist flexion is maintained by the flexor carpi radialis.

The Digits

The restoration of digital and thumb flexion requires the essential prerequisite that the wrist retain normal mobility. Finger and thumb flexion can be restored by transposition of the extensor carpi radialis longus into the long flexors and transposition of the brachioradialis into the flexor pollicis longus.

The Thumb

EXTENSION

Loss of thumb extension as an isolated event results from rupture of the extensor pollicis longus tendon. This may be a complication of a previous Colles fracture or a result of the tendon's involvement in rheumatoid arthritis. If the tendon is not amenable to suture repair, then transfer of the extensor indicis proprius tendon permits suture to the distal end of the extensor pollicis longus.

ABDUCTION AND OPPOSITION OF THE THUMB

Opposition of the thumb to the other digits is essential for the proper function of the hand. Both abduction and opposition of the thumb are lost in irreversible median nerve lesions as well as in some muscular dystrophies.

Transfer of flexor digitorum sublimis to the base of the thumb's proximal phalanx: The superficial flexor tendon is mobilized at the base of the ring finger and brought out at the wrist. It is passed through a loop and pulley created within the tendon of the flexor carpi ulnaris, and the flexor sublimis tendon is brought through a tunnel extending from the pisiform across the palm and thenar eminence for insertion into the proximal phalanx of the thumb. Alternatively, the superficial flexor tendon is left within the flexor retinaculum and brought across the palmar and thenar tunnel to the same thumb site.

Transfer of the extensor digiti minimi tendon: The tendon on the dorsum of the little finger is mobilized and divided. It is withdrawn at the wrist and brought through a tunnel extending from the ulnar side of the wrist to the base of the thumb phalanx for fixation.

Transfer of abductor digiti minimi: If the former tendons are unavailable, this hypothenar muscle is mobilized, with division of its insertion, and brought up to the carpus. It is then brought through a tunnel across the base of the palm after rotating it so that its superficial surface becomes the deep surface in its new position, thereby preventing a kink of the neurovascular bundle. If it is too short to reach the thumb phalanx, it can be attached to the tendon of the abductor pollicis brevis.

Transfer of the extensor indicis proprius: The tendon is routed around the ulnar side of the wrist and inserted at the base of the thumb.

The Clawed Hand

The main en griffe deformity is a consequence of combined median and ulnar nerve paralysis of all four fingers. A loss of flexion occurs at the metacarpophalangeal joints and loss of active extension at all the interphalangeal joints.

The long extensors and long flexors take over, in uncompensated fashion, in the functional control of the digits, with hyperextension at the metacarpophalangeal joints and flexion of the interphalangeal joints.

LOSS OF INDEX FINGER ABDUCTION

The loss of function of the first dorsal interosseous as a result of an ulnar nerve lesion results in lack of index finger abduction, which may be rectified by any of the following:

Transfer of the extensor indicis proprius tendon: After its division and proximal mobilization, the tendon is transferred and sutured into the insertion of the first dorsal interosseous tendon, with the finger abducted and the wrist in the neutral position.

Transfer of the extensor pollicis brevis

Any flexor sublimis tendon brought around the radial side of the wrist

LOSS OF THUMB ADDUCTION

There is a significant loss of power in the pinch action of the thumb. This can be improved by one of the following procedures:

The extensor carpi radialis longus tendon is divided and a free tendon graft added to it for length. This is brought through the second or third intermetacarpal space, along the line of the adductor, and inserted into its tendon.

The flexor sublimis tendon to the ring finger is detached from its insertion and retracted into the wrist. The tendon is brought around the ulnar side of the wrist and through an intermetacarpal space for suture into the adductor tendon.

Alternatively, the flexor tendon can be left within the flexor retinaculum and rerouted into the adductor tendon.

The combined improvement in the function of index abduction and thumb adduction greatly strengthens the pinch grip.

CORRECTION OF CLAWING

Replacement of the lost intrinsic muscle function and correction of hand clawing may be accomplished by tendon transfers. The extensor carpi radialis longus tendon or the flexor carpi radialis can be used for the motor drive. Tendon grafts derived from the palmaris longus, plantaris, or toe extensors are used to elongate the motor tendon and are attached to the front of the flexor retinaculum. The tendon grafts are then brought along the lumbrical canals for attachment to the extensor expansion near the proximal interphalangeal joint, using a pull-out wire for each attachment. The attachment is concluded with a degree of tension that keeps the metacarpophalangeal joint flexed at 30 to 40 degrees and the proximal interphalangeal joint extended.

THE ARTHRITIC HAND

Interference with hand function may occur because of pain or deformity attributable to destruction of a joint, its bony contours, or its synovial lining. Subsequent periarticular changes, flexor synovitis, displacement of extensor tendons, and subluxation of metacarpophalangeal joints perpetuate pain and aggravate deformity.

Clinical and radiologic examinations reveal the extent of deformity, and a general assessment of the underlying process attempts to define whether the problem is due to osteoarthritis, gout, or rheumatoid arthritis. The joint manifestations of disseminated lupus erythematosus, psoriatic arthritis, and Still's disease in the juvenile may resemble those of rheumatoid arthritis and should indicate the need for relevant diagnostic investigations before a surgical decision is made regarding treatment.

Indications for Surgery

Relief of pain: Pain limits joint function, and procedures that relieve the pain and associated hand insufficiency improve function.

Prevention of pathologic processes: Synovectomy of joints and tendons may prevent continued progression of the pathologic process with improvement of functional capacity.

Correction of deformity represents the most common indication for corrective operations.

Pathologic Conditions

OSTEOARTHRITIS

Osteoarthritis or degenerative arthritis of the hand is often superimposed on a previous traumatic event. The articular surfaces of the affected joint develop signs of wear with erosion followed by eburnation of the underlying bone and the development of osteophytes.

The most commonly affected joints are the distal interphalangeal and carpometacarpal joints of the thumb. The proximal interphalangeal joints may suffer changes, but the metacarpophalangeal and wrist joints are infrequently affected unless previous significant trauma has occurred.

Clinical Features

Heberden Nodes. Situated at the distal finger joints, these marginal osteophytes develop gradually over a period of many months. The nodules go through a phase of painful redness, with gradual resolution of the asymptomatic affliction that is aesthetically unsightly. No treatment is necessary.

Bouchard Nodes. These are similar to Heberden nodes but are located at the proximal interphalangeal joints.

Mucous Cysts. These small ganglion cysts develop over the base of the distal phalanx. The nail develops a groove. These concomitant changes are associated with degenerative changes in the distal interphalangeal joint. The cyst can be easily excised under finger-block anesthesia, and local osteophytes may be removed.

Osteoarthritis of the Thumb Carpometacarpal Joint. Although osteoarthritis of the first carpometacarpal joint occurs in both sexes, it is more common in postmenopausal women. The importance of the prehensile action of the thumb in hand manipulations means that use of the hand is seriously limited. Clinical features include weakness in exerting pinch movement and a sense of a lump at the base of the thumb. Axial pressure with gentle rotation of the metacarpal may demonstrate a positive grind sign. Radiologic examination of the joint reveals the joint space to be decreased or, in advanced disease, totally destroyed.

Surgical Management. Among the several procedures available, fusion of the joint and arthroplasty provide the main options:

Arthrodesis. Although fusion of the joint creates a small loss of thumb mobility, it achieves pain-free stability and good functional capacity. The joint surfaces are excised, and the impacted raw bone surfaces are fused by slotting the first metacarpal into the trapezium. After wire and plaster cast immobilization for up to 12 weeks, solid fusion should be complete.

   Arthroplasty. Resurfacing of the joint can be accomplished by several procedures:

Excision of the trapezium with insertion of soft tissue spacer. The flexor carpi radialis tendon is divided longitudinally, rolled up on itself based distally, and introduced into the joint space.

In *osteoarthritis of interphalangeal joints,* fusion of a single joint may restore good function. If two joints in one finger suffer osteoarthritis that requires surgical relief, there should be one normal joint between the proximal and distal affected joints.

Joint replacement either by coverage of one joint surface with a silicone implant or by total excision and implantation of an articulated stem-and-cup type of prosthesis. Joint substitutes currently available for interphalangeal joint replacement include stainless steel and Silastic rubber prostheses, although silicone enjoys wider popularity.

RHEUMATOID ARTHRITIS

   The majority of hand deformities attributable to rheumatoid arthritis are secondary to soft tissue involvement. Proliferative synovitis causes swelling and stiffness of the wrist and finger joints. Because it is a systemic disorder that involves mesenchymal tissues, tendons and their sheaths are frequently affected with the development of tenosynovitis, trigger finger, tendon rupture, and carpal tunnel syndrome.

   As the joint disease progresses, the synovial proliferation distends the joint until the intra-articular pressure disrupts the joint capsule and its surrounding ligaments. The ensuing subluxation of the metacarpophalangeal joints and the ulnar drift represent the penultimate deformity of the disease. Associated hyperextension and flexion deformities of all the joints of the fingers and thumb represent the end points of the deformation process. The rheumatoid process frequently invades the intrinsic muscles of the hand, which undergo scarring and contracture, thereby producing the classic deformities. With loss of the longitudinal arch of the hand and reversal of the arch, the fully developed swan-neck deformity causes loss of the grip (Fig. 18–12).

   Articular and periarticular erosion proceeds as the proliferative synovium and released lysozymes exert their local effects, with the formation of bony cysts and spurs and destruction and collapse of the joint.

   Clinical and radiographic examination reveal the deformities and the bony and articular changes.

   Indications for operation are failure to stop progression of the hand deformation and ulnar drift by good medical therapy, nerve entrapment, tendon rupture, severe pain, and deformity and impaired hand function.

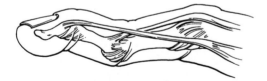

FIGURE 18–12. The swan-neck deformity characterized by hyperextension of the proximal interphalangeal joint and flexion of the distal interphalangeal joint.

Correction of Ulnar Drift. With lengthening of the radial ligamentous fibers and subluxation of the joints, the extensor and flexor tendons tend to pull the hand toward ulnar deviation. Synovectomy of the metacarpophalangeal joints is carried out and should be as complete as possible. The contracted fibers on the ulnar side of the extensor tendons are incised and released. This permits the dorsal repositioning of the extensor tendons. Plication of the radial fibers remedies the laxity of these fibers. Crossed intrinsic transfer of the extensor tendon may be added to the procedure by detaching the wing tendon distally and attaching it to the proximal phalanx of the next ulnar digit, thereby providing a radially deviating force.

Arthrodesis. Arthrodesis of the distal interphalangeal joints in a position of function may be helpful in selected instances.

Arthroplasty. In order to obtain a full range of movement and optimal functional result, arthroplasty procedures on the metacarpophalangeal joints should use prostheses. Thus joint resection and reconstruction with interposed silicone prostheses in the metacarpophalangeal and proximal interphalangeal joints attain the desired objectives of pain relief and restoration of hand function.

In selecting a prosthesis, it is vital, after excision of the joint and the bony articular ends, to use a sizer to select the prosthesis needed for each joint. The prosthesis, once inserted, must lie comfortably and permit flexion of the joint.

HAND TUMORS

Benign Tumors

Verrucae: Warts are commonly seen on the dorsal and palmar areas of the hand as well as on the nail bed regions. Caused by the human papilloma virus, they often resolve spontaneously. They may be removed by topical agents such as salicylic acid or by fulguration or freezing.

Ganglion: The most common tumor of the hand, it is usually located on the dorsum of the wrist between the extensor pollicis longus tendon and the extensor tendon to the index fingers. It is a tense, firm, cystic mass containing clear gel-like fluid. It may also present at the palmar-radial aspect of the wrist or at the palmar aspect of the base of the fingers. The cyst may be attached to tendon sheaths. Ganglia are usually attached to and communicate with the underlying joint capsule. During excision of the synovium-lined cyst, the herniated capsular component must also be removed or recurrence of the ganglion is likely. Spontaneous resolution or disintegratation after firm pressure may occur.

Giant cell tumors of the tendon sheath: Arising from tendon sheaths, these yellowish masses may be cystic, solid, or multilocular. Usually presenting over joints, they may encroach on tendons and nerves and may cause pressure erosion of the underlying bone. Histologically, they are xanthomatous. Surgical excision is indicated.

Inclusion cysts: These subcutaneous cystic masses are the result of a penetrating puncture wound that sequesters a nidus of epithelial cells below the skin surface.

Glomus tumor: These small subungual tumors arise from the glomus cells and pericytes that provide the temperature-regulating arteriovenous anastomoses. They may cause severe throbbing pain and should be resected.

Vascular masses include traumatic false aneurysms. Arteriovenous fistulae are usually congenital but may result from penetrating trauma. Various forms of hemangioma may present in the hand as elsewhere.

Mesodermal tumors include lipoma and fibroma.

Neural tumors are represented by neurofibroma and neurilemmoma.

Osseous tumors: Enchondromas, osteoid osteomas, and osteoclastomas may occur within the hand bones.

Malignant Tumors

Squamous cell carcinoma usually presents on the dorsal surface of the hand, although it may occasionally develop in the periungual area. Spread to the axillary lymph nodes may occur.

Basal cell carcinoma may present on the dorsum of the hand or on the digits.

Melanoma may present as a subungual lesion requiring ray amputation of the finger and possible axillary dissection.

Mesodermal malignancy, such as fibrosarcoma and liposarcoma, is rare in the hand. Metastic tumors of the hand bones may be due to a primary lesion of bronchus, thyroid, breast, or prostate.

CONGENITAL HAND ANOMALIES

Embryologic Development of the Upper Limb

The limb bud that first appears during the fourth week of gestation consists of an outer ectodermal layer, which gives rise to the skin and its appendages, and an inner mesodermal component that differentiates into bone, muscle, and tendon. The central nerve trunks and vascular channels give off segmental branches that sprout into the developing limb.

The upper limb bud then develops surface lines that subdivide it into a hand plate, a proximal arm, and a shoulder region.

The hand plate develops a flange, which becomes the digital plate. As digital ridges develop, indentations define the finger rays. During the sixth week of gestation the interdigital clefts and their neurovascular network become apparent.

Abnormal morphogenesis may have a genetic basis or may occur in response to teratogenic drugs, causing anomalies in limb development or degeneration of well-formed structures. Anomalies may be the result of failure of normal generation, as in syndactyly.

Swanson's classification of congenital malformations of the upper limb is the most commonly used scheme (Table 18–1).

Evaluation of children with congenital anomalies of the upper limb requires interaction with pediatricians regarding the child's general status. Clinical assessment of the anomaly should be complemented by radiologic examination of the area with study of the associated skeletal architecture. In planning surgical treat-

TABLE 18–1. Classification of Congenital Hand Deformities

I. Failure of formation of parts (arrest of development)
   A. Transverse deficiencies: amputations of arm, forearm, wrist, hand, digits
   B. Longitudinal deficiencies
      1. Phocomelia: complete, proximal, distal
      2. Radial deficiencies (radial club hand)
      3. Central deficiencies (cleft hand)
      4. Ulnar deficiencies (ulnar club hand)
      5. Hypoplastic digits
II. Failure of differentiation (separation) of parts
   A. Synostosis: elbow, forearm, wrist, metacarpals, phalanges
   B. Radial head dislocation
   C. Symphalangism
   D. Syndactyly
      1. Simple
      2. Complex
      3. Associated syndrome
   E. Contracture
      1. Soft tissue
         a. Arthrogryposis
         b. Pterygium cubitale
         c. Trigger digit
         d. Absent extensor tendons
         e. Hypoplastic thumb
         f. Thumb-clutched hand
         g. Camptodactyly
         h. Windblown hand
      2. Skeletal
         a. Clinodactyly
         b. Kirner deformity
         c. Delta bone
III. Duplication
   A. Thumb (preaxial) polydactyly
   B. Triphalangism/hyperphalangism
   C. Finger polydactyly
      1. Central polydactyly (polysyndactyly)
      2. Postaxial polydactyly
   D. Mirror hand (ulnar dimelia)
IV. Overgrowth—all or portions of upper limb, e.g., macrodactyly
V. Undergrowth
VI. Congenital constriction band syndrome
VII. Generalized skeletal abnormalities, e.g., Madelung deformity

Modified with permission from Swanson AB: Classification of congenital hand deformities. J Hand Surg 1:8–22, 1976, and Dobyns JH, Wood VE, Bayne LG, Frykman GK: Congenital hand deformities. In Orum OP (ed): Operative Hand Surgery. New York, Churchill Livingstone, 1982.

ment, if indicated, early execution before the child commences school is to the child's psychological advantage.

Failure of Differentiation

Syndactyly. The fingers are essentially normal but are joined by a web of skin, which may involve the entire length of adjacent digits or a small segment of the fingers. The condition is often familial, may be bilateral, and may be associated with webbing of the toes.

Syndactyly and polydactyly represent the two most common congenital anomalies of the hand. They are invariably present in cases of multiple hand malformations. Simple or uncomplicated syndactyly involves skin webbing only. If the epiphyseal plates are fused or there are common tendons or nerves, it is considered to be complicated.

Separation of the fingers is accomplished by division of the skin bridge and resurfacing of the fingers with local digital flaps or full-thickness skin grafts (Fig. 18–13).

Clinodactyly. This is an angulation deformity affecting the distal interphalangeal joint of the little finger, which is usually present at birth or may appear soon after. Similar involvement of the index finger is defined as the delta phalanx. Mild deformity is best left alone. Removal of a wedge of cartilage from the head of the middle phalanx, before ossification at 18 months, restores the normal alignment. In childhood a wedge osteotomy may be appropriate.

Camptodactyly. The crooked finger is caused by a contracture deformity, most commonly of the little finger. A flexion contracture with supination occurs at the proximal interphalangeal joint. Surgical treatment provides disappointing results.

Arrested Development

Radial Club Hand. Absence of the radius is also known as radial dysplasia or radial hemimelia. The radius may be totally or partially absent and the condition occurs more often in males. It is usually unilateral and may be accompanied by absence of the thumb. Absence of the first metacarpal is referred to as pouce flottant.

The radial carpal bones may be fused or absent, and the shortened, curved ulna causes the hand to deviate radially until it lies at an angle to the long axis of the forearm.

Treatment requires the centralization of the hand on the ulnar axis. This requires serial casting after release of the tightened radial volar structures, excision of the central carpal bones, and wire fixation of the ulna in a central position within the residual carpal bones. An osteotomy of the ulna may become necessary to relieve its bowing and may produce up to 3 cm of lengthening.

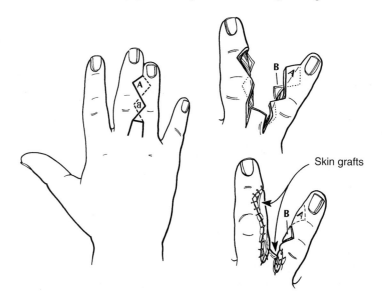

FIGURE 18–13. Design and release of a syndactyly. Release requires a full-thickness skin graft to at least one and sometimes both digits.

Thumb Aplasia. Either pollicization of the index finger or toe-to-hand transfer by microsurgical technique may be appropriate.

Ulnar Club Hand. In the ulnar deficiency state, which occurs at an earlier stage than radial club hand, development of the hand occurs toward the ulnar border. There is associated bowing of the radius. If the radial head is dislocated, proximal radioulnar fusion may be done.

Dynamic splinting at an early age may minimize the radial bowing so that by 6 months of age the residual distal ulnar fibrocartilaginous remnant can be removed. The radius can later be transposed and arthrodesis to the proximal ulnar remnant performed.

Cleft Hand. Absence of all or part of the central ray form is characterized by a defect in the central part of the hand, which is divided into radial and ulnar components, each carrying two digits. In the atypical form only two rays are present, a radial and an ulnar.

Treatment of the anomaly requires the development of a small flap at the base of the ulnar side of the index finger, with the incision extending onto the base of the ring finger. The adjacent metacarpals of the index and ring fingers are exposed and realigned by the insertion and tying of stainless steel wires. The skin flap is then aligned so as to restore the web.

In the atypical form the web between the two digits can be lengthened by a Z-plasty, thereby improving their grasping function.

Duplication

Polydactyly. The normally shaped hand has an extra small digit growing from the fifth metacarpal (postaxial). It may, however, present on the radial border of the hand with duplication of the thumb. Involvement of the middle and ring fingers may be accompanied by syndactyly.

Polydactyly of the thumb, which is the preaxial form, may be of several varieties. It may present as a broadening of the distal phalanx or as a distinct bifurcation at the tip. There is often a common base with duplication of the distal two thirds of the thumb. Another variety is represented by two distal phalanges or by a rudimentary thumb attached near the base of the proximal phalanx or even articulating with the head of the metacarpal. Thumb duplication is best classified by Wassel, who lists seven types (Fig. 18–14). Type IV is the most common type, characterized by a single metacarpal with duplication of the proximal and distal phalanges.

Surgical management is directed toward providing cosmetic improvement. In simple cases, amputation of the supernumerary digit is readily accomplished. In complex circumstances, the aim is restoration of the morphologic and functional status. This requires proper assessment of the bony structure and tendon function.

The Mirror-Image Hand or Ulnar Dimelia. This is a form of duplication in that the normal preaxial structures are replaced by a mirror image of the postaxial digits with duplication of the ulna. The extraradial digits are amputated, leaving one for pollicization.

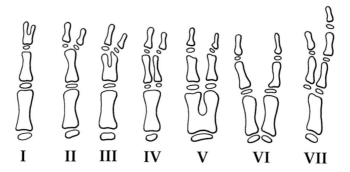

FIGURE 18–14. Wassel's classification of thumb duplication. Type IV is the most common form of bifid thumb.

The Triphalangeal Thumb. In this form of duplication, the thumb consists of three phalanges. The anomalous phalanx may be removed, with correction of the associated angulation deformity.

Macrodactyly. This rare condition is characterized by gigantism of a finger with overgrowth of all the finger elements, including the phalanges, nails, nerves, vessels, and integuments, with marked increase in the subcutaneous fibrofatty tissue.

Operations to reduce the fibrofatty components may be complemented by removal of bone or by stapling the epiphysis to stop growth. Amputation of a deformed finger may be indicated.

Ring Constrictions

Annular bands may occur at any level of the upper limb, with the fingers, wrist, and forearm being the most common sites. Shallow grooves may be left alone, but deeper constrictions cause edema of the distal limb or digit. Excision of the annular groove should be complemented by undermining of the inverted skin edges and transposition of single or multiple Z-plasty flaps.

Suggested Reading

Brand PW: Biomechanics of tendon transfer. Hand Clin 4:205, 1988

Bruner JM: The zig-zag volar digital incision for flexor-tendon surgery. Plast Reconstr Surg 40:571, 1967

Burkhalter WE: Deep space infections. Hand Clin 5:553, 1989

Doyle JR, Blythe WF: Anatomy of the flexor tendon sheath and pulleys of the thumb. J Hand Surg 14A:949, 1989

Green DP: Complications of phalangeal and metacarpal fractures. Hand Clin 2:307, 1986

Kleinert HE, Kutz JE, Atasoy E, Stormo A: Primary repair of flexor tendons. Orthop Clin North Am 4:865, 1973

Lister G: Local flaps to the hand. Hand Clin 1:621, 1985

Millender LH, Nalebuff EA: Reconstructive surgery in the rheumatoid hand. Orthop Clin North Am 6:709, 1975

Spinner M, Spencer PS: Nerve compression lesions of the upper extremity: A clinical and experimental review. Clin Orthop 104:46, 1974

Swanson AB: A classification for congenital limb malformations. J Hand Surg 1:8, 1976

Index

Note: Page numbers in *italics* refer to illustrations; page numbers followed by t refer to tables.

Abbé flap, in reconstruction of lips, 240–241, *241*
Abdomen, body contouring of, 325–329
    abdominal dermolipectomy in, 326–327, *328*
    abdominoplasty in, 326, *327–328*
    complications due to, 329
    mini-abdominoplasty in, 327, 329
Abdominal dermolipectomy, 326–327, *328*
    complications of, 329
Abdominal tube pedicle flap, in reconstruction of penis, 341
Abdominal wall, defects of, 313–314
    acquired, reconstruction of, 314, *315*
    weakness of, as complication of TRAM flap, 299
Abdominoplasty, 326, *327–328*
    complications of, 329
Abduction, loss of, of index finger, 375
    of thumb, 375
Abductor digiti minimi, transfer of, for abduction and opposition of thumb, 375
Abscess, breast, 293
Acid burn, 61
Acinic cell carcinoma, of parotid gland, 189
Acquired immunodeficiency syndrome (AIDS), Kaposi sarcoma in, 30–31
Acrocephaly, *140,* 141t
Actinic (solar) keratosis, 22, *23,* 32
Adamantinoma, 178
Adductor pollicis muscle, 370–371
Adenocarcinoma, of parotid gland, 189
Adenoma, of face or scalp, sebaceous, 26
    of parotid gland, pleomorphic, 188
    of thyroid gland, 196
Adhesive, tissue, 12
Advancement skin flap, 86, *86*
    for fingertip injury, 362, *363*
Aesthetic facial surgery, 257–281. See also specific surgery, e.g., *Rhytidectomy.*
    ancillary procedure(s) in, 275–277
        chemical peels as, 276–277
        collagen injection as, 275–276
        dermabrasion as, 277
        laser resurfacing as, 277
        liposuction as, 275, *276*
Agenesis, vaginal, 344–345
Aging, of skin, 8
AIDS (acquired immunodeficiency syndrome), Kaposi sarcoma in, 30–31
Airway, maintenance of, in soft tissue trauma, 203
Alar deformity, secondary rhinoplasty for, 264
Alkali burn, 61. See also *Burn(s).*
Allograft(s). See also *Graft(s).*
    bone, 76
    cartilage, 73
    skin, 67

Alloplastic material(s), 76–77
    in reconstruction of skull defects, 206
Alopecia (baldness), 277
Alpha-hydroxy acids, as chemical peels, 276
Alveolar reconstruction, for cleft palate, 171–172, *172*
Amastia, 289
Ameloblastoma, 178
Amnion, as allogeneic replacement material, 72
Amputation, of thumb, 364, *365*
Anaplastic carcinoma, of thyroid gland, 197
Anastomosis, 115–117
    faciohypoglossal and facioaccessory, for facial paralysis, 251–252
    patency of, 115–116, *117*
    preparation for, 115
    technique of, 115, *116*
Anesthesia, for excision of lesions, 13
    for rhytidectomy, 266–267
    regional, for periorbital reconstruction, 232–234, *233*
Aneurysmal bone cyst, 178
Angiosarcoma, 30
Angle classification, of dental occlusion, 146–147, *148*
Angle fracture, mandibular, treatment of, 226
Ankle, fracture of, management of, 317
Ankylosis, of temporomandibular joint, 227
Annular bands, of upper extremity, 384
Antibiotics, topical, for burns, 56–57
Antrum, mastoid and maxillary, development of, 133
Apert syndrome, 141
Aponeurosis, palmar, 352–353
Arachnoid nevus, 29
Arch bars, for mandibular fractures, 225
Areola, reconstruction of, after mastectomy, 302
Argon laser, 45
Arm, upper, body contouring of, 329–330
Arm flap, lateral, tissue transfer of, 123
Arterial insufficiency, of lower extremity, 317
Arterial malformation, 29
Arthritis, of hand, 376–379
    indications for surgery in, 376–377
    pathologic conditions in, 377–378
    rheumatoid, of interphalangeal joints, *378,* 378–379
Arthrodesis, 377–378
    of interphalangeal joints, 379
Arthroplasty, 378
    of interphalangeal joints, 379
Ascorbic acid deficiency, wound healing and, 6
Aspiration, fine-needle, of breast lump, 295
Atasoy-Kleinert volar advancement flap, for fingertip injury, 362, *363*
Athelia, 289
Augmentation, of malar prominence, 275
Augmentation mammoplasty, 287–289, *288*

Augmentation mammoplasty (Continued)
   complications of, 288–289
Auricle, accessory, 244
   anatomy of, 243, 243
Autograft(s). See also Graft(s).
   bone, 73–75
   cartilage, 73
   skin, 67
Avulsion, of ears, 246
   of penis and scrotum, 340
   of scalp, 206
Axonotmesis, 127–128

Back defect(s), 311–313
   acquired, 312–313
   spina bifida as, 311–312, 312
Baldness (alopecia), 277
Banner flap, for closure of nasal defect, 246, 247
Basal cell carcinoma, 32–34
   clinical varieties of, 33, 33–34
   histologic identification of, 34
   of hand, 380
   treatment of, 34
Basal cell nevus syndrome (Gorlin syndrome), 33
Bennett fracture, 367
Bilobed flap, for closure of nasal defect, 246, 247
Biopsy, of breast lump, 295
Bladder, exstrophy of, 340
Blepharophimosis, 239
Blepharoplasty, 271–274
   complications of, 273–274
   lower lid, 273, 273–274
      transconjunctival, 273
      transpalpebral, 273, 273–274
   upper lid, 272, 272
Blood supply, lingual, 179
Blow-out fracture, 219, 220
Blue nevus, 24
Body contouring, 325–332
   by suction lipectomy, 330–331, 331–332
      tumescent technique in, 331–332
   of abdomen, 325–329
      abdominal dermolipectomy in, 326–327, 328
      abdominoplasty in, 326, 327–328
      complications due to, 329
      mini-abdominoplasty in, 327, 329
   of thigh, 329, 330
   of upper arm, 329–330
Bone(s). See also named bones, e.g., Carpal bone(s).
   long, layers and blood supply to, 73, 74
   wormian, 133
Bone allograft, 76
Bone cyst, aneurysmal, 178
Bone flap, tissue transfer of, 123, 125, 125
Bone graft, 73–76
   in reconstruction of skull defects, 206
   nonvascularized, 73–74, 75
   vascularized, 75
Bony skeleton, of nose, narrowing of, 262, 262
Bouchard nodes, of arthritic hand, 377
Boutonniere deformity, 361, 361
Bowen disease, 32
Brachioplasty, 329–330
Brachycephaly, 141t
Branchial arch syndrome, first and second, correction of, 151–152
Branchial cysts, 193–195, 194
Breast, 285–302

Breast (Continued)
   accessory, 285
   benign lesions of, 291–293
      in adult, 292–293
      prepubertal, 291
      pubertal, 291–292
   cancer of, 294–295
      diagnosis of, 294–295
      histologic types of, 294
      treatment of, 295
   development of, 285
   ptosis of, 290, 290–291
   reconstruction of, after mastectomy, 295–302. See also
      Mastectomy, breast reconstruction after.
   shape of, abnormalities in, 289–290, 290
   size of, abnormalities in, 285–289, 286–288
   surgical removal of. See Mastectomy.
Breast abscess, 293
Breast cyst, 292
Breast deformity, tuberous, 289, 290
Breast prosthesis, implantable, after mastectomy, 296–297
   types of, 287–288
Breast tissue, ectopic, 285
   expansion of, 105–106, 106
      after mastectomy, 296, 296–297
Breslow's classification, of melanoma, 39
Brooke formula, of fluid resuscitation, 55t
Burn(s), 51–62
   chemical, 61
   depth of, 53, 53
   electrical, 60, 61
   extent of, 51–52, 51–52, 52t
   inhalation, 55
   medical treatment of, 55–58
      fluid requirements in, 55t, 55–56
      metabolic requirements in, 58
      prevention of infection in, 56–57
      shock in, 55
   pathophysiology of, 54
   rehabilitation following, 62
   severity of, 54, 54t
   surgical treatment of, 58–60
      débridement in, 58
      escharotomy in, 58, 59
      excision and grafting in, 58–60
      to specific areas, 60
   unstable, 62
Bursa, 354, 354

Calcifying epithelioma of Malherbe (pilomatrixoma), 26
Calorie intake, daily, for burn patient, 58
Calvarial graft, 74, 75
   split, for saddle nose deformity, 264
Camptodactyly, 382
Canine, anatomy of, 177, 177
Canthus, medial or lateral, reconstructive surgery of, 237
Cap splints, for mandibular fractures, 225
Capillary lymphangioma, 30
Capillary malformation, 29
Capsular contracture, as complication of augmentation mammoplasty, 288–289
Carbon dioxide (CO_2) laser, 44–45
Carcinoma. See also specific neoplasm.
   basal cell. See Basal cell carcinoma.
   breast, 294–295
   hypopharyngeal, 185–186
   intraepidermal (Bowen disease), 32
   maxillary, 184–185

Carcinoma (Continued)
  nasopharyngeal, 183–184
  oral, 181–183
    staging of, 181t
    TNM classification of, 180t
  oropharyngeal, 183
  squamous cell. See Squamous cell carcinoma.
  thyroid, 196–197
  vulvar, resection of, reconstruction following, 344, 345
Carpal bone(s), injury to, 349–351
  lunate dislocation as, 350–351
  scaphoid fracture as, 349–350
  trans-styloid radiocarpal dislocation as, 351
Carpal tunnel syndrome, 371–372
  treatment of, 372
Carpenter syndrome, 142
Carpometacarpal joint, osteoarthritis of, 377
Cartilage, types of, 73
Cartilage graft, 73
"Cauliflower ears," 210
Cavernositis, indurative, 341
Cavernous hemangioma, 28, 28
Cavernous lymphangioma, 30
Cementoma, 178
Cephalometrics, in maxillary reconstruction, 146, 147
Cervical. See also Neck.
Cervical lymph node(s), swelling of, 195
Cervical plexus graft, for facial paralysis, 251
Cervical webs, 193
Charles procedure, for lymphedema, 318
Chemical burn, 61. See also Burn(s).
Chemical facial peel(s), 276–277
  deep peeling agents in, 277
  superficial peeling agents in, 276
Chemotherapy, for breast cancer, 295
  for melanoma, 40
Chest wall, acquired defect(s) of, 309–311
  empyema causing, 309, 311
  malignancy causing, 309, 310
  post-median sternotomy infection causing, 309
  radiation wounds causing, 311
  congenital malformation(s) of, 302–305
    pectus carinatum as, 303
    pectus excavatum as, 303, 304
    Poland syndrome as, 304–305, 305
    sternal clefts as, 303–304
  embryonic development of, 302
Chin implant, for microgenia, 275
Chordee, 338
Chromosome(s), sex, 343
Clark levels of invasion, of melanoma, 38, 38
Clawed hand, 375–376
  correction of, 376
Cleft(s), craniofacial, 155–172. See also Cleft lip; Cleft
    palate.
    Tessier's classification of, 136–138, 137
  sternal, 303–304
Cleft hand, 383
Cleft lip, bilateral, repair of, 160–161
    Millard, 161, 161–162
  classification of, 155, 155–157, 157
  etiology of, 158
  microform, repair of, 158–159
  prealveolar, bilateral, 162–163
    secondary procedures for, 161–163
    unilateral, 161–162, 162
  prerepair management of, 158
  repair of, guides to, 158–161
    principles of, 157
    timing of, 157–158

Cleft lip (Continued)
  unilateral complete, repair of, 159–160
    lip adhesion in, 159
    Millard, 159–160, 160
    Randall, 160, 160
  unilateral incomplete, repair of, 159
Cleft palate, 163–167
  classification of, 156–157, 157
  complete, 164
    repair of, 166–167, 168
    Veau-Wardill-Kilner palatoplasty repair of, 167, 169
    Von Langenbeck palatoplasty repair of, 167, 168
  developmental basis of, 164
  effects of, 164–165
  incomplete, 164
  repair of, 165–167
    Furlow, 166, 167
    intravelar veloplasty, 166, 166
    objectives in, 165
    technique(s) in, 166–167, 166–169
    timing of, 165
  submucous, 164
Clinodactyly, 382
Clips, skin, 12
Cloaca, development of, 335–336
Club hand, radial, 382
  ulnar, 383
Cold injury, 61
Collagen, grafting of, 76
Collagen injection(s), 275–276
Collagen synthesis, disorders of, in wound healing, 7–8
Color change, in skin grafts, 70
Compartment syndrome, of lower extremity, 314
Composite flap(s), 87, 90, 90
Composite graft(s), transplantation of, in hair replacement
    therapy, 278
Compound nevus, 24
Computed tomography (CT), of face, 203, 204
Condylar neck fracture, treatment of, guidelines in,
    225–226
Congenital anomaly(ies), of hand, 380–384. See also
    Hand(s), congenital anomaly(ies) of.
Conjunctiva, 232
Connective tissue disorder, as complication of augmentation
    mammoplasty, 289
Continuous over-and-over suture, 10, 12, 12
Continuous-wave infrared laser(s), 44–45
Continuous-wave visible light laser(s), 45–46
Contraction, in wound healing, 6
Contracture(s), scar, 62
Copper vapor laser, 46
Coronal suture, premature closure of, 139, 141–142
Cranial aplasia, congenital, 138
Craniofacial cleft(s), 155–172. See also Cleft lip; Cleft
    palate.
Craniofacial deformity(ies), 142–150
  clinical evaluation of, 143
  definitive correction of, principles of, 143–150
  surgical intervention for, dysostosis and, 144, 144
    early, 143
    mandibular correction in, 149–150, 151
    maxillary reconstruction in, 146–147, 147–150, 149
    orbital advancement in, 144–146, 145–146
    principles of, 143–144
Craniofacial development, anomaly(ies) of, 135–139
  congenital cranial aplasia as, 138
  congenital dermal sinus as, 139
  encephalocele as, 138–139
  failure of skull ossification as, 138–139
  premature closure of cranial sutures as, 139

Craniofacial development (Continued)
  residual clefts as, 136–138, 137. See also Cleft lip;
    Cleft palate.
    Tessier's classification of, 136–138, 137
Craniofacial dysostosis, 144, 144
Craniofacial trauma, 205–211. See also Soft tissue trauma.
Craniosynostosis, 139–142, 140
  effects of, 139, 140
  patterns in, 139, 141t, 141–142
Cranium. See Skull.
Crile incision, for radical neck dissection, 198
Cross-facial graft, for facial paralysis, 251, 252
Cross-finger flap, for fingertip injury, 362, 363
Cross-leg flap, 87
Crouzon syndrome, 141
Cryptorchism, 337
Cryptotia, 244
CT (computed tomography), of face, 203, 204
Cubital tunnel syndrome, 373
Cutaneous nerve(s), antebrachial, grafting of, 130
Cutaneous T-cell lymphoma (mycosis fungoides), 32
Cutis laxa, associated with collagen disorders, 7
Cylindroma (turban tumor), 25
  of parotid gland, 189
Cyst(s), bone, aneurysmal, 178
  branchial, 193–195, 194
  breast, 292
  dermoid, 21, 22
  inclusion, 379
    epidermal, 21
  mucous, of arthritic hand, 377
  odontogenic, 177
  sebaceous, 21
Cystadenoma, 25
Cystic hygroma, 30
Cystic lobular hyperplasia, 293
Cystic lymphangioma, 30
Cystosarcoma phylloides, 294
Cytotoxic drugs, wound healing and, 7

Dacryocystorhinostomy, 237, 237
Darier disease (keratosis follicularis), 22
De Quervain disease, 360
Débridement, of burns, 58
Decubitus ulcers. See Pressure sores.
Deltopectoral flap, 82
Dental malocclusion, 172
Dental occlusion, 146–147, 148
Dentigerous cyst, 177
Dermabrasion, 277
Dermal sinus, congenital, 139
Dermatofibroma, 26
Dermatofibrosarcoma protuberans, 27
Dermatome(s), for cutting grafts, 70–71
Dermis, 4, 4–5
Dermofasciectomy, for Dupuytren contracture, 353
Dermoid cyst, 21, 22
Dermolipectomy, abdominal, 326–327, 328
  complications of, 329
  thigh, 329, 330
Diabetes mellitus, leg ulcers due to, 318
Digastric muscle, 223
Digit(s). See also Finger(s); Toe(s).
  flexion of, restoration of, 374
  joints of, 366
  replantation of, elective, contraindications to, 118–119
    salvage, justification for, 119, 119
    technical considerations in, 119–120, 120

Digital tenosynovitis, stenosing (trigger finger), 359
Diplopia (double vision), 219
Disarticulation, hip, for pressure sores, 325
Dislocation, lunate, 350–351
  mandibular, 226
  of interphalangeal joints, 366
  of metacarpophalangeal joints, 366
  radiocarpal, trans-styloid, 351
Distocclusion, 147, 148
Distraction osteogenesis, 150, 151
Donor sites, for skin grafts, 70
  cutting grafts from, 70–71
Dosage equation, in laser therapy, 44
Drug(s). See also Chemotherapy.
  cytotoxic, wound healing and, 7
Drum dermatome, for cutting grafts, 71
Dry eye syndrome, caused by blepharoplasty, 273
Ductal carcinoma, of breast, 294
Ductal papilloma, of breast, 292
Dupuytren contracture, 353
Dysostosis, craniofacial, 144, 144
Dysplasia, fibrous, correction of, 152
  of jaw, 178
Dysplastic nevus, 24

Ear(s), acquired deformities of, 246
  avulsion of, 246
  burns to, management of, 60
  congenital abnormalities of, 244
  external anatomy of, 243, 243
  injury to, treatment of, 210
  lop or cup, 244
  microtic, 244
    reconstruction of, 245
  misshapen, 244
  protruding, 244
    reconstruction of, 244–245
  tissue expansion of, 109
Ectopic testes, 337
Ectropion, caused by blepharoplasty, 274
  causes of, 237–238
  treatment of, 238
Ehlers-Danlos syndrome, associated with collagen
    disorders, 7
Elastic cartilage, 73
Elbow, 373–374
  extension of, restoration of, 374
  flexion of, restoration of, 373–374
Electrical burn, 60, 61. See also Burn(s).
Embolus, pulmonary, as complication of abdominoplasty
    and abdominal dermolipectomy, 329
Empyema, treatment of, 309, 311
En griffe deformity, 375
Encephalocele(s), 138–139
  frontoethmoidal (nasal), 139
Enophthalmos, 220
Entrapment neuropathy(ies), of upper limb, 373
Entropion, 238
Ephelis (freckle), 25
Epidermal appendages, tumors of, 25–26
Epidermal inclusion cyst, 21
Epidermal lesions, 21–22, 23
Epidermis, 3–4, 4
Epiphyseal fracture(s), Salter-Harris classification of, 366,
    367
Epispadias, 336, 339–340
  repair of, 339–340
Epithelialization, in wound healing, 6

Epithelioma adenoides cysticum, 31
Escharotomy, of burns, 58, *59*
Excision, of necrotic material, in burn patient, 58
Expander prosthesis, 103, *104*
Exstrophy of bladder, 340
Extensor tendon(s), 359–362
　anatomy of, 359, *360*
　injury to, *361,* 361–362
　rupture of, 360
　transfer of, for abduction and opposition of thumb, 375
Extremity(ies), lower. See *Lower extremity.*
　upper. See *Upper extremity.*
Eye(s). See also *Orbital* entries.
　burns to, management of, 60
Eye socket, contraction of, 238
Eyelid(s), anatomy of, *231,* 231–232
　lower, blepharoplasty for, 273, *273–274*
　　reconstructive surgery of, 234–235, *234–236*
　muscles of, *231,* 231–232
　skin of, 231
　upper, blepharoplasty for, 272, *272*
　　reconstructive surgery of, 235–240, *236–237*

Face, burns to, management of, 60
　reconstruction following, 62
　CT scan of, 203, *204*
　development of, 134–135, *136*
　reconstruction of, 231–253
　　involving ears, 243–246
　　involving eyelids, 231–240
　　involving lips, 240–243
　　involving nose, 246–249
　　involving paralysis, 249–253
　skeletal deformities of, correction of, 151–152
　soft tissue wounds of, treatment of, 207–209
　tissue expansion of, 109, *110*
Face lift. See *Rhytidectomy.*
Facial bipartition, 146, *146*
Facial bones, fractures of, 211–226
Facial buttress(es), 212, *213*
Facial nerve, 266
　branches of, 250
　central nuclei of, 250
Facial osteotomy, 147, 149, *149–150*
Facial paralysis, 249–253
　causes of, 250–251
　　acquired, 250–251
　　congenital, 250
　clinical features of, 251
　operative treatment of, 251–253
　　dynamic reconstruction in, 252–253
　　restoration of neural pathway in, 251–252, *252*
　　static reconstruction in, 253
Facial peels, chemical, 276–277
Facial surgery, aesthetic, 257–281. See also specific
　　surgery, e.g., *Rhytidectomy.*
　ancillary procedure(s) in, 275–277
　　chemical peels as, 276–277
　　collagen injection as, 275–276
　　dermabrasion as, 277
　　laser resurfacing as, 277
　　liposuction as, 275, *276*
Facioaccessory anastomosis, for facial paralysis, 251–252
Faciohypoglossal anastomosis, for facial paralysis, 251–252
Fan flap, in reconstruction of lips, 241, 243
Fascia, of hands, deep, 352–353
　superficial, 352
Fascia lata slings, for facial paralysis, 253

Fasciectomy, for Dupuytren contracture, 353
Fasciocutaneous flap, 97–99
　axial, *98,* 98–99
　expansion of, 109, 111
　random, 98, *98*
　tissue transfer of, 123, *124*
Fasciotomy, for Dupuytren contracture, 353
Fat, grafting of, 76
Fat necrosis, as complication of reduction mammoplasty,
　　287
　of breast, 292–293
Feeding, difficulties of, cleft palate and, 165
Ferris-Smith knife, for cutting grafts, 71
Fibroadenoma, of breast, 292
　juvenile, 291
Fibrocartilage, 73
Fibrocystic disease, 293
Fibrocystic mastopathy, 293
Fibroplasia, in wound healing, 5, 6
Fibrosis, of tunica albuginea, 341
Fibrous dysplasia, correction of, 152
　of jaw, 178
Fibrous lesions, of skin, 26–27
Fibular flap, tissue transfer of, 123, 125, *125*
Fine-needle aspiration, of breast lump, 295
Finger(s), 349
　index, loss of abduction of, 375
　　pollicization of, 364
　mallet, 361
　ring, pollicization of, 364
　trigger (stenosing digital tenosynovitis), 359
Fingertip(s), injuries to, 362–363, *363*
Finklestein sign, 360
First-degree burn, 53
Fistula, cervical, 193–195
　palatal, 171
Flap(s), 81–99. See also named flap, e.g., *Abbé flap.*
　composite, 87, 90, *90*
　definition of, 81
　fasciocutaneous, 97–99
　　axial, *98,* 98–99
　　expansion of, 109, 111
　　random, 98, *98*
　　tissue transfer of, 123, *124*
　for fingertip injuries, 362, *363*
　in closure of nasal defects, 246, *247*
　in hair replacement therapy, 280, *280–281*
　in reconstruction of lips, 240–243, *241–242*
　in reconstruction of nipple, 299, *301,* 302
　in reconstruction of nose, *248,* 248–249
　muscle and musculocutaneous, 90–97. See also *Musculo-
　　cutaneous flap(s).*
　pedicle, in reconstruction of penis, 341
　radial forearm, 123, 125
　　in reconstruction of penis, 341, *342*
　skin, 81–87. See also *Skin flap(s).*
　tongue, 179
　types of, 81
"Flash burns," 60
Flash lamp–pumped pulsed dye laser, 46, *47*
Fleur-de-lis dermolipectomy, 326, *328*
Flexor retinaculum, of hands, 352
Flexor tendon(s), anatomic zones of, 355, *356*
　grafting of, 358–359
　　staged, 358
　injury to, 355–359
　　zone I repair of, 355–356
　　zone II repair of, 356–357, *357*
　　zone III repair of, 357
　　zone IV repair of, 357

Flexor tendon(s) (Continued)
  zone V repair of, 357
  of hand, 353–359
  of thumb, 358–359
  pulley mechanism of, 357, 357–358
  transfer of, for abduction and opposition of thumb, 375
Fluid requirement(s), estimation of, in burn patient, 55t, 55–56
Follicular carcinoma, of thyroid gland, 196–197
Foot, fracture of, management of, 317
Forearm flap, radial, in reconstruction of penis, 341, 342
  tissue transfer of, 123
Forehead, tissue expansion of, 107, 109
Forehead flap, 82, 89
  in reconstruction of nose, 248, 248–249
Forehead-brow lift, 270–271
  coronal, 270–271, 271
  endoscopic, 271
Fracture(s), Bennett, 367
  epiphyseal, Salter-Harris classification of, 366, 367
  etiology of, 212
  facial, 211–226
  frontal sinus, 221–222
  hand, 366–368
  intra-articular, 367
  lower extremity, management of, 316, 316–317
    osteomyelitis complicating, 317
  management of, 212
  mandibular, 223–226, 224
  maxillary, 213–217, 214, 216
  metacarpal, 367–368
  nasal, 217
  nasoethmoid, 221, 221
  orbital, 219–220, 220
  penile, 340
  phalangeal, 368
  Rolando, 367
  scaphoid, 349–350
  thumb, 367
  zygomatic, 217–219, 217–220
Freckle (ephelis), 25
Frey syndrome, 190
Frontal nerve, 233
Frontal sinus, development of, 133
  fractures of, 221–222
Frontoethmoidal encephalocele, 139
Frontofacial advancement, monoblock, 145, 145
Frontonasal process, surrounding stomodeum, 134–135
Frostbite, 61
Full-thickness burn, 53
Funnel chest (pectus excavatum), 303, 304
Furlow repair, of cleft palate, 166, 167

Ganglion, 379
Gastrocnemius muscle, for reconstruction of lower extremity, 97
Gastroschisis, 313
Gender, 342–343
Genioglossus muscle, 223
Geniohyoid muscle, 223, 223
Genital tubercle, 336–337
Genitalia, male, injuries to, 340–341
Genitourinary system, 335–345. See also specific part.
  development of, 335
Giant cell tumor, of tendon sheath, 379
Giant pigmented nevus, 24, 25
Glands of Moll, 231
Glands of Zeiss, 231

Glomus tumor, 31, 380
Gluteus maximus muscle, for reconstruction of trunk, 94, 96
  tissue transfer of, 122–123
Gorlin syndrome (basal cell nevus syndrome), 33
Gracilis muscle, for reconstruction of lower extremity, 96
  tissue transfer of, 122
Graft(s), bone, 73–76
  for saddle nose deformity, 263, 263–264
  nonvascularized, 73–74, 75
  vascularized, 75
  cartilage, 73
  collagen, 76
  composite, transplantation of, in hair replacement therapy, 278
  fat, 76
  flexor tendon, 358–359
    staged, 358
  muscle, for facial paralysis, 253
  nerve, 129, 129–130
    for facial paralysis, 251–252, 252
  nipple, contralateral, 302
  skin, 67–72. See also Skin graft(s).
Granular cell myoblastoma, 31
Granulation, in wound healing, 6
Groin flap, 82, 83, 87, 88
  tissue transfer of, 123
Guerin fracture. See Le Fort I fracture.
Gunning splints, for mandibular fractures, 225
Gynecomastia, 292

Hair follicle nevus, 31
Hair replacement, 277–281
  scalp expansion in, 280–281
  scalp flaps in, 280, 280–281
  scalp reduction in, 278–279, 279
  transplantation of composite grafts in, 278
Hand(s), 351–373
  arthritic, 376–379
    indications for surgery of, 376–377
    pathologic conditions of, 377–378
  burns to, management of, 60
    reconstruction following, 62
  clawed, 375–376
    correction of, 375–376
  congenital anomaly(ies) of, 380–384, 381t
    arrested development and, 382–383
    camptodactyly as, 382
    cleft hand as, 383
    clinodactyly as, 382
    duplication as, 383–384
    failure of differentiation and, 381–382
    macrodactyly as, 384
    polydactyly as, 383, 384
    radial club hand as, 382
    ring constrictions as, 384
    syndactyly as, 381–382, 382
    thumb aplasia as, 383
    triphalangeal thumb as, 384
    ulnar club hand as, 383
    ulnar dimelia as, 383
  embryologic development of, 380
  fascia of, deep, 352–353
    superficial, 352
  flexor tendons of, 353–359
  fracture of, 366–368
  infections of palm of, 354, 354–355
  muscles of, 370–371

Hand(s) *(Continued)*
  nerves of, 368–370
  skin of, 352
  soft tissue lacerations of, 362
  structural and functional elements of, 349
  surface anatomy of, *351,* 351–352
  tumors of, benign, 379–380
    malignant, 380
Head and neck, carcinoma of, 180–184
  involving hypopharynx, 185–186
  involving maxilla, 184–185
  involving mouth, 181–183
  involving nasopharynx, 183–184
  involving oropharynx, 183
  involving salivary glands, 189
  radical neck dissection for, 197–198, *198*
  staging of, 181t
  TNM classification of, 180t
  lymphatic drainage from, 192, *192*
  reconstruction of, muscle/musculocutaneous flaps for,
    92–93
Heat energy, conversion of light to, in laser therapy, 43–44
Heberden nodes, of arthritic hand, 377
Hemangioma, *28,* 28–29
  of breast, 291
Hematoma, caused by abdominoplasty, 329
  caused by blepharoplasty, 273
  caused by rhytidectomy, 270
Hemicircumoral loop, for facial paralysis, 253
Hemifacial microsomia, correction of, 151–152
Hemorrhage, control of, in soft tissue trauma, 203
Heterograft(s), skin, 67
Hip disarticulation, for pressure sores, 325
Holevich flap, for fingertip injury, 362
Homograft(s). See *Allograft(s).*
Hordeolum (stye), 231
Horizontal mattress suture, 10, *11*
Horseshoe kidney, 335
Hueston flap, for fingertip injury, 362
Humby knife, for cutting grafts, 71
Hürthle cell carcinoma, of thyroid gland, 197
Hyaline cartilage, 73
Hydradenitis suppurativa, 31
Hydroxyapatite, as alloplastic material, 76
Hygroma, cystic, 30
Hyoid arch, 194
Hypertelorism, orbital, 142
Hypogastric flap, 82
Hypomastia, 287–289, *288*
Hypopharynx, anatomic landmarks of, 180, *180*
  carcinoma of, 185–186
Hypoplasia, maxillary, associated with facial clefts,
    136–138, *137*
Hypospadias, 336, 337–339
  anatomy of, 338
  surgical repair of, 338
    complications after, 339
    one-stage, 339
Hypothenar eminence, 371

Iliac bone, graft from, 74
Iliac crest autograft, for saddle nose deformity, 263
Iliac crest–circumflex iliac artery flap, tissue transfer of,
    125
Implant(s), breast, after mastectomy, 296–297
    types of, 287–288
  chin, for microgenia, 275
  penile, for impotence, 341–342

Impotence, penile implants for, 341–342
Incision(s), Crile, 198
  MacFee, 198, *198*
  rhinoplasty, *259,* 259–260
  Weber-Fergusson, 185, *185*
Inclusion cyst, 379
  epidermal, 21
Incontinence, urinary, control of, 339
Infection(s), as complication of augmentation
    mammoplasty, 288
  in burn patient, prevention of, 56–57
  of palm of hand, *354,* 354–355
  sternotomy, post-median, treatment of, 309
Inferior pedicle technique, for reduction mammoplasty, 286,
    287
Inflammation, in wound healing, *5,* 5–6
Inflammatory carcinoma, of breast, 294
Infrared laser(s), continuous-wave, 44–45
Inhalation burn, 55. See also *Burn(s).*
Interdental eyelet wiring, of mandibular fractures, 225
Interosseous muscles, of hand, 371
Interosseous nerve, posterior, grafting of, 130
Interphalangeal joint(s), 366
  rheumatoid arthritis of, *378,* 378–379
Interpolation skin flap, 85
Interrupted suture, 10, *11*
Intradermal nevus, 24
Intraepidermal carcinoma (Bowen disease), 32
Intravelar veloplasty repair, of cleft palate, 166, *166*
Ischial pressure sores, closure of, 322, 324, *324*
Island forehead flap, in reconstruction of nose, 249

Jadassohn tumor (nevus sebaceus), 26, *26*
Jaw. See also *Mandibular; Maxillary* entries.
  nonodontogenic tumors of, 178
Jejunum, transfer of, 126
Jessner's solution, as chemical peel, 276
Joint(s). See also named joint, e.g., *Wrist.*
  carpometacarpal, osteoarthritis of, 377
  interphalangeal, 366
    rheumatoid arthritis of, *378,* 378–379
  metacarpophalangeal, 366
  replacement of, 378
  spraining of, 366
  temporomandibular, 226–227
Junctional nevus, 24
Juri flap (temporo-parietal-occipital flap), in hair
    replacement therapy, 280
Juvenile fibroadenoma, of breast, 291
Juvenile thelarche, 291

Kaposi sarcoma, 30–31
Karapandzic flap, in reconstruction of lips, 241–242, *242*
Kasabach-Merritt syndrome, 29
Keloid(s), 8, *9*
Keratinocytes, cultured, as skin substitute, 72, *72*
Keratoacanthoma, 22, *23*
Keratocyst, 177
Keratosis, actinic (solar), 22, *23,* 32
  seborrheic, 21–22
Keratosis follicularis (Darier disease), 22
Keratosis palmaris, 22
Keratosis plantaris, 22
Keyhole pattern, for reduction mammoplasty, 286, *286*
Kidney(s), congenital malformations of, 335
  development of, 335

Kleeblattschädel, *140,* 141t
Klippel-Feil syndrome, 193
Klippel-Trenaunay syndrome, 30
Knives, for cutting grafts, 71
Krypton laser, 45–46
Kutler lateral advancement flap, for fingertip injury, 362, *363*

Lacerations, nasal, treatment of, 210
  soft tissue, of hand, 362
Lacrimal apparatus, 232
  reconstructive surgery of, 237, *237*
Lacrimal nerve, 233
Laser(s), 43–47
  argon, 45
  carbon dioxide, 44–45
  classification of, by source of light, 45t
  conversion of, to heat energy, 43–44
  copper vapor, 46
  effect of, 43
  energy delivered by, components of, 44
  flash lamp–pumped pulsed dye, 46, *47*
  hazards of, 46–47
  krypton, 45–46
  neodymium-YAG, 45
  physics of, 43–44
  Q-switched, 46
Laser resurfacing, of facial skin, 277
Lateral arm flap, tissue transfer of, 123
Lathyrism, 7
Latissimus dorsi muscle, in reconstruction of breast, 297, *298*
  in reconstruction of chest wall defects, 309, *310,* 311
  in reconstruction of trunk, 93–94
  tissue transfer of, 121
Le Fort I fracture, 214
  malunion of, management of, 216–217
  management of, 215–216, *216*
Le Fort I osteotomy, 149, *150*
Le Fort II fracture, 214
  malunion of, management of, 217
  management of, 215–216, *216*
Le Fort II osteotomy, 149, *149*
Le Fort III fracture, 214
  malunion of, management of, 217
  management of, 216
Le Fort III osteotomy, 147, 149, *149*
Lentigo maligna (melanotic freckle of Hutchinson), 24
Lentigo senilis, 24
Levator palati muscle, 163
Levator palpebrae superioris muscle, *231,* 231–232
Ligament(s), facial, 266
Light, conversion of, to heat energy, in laser therapy, 43–44
Lip(s), aesthetic procedures for, 275
  anatomy of, 240
  carcinoma of, 181–182
  cleft of. See *Cleft lip.*
  injury to, treatment of, 211
  lower, reconstructive surgery of, 241–243, *242*
  upper, reconstructive surgery of, 240–241, *241*
Lip adhesion, in unilateral complete cleft lip repair, 159
Lipoma, of parotid gland, 188
Liposuction, 275, *276*
  body contouring by, 330–331, *331–332*
  tumescent technique in, 331–332
Littler island transfer flap, for fingertip injury, 362, *363*
Lobular carcinoma, of breast, 294
Lower extremity, 314–320. See also specific part, e.g., *Foot.*

Lower extremity *(Continued)*
  fractures of, management of, *316,* 316–317
    osteomyelitis complicating, 317
  lymphedema of, 318–320
    primary, 318, *319*
    secondary, 318, 320
  reconstruction of, muscle/musculocutaneous flaps for, 96–97
  trauma to, 314, 316–317
  ulceration of, chronic, 317–318
Lumbrical muscles, 371
Lumpectomy, 295
Lunate dislocation, 350–351
Lund-Browder chart, in estimation of burn surface area, 51–52, *52,* 52t
Lymph node(s), cervical, swelling of, 195
Lymphangioma, 30
  of breast, 291
Lymphangiosarcoma, 30
Lymphatic drainage, from head and neck, 192, *192*
Lymphatic malformation(s), 30
Lymphedema, of lower extremity, 318–320
  primary, 318, *319*
  secondary, 318, 320
Lymphedema praecox, 318, *319*
Lymphedema tarda, 318
Lymphoma, cutaneous T-cell (mycosis fungoides), 32
  in thyroid gland, 197

MacFee incision, for radical neck dissection, 198, *198*
Macrodactyly, 384
Macromastia, 285–287, *286–287*
Macrotia, 244
Mafenide acetate (Sulfamylon), for burns, 57
Maffucci syndrome, 30
Malar prominence, augmentation of, 275
Malignant melanoma. See *Melanoma.*
Mallet finger, 361
Malocclusion, dental, 172
Malunion, of Le Fort fractures, management of, 216–217
Mammogram(s), obscuring of, as complication of augmentation mammaplasty, 289
Mammography, for breast cancer, 295
Mammaplasty, augmentation, 287–289, *288*
  complications of, 288–289
  reduction, 285–287
    complications of, 287
    free nipple graft technique for, 286–287
    inferior pedicle technique for, 286, *287*
    keyhole pattern for, 286, *286*
Mandibular arch, 194
Mandibular correction, for craniofacial deformities, 149–150, *151*
Mandibular defects, asymmetric, 150
  correction of, 149–150, *151*
  symmetric, 150
Mandibular dislocation, 226
Mandibular fracture(s), 223–226
  displacement in, factors influencing, 224, *224*
  fixation of, methods of, 225
  reduction of, 225
  treatment of, guidelines to, 225–226
Mandibular loop, for facial paralysis, 253
Mandibular muscle, insertions of, 222–223, *223*
Mandibular process, surrounding stomodeum, 135
Marcus Gunn syndrome, 239–240
Marfan syndrome, associated with collagen disorders, 8
Masseter muscle, 222, *223*

Masseter muscle *(Continued)*
  transfer of, for facial paralysis, 252
Mastectomy, breast reconstruction after, 295–302
    implant in, 296–297
    musculocutaneous flaps for, 297–299, *298–300*
      complications of, 299
      latissimus dorsi muscle in, 297, *298*
      transverse rectus abdominis muscle in, 297–298,
        299–300
    of areola, 302
    of contralateral breast, 302
    of nipple, 299, *301, 302*
    surgical techniques in, 296–302
    timing of, 296
    tissue expansion in, 296, *296–297*
  radical, 295
  simple, 293
  subcutaneous, 293–294
Mastication, muscles of, 222, *223*
Mastoid antrum, development of, 133
Mastopathy, fibrocystic, 293
Mattress suture(s), 10, *11*
Maturation, in wound healing, *5, 6*
Maxillary antrum, development of, 133
Maxillary carcinoma, 184–185
  clinical features of, 184
  treatment of, 185, *185*
Maxillary defects, reconstruction of, 146–147, *147–150,*
  149
Maxillary fracture(s), 213–217
  clinical features of, 215
  Le Fort classification of, 214, *214*
  management of, 215–217, *216*
  mechanism of injury in, 214–215
Maxillary hypoplasia, associated with facial clefts,
  136–138, *137*
Maxillary nerve, 233
Maxillary process, surrounding stomodeum, 135
Maxillectomy, 185, *185*
Maxillofacial trauma, fractures as, 211–226. See also
  Fracture(s).
  involving temporomandibular joint, 226–227
  soft tissue injury in, 203–211. See also *Soft tissue
    trauma.*
Median forehead flap, in reconstruction of nose, 248, *248*
Median nerve, 368–369
Medullary carcinoma, of thyroid gland, 197
Meibomian glands, 231
Melanoma, 36–40
  acral lentiginous, 37–38
  Breslow's classification of, 39
  chemotherapy for, 40
  examination of, 39
  invasion of, Clark levels of, 38, *38*
  nodular, 37, *37*
  of hand, 380
  prognosis of, 38–39
  superficial spreading, 36–37, *37*
  surgical excision of, 39
  treatment of, 39–40
    metastatic disease and, 40
    regional lymph node involvement and, 39–40
  varieties of, 36–38
Melanotic freckle of Hutchinson (lentigo maligna), 24
Meningocele, 138, 311
Meningoencephalocele, 138–139
Meningoencephalocystocele, 139
Meningomyelocele, 311–312
  closure of, 312, *312*
Merkel cell tumor, 35–36

Mesiocclusion, 147, *148*
Mesodermal malignancy, of hand, 380
Mesodermal tumor(s), 380
Metabolic requirements, of burn patient, 58
Metacarpal bone(s), *351*
  fracture of, 367–368
Metacarpophalangeal joint(s), 366
Methyl methacrylate, as alloplastic material, 76
Microgenia, chin implant for, 275
Micrograft(s), in hair replacement therapy, 278
Microneurovascular muscle transfer, for facial paralysis,
  253
Microsomia, hemifacial, correction of, 151–152
Microvascular surgery, 115–130
  failure of, pathogenesis of, 117–118
  in free tissue transfer, *121–122,* 121–123, *124–125,* 125–
    126
  in microneural repair, *126,* 126–129, *128*
  in nerve grafting, *129,* 129–130
  in replantation of digits, 118–120, *119–120*
  postoperative care following, 117
  techniques in, 115–118, *116–117*
Middle ear disease, cleft palate and, 165
Midpalmar space of Kanavel, 355
Milia, 21
Millard repair, of bilateral cleft lip, 161, *161–162*
  of unilateral complete cleft lip, 159–160, *160*
Milroy disease, 318
Mini-abdominoplasty, 327, 329
  complications of, 329
Mirror-image hand (ulnar dimelia), 383
Moberg volar advancement flap, for fingertip injury, 362,
  363
Mohs excision, of squamous cell carcinoma, 35, *36*
Molecular cross-linkage, impedance to, 7
Mondor's disease (thrombophlebitis), 293
Monoblock frontofacial advancement, 145, *145*
Mouth floor, carcinoma of, 182–183
Mucous cyst(s), of arthritic hand, 377
Muller's muscle, 232
Muscle(s). See also named muscle.
  of eyelids, *231,* 231–232
  of hand, 370–371
  of mastication, 222, *223*
  paralysis of, tendon transfer for, 373–376
Muscle graft, free, for facial paralysis, 253
Musculocutaneous flap(s), 90–97, *91*
  classification of, 92
  expansion of, 109, 111
  for reconstruction of breast, 297–299
    latissimus dorsi muscle in, 297, *298*
    transverse rectus abdominis muscle in, 297–298, *299–
      300*
    complications of, 299
  for reconstruction of chest wall defects, 309, *310,* 311
  for reconstruction of head and neck, 92–93
    temporalis muscle in, 92
    trapezius muscle in, 93
  for reconstruction of lower extremity, 96–97
    gastrocnemius muscle in, 97
    gracilis muscle in, 96
    rectus femoris muscle in, 96–97
    soleus muscle in, 97
    tensor fasciae latae muscle in, 96
  for reconstruction of trunk, 93–96
    gluteus maximus muscle in, 94, 96
    latissimus dorsi muscle in, 93–94
    pectoralis major muscle in, 93
    rectus abdominis muscle in, 94, *95*
  tissue transfer of, 121–123, *122*

Mycosis fungoides (cutaneous T-cell lymphoma), 32
Mylohyoid muscle, 222–223, *223*
Myoblastoma, granular cell, 31
    pyogenic, 31
Myocutaneous flap, expansion of, 109, 111

Nasal. See also *Nose.*
Nasal bridge depression, correction of, in adults, 263–264
        in children, 262–263
Nasal encephalocele, 139
Nasal hump, removal of, 261
Nasal recesses, 258
Nasal septum, straightening of, 262
Nasal tip, 260, *260*
    deformities of, corrective rhinoplasty for, 260, *260–261*
        secondary rhinoplasty for, 264
Nasociliary nerve, 233
Nasoethmoid fracture, 221, *221*
Nasofrontal buttress, 212, *213*
Nasolabial transposition flap, for closure of nasal defect,
        246, *247*
Nasopharynx, carcinoma of, 183–184
Neck, 191–196. See also *Head and neck.*
    anatomy of, 191–192
    correction of, in rhytidectomy, 268, *269*
    cysts and fistulae of, 193–195, *194*
    developmental disorders of, 192–193, *193*
    dissection of, radical, 197–198, *198*
        modified, 198
    mass in, solitary, 196
    swellings in, 195–196
    tissue expansion of, 109, *110–111*
Neodymium-YAG laser, 45
Nerve(s). See also named nerve, e.g., *Facial nerve.*
    cross-section of, *126*
    direct suturing of, in facial paralysis, 251
    functional recovery of, factors determining, 129
    grafting of, *129,* 129–130
        in facial paralysis, 251–252, *252*
    of hand, 368–370
    repair of, *28,* 128–129
        epineural, 128
        perineural, 128–129
    structure of, 126–127
    tissue damage to, 127–128
        Seddon's classification of, 127–128
        Sunderland's grading of, 127
    trauma to, caused by rhytidectomy, 270
Nerve compression syndrome(s), 371–373
    of carpal tunnel, 371–372
    of cubital tunnel, 373
    of radial tunnel, 373
    of ulnar tunnel, 372
Neural tumor(s), 380
Neurapraxia, 127
Neurilemmoma, 27
Neurocclusion, 147, *148*
Neurofibroma, 27
    of breast, 291
Neuropathy(ies), entrapment, of upper limb, 373
Neurotmesis, 128
Nevus(i), hair follicle, 31
    pigmented, types of, 24–25, *25*
    spider (arachnoid), 29
Nevus of Ota, 24
Nevus sebaceus (Jadassohn tumor), 26, *26*
Nevus verrucosus, 22, *23*
Newborn, sex of, 343

Nipple(s), accessory, 285
    inverted, 290
    loss of sensation of, as complication of reduction mam-
        moplasty, 287
    Paget's disease of, 294
    reconstruction of, after mastectomy, 299, *301, 302*
Nipple graft, contralateral, 302
Nipple graft technique, free, reduction mammoplasty,
        286–287
Nipple-areola loss, as complication of reduction
        mammoplasty, 287
Nitrofurazone (Furacin), for burns, 57
Noninnervated regional flap, for fingertip injury, 362, *363*
Nose, 257–264. See also *Nasal; Naso-* entries.
    anatomy of, 257, *257*
    bony skeleton of, narrowing of, 262, *262*
    burns to, management of, 60
    congenital anomalies of, 258
    defects of, reconstruction of, 246–249
        forehead flaps in, *248,* 248–249
        local flaps in, 246, *247*
    fractures of, 217
    lacerations of, 210
    proportions of, 257–258
    reconstructive operations on, 258–264. See also *Rhino-
        plasty.*
    shortening of, 261–262
Nostril deformity, secondary rhinoplasty for, 264
Nutrition, in wound healing, 6–7

Occipitoparietal flap, in hair replacement therapy, 280
Occlusion, dental, 146–147, *148*
Odontogenic cysts, 177
Odontogenic tumors, 177–178
Odontoma, 178
Omentum, transfer of, 126
Omphalocele, 313
Oncocytoma, of parotid gland, 188
Ophthalmic nerve, 233
Ophthalmoplegia, 239
Oral cavity, anatomic landmarks of, 180, *180*
    carcinoma of, 181–183
        TNM classification of, 180t
Oral commissure, deformity of, repair of, 243
Orbicularis oculi muscle, 231, *231*
Orbital advancement, for craniofacial deformities, 144–146,
        145–146
Orbital exenteration, 238
Orbital fracture, 219–220, *220*
Orbital hypertelorism, 142
Orbital soft tissue, entrapment of, 219–220
Oromandibular disorder(s), affecting teeth, *177,* 177–178
    affecting tongue, 178–179
Oropharynx, anatomic landmarks of, 180, *180*
    carcinoma of, 183
Osseocutaneous flap, tissue transfer of, 123, 125, *125*
Osseous tumor(s), 380
Ossification, of skull, failure of, 138–139
Osteoarthritis, clinical features of, 377
    of hand, 377–378
    of thumb, 377
    surgical management of, 377–378
Osteogenesis, distraction, 150, *151*
Osteomyelitis, lower extremity fracture complicated by, 317
Osteotomy(ies), facial, 147, 149, *149–150*
    vertical ramus, 150, *151*
Ovaries, development of, 337
Oxycephaly, 141t

Paget's disease, of nipple, 294
Palate, 155, *155*
  hard, 163
  primary, cleft of. See *Cleft lip.*
  secondary, cleft of. See *Cleft palate.*
    dental malocclusion and, 172
    lengthening of, 169–170
    problem(s) of, 169–172
      alveolar reconstruction for, 171–172, *172*
      dental malocclusion and, 172
      fistulae as, 171
      velopharyngeal insufficiency as, 169–171, *170–171*
  soft, 163
    muscles of, 163–164
Palatoglossus muscle, 164
Palatopharyngeus muscle, 163–164
Palatoplasty, Furlow double reverse, 170
  pushback, 169
Palmar aponeurosis, 352–353
Palmar bursa, 354, *354*
Palmaris brevis muscle, 352–353
Papillary carcinoma, of thyroid gland, 196
Papillary cystadenoma lymphomatosum, of parotid gland, 188, *189*
Papillary syringocystadenoma, 25
Papilloma, ductal, of breast, 292
Paralysis, facial, 249–253. See also *Facial paralysis.*
  muscle, tendon transfer for, 373–376
Parasymphyseal fracture, treatment of, 226
Parkland formula, of fluid resuscitation, 55t
Parotid (Stensen) duct, 187
  transposition of, 190
Parotid gland, anatomy of, 186–187, *187*
  benign tumors of, 188, *189*
    surgical treatment for, 189–190
  malignant tumors of, 189
    surgical treatment for, 189–190
  pathologic conditions of, non-neoplastic, 188
  structures within, 187–188
Parotidectomy, superficial, 189
  total, 190
Parrot beak (supratip deformity), secondary rhinoplasty for, 264
Partial-thickness burn, 53
PDGF (platelet-derived growth factor), in wound healing, 6
Pectoralis major muscle, for reconstruction of trunk, 93
Pectoralis minor muscle, tissue transfer of, 122
Pectus carinatum (pigeon breast), 303
Pectus excavatum (funnel chest), 303, *304*
Pedicle technique, inferior, for reduction mammoplasty, 286, *287*
Peeling agents, deep, 277
  superficial, 276
Penile implant(s), for impotence, 341–342
Penile prosthesis, inflatable, 342
Penis, avulsion injuries of, 340
  fracture of, 340
  loss of, 341
  reconstruction of, 341, *342*
Periorbital reconstruction procedure(s), 231–240
  involving eyelids, *231,* 231–232
    lower, 234–235, *234–235*
    upper, 235–240, *236–237*
  regional anesthesia for, 232–234, *233*
Periorbital trauma, treatment of, 209, *209–210*
Peyronie disease, 341
Pfeiffer syndrome, 141
Phalangization, 364
Phalanx (phalanges), fracture of, 368
  of hand, *351*

Phalen wrist flexion test, 372
Pharyngeal flap pharyngoplasty, 170, *170*
Pharyngoplasty, pharyngeal flap, 170, *170*
Phenol, as chemical peel, 277
Phonation, cleft palate and, 164–165
Phosphorus burn, 61
Physics, laser, 43–44
Pierre Robin syndrome, 164
Pigeon breast (pectus carinatum), 303
Pigmented skin lesions, benign, 22, 24–25, *25*
Pilomatrixoma (calcifying epithelioma of Malherbe), 26
Pilonidal sinus, 31–32
Pinna, congenital absence of, 244
Plagiocephaly, *140,* 141t
Platelet-derived growth factor (PDGF), in wound healing, 6
Platysma muscle, anatomy of, 191
  patterns of insertion of, 266, *266*
Pleomorphic adenoma, of parotid gland, 188
Poland syndrome, 304–305, *305*
Pollicization, of fingers, 364
Polydactyly, 383, *384*
Polymastia, 285
Polymorphonuclear leukocytes, in wound healing, 5
Polythelia, 285
Porcine skin, as xenogenic replacement material, 72
Poroma, 25
Port wine stain, 29
  laser therapy for, 46, *47*
Pressure sores, 320–325
  development of, 320
  etiology of, 320
  grading of, 321, *321*
  hip disarticulation for, 325
  ischial, closure of, 322, 324, *324*
  prevention of, 320
  recurrent wound breakdown of, 325
  sacral, closure of, 322, *323*
  surgical management of, 321–325
    closure of specific ulcers in, 322, *323–325,* 324
    indications for flap coverage in, 322
    postoperative care following, 324–325
    principles of, 322
  trochanteric, closure of, 324, *325*
Progeria, associated with collagen disorders, 8
Pronator teres syndrome, 373
Proplast, as alloplastic material, 76–77
Prosthesis, breast, after mastectomy, 296–297
    types of, 287–288
  expander, 103, *104*
  extrusion of, as complication of tissue expansion, 105
  penile, inflatable, 342
Protein deficiency, wound healing and, 7
Prune-belly syndrome, 313–314
Pseudoptosis, of breast, *290,* 291
Pseudoxanthoma elasticum, associated with collagen disorders, 7
Pterygoid muscle, 222, *223*
Pterygomaxillary buttress, 212, *213*
Ptosis, of breast, *290,* 290–291
  skin, 264–265, *265*
  upper eyelid, 238–240
    acquired, 240
    caused by blepharoplasty, 274
    congenital, 239t, 239–240
    severity of, 239t
Pulley mechanism, of flexor tendons, *357,* 357–358
Pulmonary embolus, as complication of abdominoplasty and abdominal dermolipectomy, 329
Pulsed laser(s), 46

Punch graft(s), in hair replacement therapy, 278
Pyogenic myoblastoma, 31

Q-switched laser(s), 46
Quadripod flap, in reconstruction of nipple, 299, *301,* 302

Radial bursa, 354, *354*
Radial club hand, 382
Radial forearm flap, in reconstruction of penis, 341, *342*
   tissue transfer of, 123, 125
Radial nerve, 369–370
   injury to, wrist drop due to, 374
   superficial, grafting of, 130
Radial tunnel syndrome, 373
Radiation therapy, for breast carcinoma, 295
   for keloids, 8
   for tongue carcinoma, 182
Radiation wounds, chest wall, treatment of, 311
Radiocarpal joint. See *Wrist.*
Radiography, of skull, 203–205, *204–205*
Ramus fracture, treatment of, guidelines in, 226
Randall repair, of unilateral complete cleft lip, 160, *160*
Rectus abdominis muscle, in reconstruction of abdominal
      wall defects, 314, *315*
   in reconstruction of breast, 297–298, *299–300*
      complications of, 299
   in reconstruction of chest wall defects, 309, *310,* 311
   in reconstruction of trunk, 94, *95*
   tissue transfer of, 121, *122*
Rectus femoris muscle, in reconstruction of lower
      extremity, 96–97
Reduction mammoplasty, 285–287
   complications of, 287
   free nipple graft technique for, 286–287
   inferior pedicle technique for, 286, *287*
   keyhole pattern for, 286, *286*
Rehabilitation, of burn victim, 62
Reiger glabella flap, for closure of nasal defect, 246, *247*
Rendu-Osler-Weber syndrome, 30
Replantation, of digits, contraindications to, 118–119
      justification for, 119, *119*
      technical considerations in, 119–120, *120*
   of thumb, 364
Retin A (trans-retinoic acid), 276
Retractile testes, 337
Retrobulbar hematoma, caused by blepharoplasty, 273–274
Rheumatoid arthritis, of interphalangeal joints, *378,*
      378–379
Rhinophyma, 26, *27*
Rhinoplasty, 258–263
   corrective, 260–264
      for narrowing of bony skeleton, 262, *262*
      for nasal bridge depression or saddle nose deformity,
         in adults, *263,* 263–264
         in children, 262–263
      for nasal shortening, 261–262
      for nasal tip deformities, 260, *260–261*
      for removal of nasal hump, 261
      for septal straightening, 262
   incisions in, *259,* 259–260
   secondary, 264
Rhomboid skin flap, 85, *85*
Rhytidectomy, 264–270
   anesthesia for, 266–267
   complications of, 270
   correction of neck in, 268, *269*

Rhytidectomy *(Continued)*
   elevation of skin flaps in, 267, *268*
   elevation of SMAS in, 267–268, *268*
   liposuction as adjunct to, 275, *276*
   subperiosteal, 268, 270
   technique of, 267–270
Rib(s), bone graft from, 74
Rolando fracture, 367
Rotation skin flap, *84,* 84–85

Sacral pressure sores, closure of, 322, *323*
Saddle nose deformity, correction of, in adults, *263,*
      263–264
   in children, 262–263
Saethre-Chotzen syndrome, 142
Salivary gland(s), 186–191
   parotid, 186–190. See also *Parotid gland.*
   submandibular, anatomy of, 190, *191*
      disorder of, 191
Salter-Harris classification, of epiphyseal fractures, 366, *367*
Sarcoma, chest wall, resection of, 309, *310*
   Kaposi, 30–31
Scalp, anatomic layers of, 205
   avulsion of, 206
   closed wounds of, 205–206
   defects of, reconstruction of, 206, *207–208*
   expansion of, in hair replacement therapy, 280–281
   open wounds of, 205
   reduction of, in hair replacement therapy, 278–279, *279*
   tissue expansion of, 107, *108*
Scalp flap, in hair replacement therapy, 280, *280–281*
Scalping forehead flap, in reconstruction of nose, 249
Scaphocephaly, *140,* 141t
Scaphoid fracture, 349–350
Scapular flap, tissue transfer of, 123, *124,* 125
Scar(s), depressed, 15
   dirt-ingrained, 15
   hypertrophic, 8, *9,* 15
   irritable or painful, 14
   management of, 14–17
      W-plasty technique in, 17
      Z-plasty technique in, 15, *15–17,* 17
   unsightly appearance of, 15
Scar contracture(s), 62
Schiff base, 4–5
Scrotum, avulsion injuries of, 340
Sebaceous adenoma, 26
Sebaceous cyst, 21
Sebaceous hyperplasia, senile, 26
Seborrheic keratosis, 21–22
Second-degree burn, 53
Seddon's classification, of nerve damage, 127–128
Senile sebaceous hyperplasia, 26
Sensation, in skin grafts, 70
Sepsis, wound healing and, 7
Septum, nasal, straightening of, 262
Seroma, as complication of abdominoplasty, 329
Serratus anterior muscle, tissue transfer of, 121–122
Sex, of newborn, 343
Sex identification, 342–343
Shock, control of, in soft tissue trauma, 203
   in burn patient, anticipation and treatment of, 55
Sialectasis, chronic, 188
Silicone, as alloplastic material, 77
Silicone gel breast implant(s), 287–288
   in breast reconstruction, 296–297
Silver nitrate, for burns, 56–57
Silver sulfadiazine (Silvadene), for burns, 56

Sinus(es), dermal, congenital, 139
  frontal, development of, 133
Sipple syndrome, 197
Sjögren syndrome, 188
Skate flap, in reconstruction of nipple, *301, 302*
Skeleton, facial, deformities of, 151–152
Ski-jump nasal deformity, secondary rhinoplasty for, 264
Skin, adnexal structures of, 4–5
  aging of, 8
  anatomy of, 265–266, *266*
  biologic replacement of, 71–72, *72*
  epidermal appendages of, tumors of, 25–26, *26–27*
  for full-thickness grafts, 71
  normal, 3–5, *4*
  of hand, 352
  porcine, as xenogenic replacement material, 72
  ptosis and wrinkling of, 264–265, *265*
  subcutaneous layer of, 5
Skin clips, 12
Skin flap(s), 81–87
  advancement, 86, *86,* 362, *363*
  axial pattern, 81–82, *82*
  deltopectoral, 82
  direct transfer, 87, *88*
  distant, 87, *88–89*
  elevation of, in rhytidectomy, 267, *268*
  failure of, prevention of, 84
  forehead, 82
  groin, 82, *83*
  hypogastric, 82
  indications for, 82
  indirect transfer, 87, *89*
  interpolation, 85
  island, 82
  local, 84–86
  necrosis of, as complication of reduction mammoplasty, 287
  random pattern, 81, *81*
  repair by, principles of, 83–84
  rhomboid, 85, *85*
  rotation, *84,* 84–85
  size of, 84
  successful, postoperative characteristics of, 87
  survival of, 82–83, *83*
  transposition, 84–85, *85*
  types of, 84–87
  vascular determination of, 81–83
Skin graft(s), 67–72
  changes in, 70
  composite, 68–69, *69*
  donor sites for, 70
    cutting grafts from, 70–71
    full-thickness, 71
  for burns, 58–60
  full-thickness, 67–68, *68*
    pre-expansion of, 111
  split-thickness, 67, *67–68*
  survival of, 69–70
  types of, 67–70
Skin lesion(s), 21–40
  cystic, benign, 21, *22*
  epidermal, 21–22, *23*
  excision of, 13–14, *14*
    anesthesia for, 13
    preparation for, 13, *13*
  fibrous, 26–27
  infectious, 31–32
  lymphatic, 30
  malignant, 32–40
    basal cell carcinoma as, 32–34, *33–34*

Skin lesion(s) *(Continued)*
    melanoma as, 36–40, *37–38*
    Merkel cell tumor as, 35–36
    squamous cell carcinoma as, 34–35, *35*
  miscellaneous, 31
  of neural origin, 27
  pigmented, benign, 22, 24, *25*
  vascular, 27–30, *28*
    malignant, 30–31
Skin loss, caused by rhytidectomy, 270
Skin slough, as complication of abdominoplasty, 329
Skin staples, 12
Skin sutures, 9–10
  choice of, 10
  subcutaneous, 10, *10*
  types of, 10, *10–12,* 12
Skull, 133–135. See also *Cranial; Cranio-* entries.
  anatomy of, 133, *134–135*
  base of, 133
  defects of, treatment of, 206
  development of, 133
    abnormalities in, 138–139
  ossification of, failure of, 138–139
  radiographic views of, 203–205, *204–205*
  sutures of, 133, *134–135*
    premature closure of. See *Craniosynostosis.*
SMAS (superficial musculoaponeurotic system), 265
  elevation of, in rhytidectomy, 267–268, *268*
Soft tissue, of hand, lacerations of, 362
Soft tissue trauma, 203–211
  craniofacial, immediate priorities in, 203–205, *204–205*
    involving ear, 210
    involving eyes, 209, *209–210*
    involving face, 207–209
    involving lips, 211
    involving nose, 210
    involving scalp, 205–206, *207–208*
    involving skull, 206
    treatment of, 205–211
Solar (actinic) keratosis, 22, *23,* 32
Soleus muscle, for reconstruction of lower extremity, 97
Sphincteroplasty, dynamic, 170–171, *171*
Spider nevus, 29
Spina bifida cystica, 311–312, *312*
Spina bifida occulta, 311
Spiradenoma, 25
Splint(s), for mandibular fractures, 225
Sprain, joint, 366
Squamous cell carcinoma, 34–36, *35*
  Mohs excision of, 35, *36*
  of hand, 380
  of parotid gland, 189
Staging, of head and neck carcinoma, 181t
Staples, skin, 12
Stenosing digital tenosynovitis (trigger finger), 359
Stensen (parotid) duct, 187
  transposition of, 190
Sternal clefts, 303–304
Sternomastoid muscle, anatomy of, 191–192
Sternotomy infection, post-median, treatment of, 309
Steroids, wound healing and, 7
Stomodeum, processes surrounding, 134–135
Strawberry hemangioma, 28, *28*
Strip graft(s), in hair replacement therapy, 278
Sturge-Weber syndrome, 30
Stye (hordeolum), 231
Subcutaneous layer, of skin, 5
Submandibular salivary gland, anatomy of, 190, *191*
  disorder of, 191
Suction lipectomy, body contouring by, 330–331, *331–332*

Suction lipectomy *(Continued)*
  tumescent technique in, 331–332
Sunderland's grading, of nerve damage, 127
Superficial musculoaponeurotic system (SMAS), 265
  elevation of, in rhytidectomy, 267–268, *268*
Suprahyoid neck dissection, 197
Supraomohyoid neck dissection, 198
Supratip deformity (parrot beak), secondary rhinoplasty for, 264
Sural nerve, grafting of, 129, *129*
Surgical excision, of melanoma, 39
Surgical planing (dermabrasion), 277
Suture(s), 9–10
  choice of, 10
  cranial, 133, *134–135*
    premature closure of. See *Craniosynostosis.*
  subcutaneous, 10, *10*
  types of, 10, *10–12,* 12
Swan neck deformity, of interphalangeal joint, 378, *378*
Swanson's classification, of congenital anomalies of hand, 381t
Symblepharon, 238
Symphyseal fracture, treatment of, 226
Syndactyly, 381–382, *382*
Synostosis, bilateral, 139, 141
  metopic, 142
  multiple, 142
  sagittal, 142
  unilateral, 139
Syringocystadenoma, papillary, 25
Syringoma, 25
Systemic disease, wound healing and, 7

Tagliacozzi flap, 87
Tamoxifen, for breast cancer, 295
Tarsal plates, of eyelid, 232
Temporal vertical flap, in hair replacement therapy, 280
Temporalis muscle, for reconstruction of head and neck, 92
  transfer of, for facial paralysis, 253
Temporomandibular joint, 226–227
  ankylosis of, 227
  internal derangement of, 227
Temporoparietal flap, tissue transfer of, 123
Temporo-parietal-occipital flap (Juri flap), in hair
    replacement therapy, 280
Tendon(s), extensor, 359–362. See also *Extensor tendon(s).*
  flexor, 355–359. See also *Flexor tendon(s).*
  transfer of, for muscle paralysis, 373–376
Tendon sheath, giant cell tumors of, 379
Tenosynovitis, 360
  stenosing digital (trigger finger), 359
Tenotomy, lower, for torticollis, 193
Tensor fasciae latae muscle, for reconstruction of lower
    extremity, 96
Tensor palati muscle, 163
Tessier's classification, of residual craniofacial clefts,
    136–138, *137*
Testes, descent of, 337
  development of, 337
Tetanus, prevention of, in burn patient, 57
Tetanus immune globulin, 57
Tetanus toxoid, 57
Thelarche, juvenile, 291
Thenar eminence, 370
Thenar space, 355
Thermal relaxation time, in laser therapy, 44
Thigh dermolipectomy, 329, *330*
Third-degree burn, 53, *53*

Thoracic outlet syndrome, 373
Thrombophlebitis (Mondor's disease), 293
Thumb, 349
  abduction of, 375
  adduction of, loss of, 376
  amputation of, 364, *365*
  aplasia of, 383
  duplication of, 383–384
    Wassel's classification, 383, *384*
  extension of, restoration of, 374
  flexor tendon of, 358–359
  fracture of, 367
  metacarpophalangeal joint of, 366
  opposition of, 375
  osteoarthritis of, 377
  triphalangeal, 384
Thyroglossal duct cyst, surgical approach to, *194,* 195
Thyrohyoid arch, 194
Thyroid gland, tumors of, 196–197
Tinel sign, 372
Tissue(s), loss of, as complication of TRAM flap, 299
  replanted, postoperative management of, 117
  response of, to expansion, 105
  soft. See *Soft tissue* entries.
Tissue adhesive, 12
Tissue expansion, 103–111
  complications of, 105
  of breast, 105–106, *106,* 296, *296–297*
  of ear, 109
  of extremities, 106–107
  of face, 109, *110*
  of forehead, 107, 109
  of neck, 109, *110–111*
  of scalp, 107, *108*
  of trunk, 106, *107*
  prosthesis for, 103, *104*
  regional, 105–111
  technique of, 103, *104,* 105
Tissue transfer, *121,* 121–126
  of bone and osseocutaneous flaps, 123, 125, *125*
  of fasciocutaneous flaps, 123, *124*
  of muscle/musculocutaneous flaps, 121–123, *122*
  specialized, 125–126
TNM classification, of head and neck carcinoma, 180t
Toe(s), transfer of, 125–126
  transplantation of, 364, *365*
Tongue, 178–179
  blood supply to, 179
  carcinoma of, 182
  developmental abnormalities of, 179
  oromandibular disorders affecting, 178–179
Tongue flaps, 179
Tooth (teeth), anatomy of, 177, *177*
  oromandibular disorders affecting, *177,* 177–178
Torticollis, congenital, 192–193, *193*
Tourniquet test, 372
Toxoid, tetanus, 57
TRAM (transverse rectus abdominis muscle) flap, in
    reconstruction of breast, 297–298, *299–300*
  complications of, 299
Transplantation, of toe, 364, *365*
Transposition skin flap, 84–85, *85*
Trans-retinoic acid (Retin A), 276
Transverse rectus abdominis muscle (TRAM) flap, in
    reconstruction of breast, 297–298, *299–300*
  complications of, 299
Trapezium, excision of, for osteoarthritis, 378
Trapezius muscle, for reconstruction of head and neck, 93
Trauma. See also specific trauma, e.g., *Fracture(s).*
  to carpal bones, 349–351

Trauma *(Continued)*
 to fingertips, 362–363, *363*
 to flexor tendons, 355–359
 to lower extremity, 314, 316–317
 to male genitalia, 340–341
 to radial nerve, wrist drop due to, 374
 to soft tissue, 203–211. See also *Soft tissue trauma.*
Treacher Collins syndrome, 138
 correction of, 152
Triamcinolone, hypertrophic scar reduction with, 8
Trichloroacetic acid, as chemical peel, 277
Trichoepithelioma, 26
Tricholemmoma, 26
Trigeminal nerve, maxillary and mandibular branches of, 232, *233*
Trigger finger (stenosing digital tenosynovitis), 359
Trigonocephaly, *140,* 141t
Trilobed flap, in reconstruction of nipple, *301,* 302
Triphalangeal thumb, 384
Trochanteric pressure sores, closure of, 324*325*
Trunk, burns to, management of, 60
 reconstruction of, muscle/musculocutaneous flaps for, 93–96
 tissue expansion of, 106, *107*
Trunk flap, 87
Tumor(s). See also named tumor, e.g., *Glomus tumor.*
 benign, of breast, 291–293
  of hand, 379–380
  of parotid gland, 188, *189*
 malignant. See *Carcinoma.*
 neural, 380
 nonodontogenic, 178
 odontogenic, 177–178
 of epidermal appendages, 25–26
 osseous, 380
Tunica albuginea, fibrosis of, 341
Turban tumor (cylindroma), 25
 of parotid gland, 189
Turner syndrome, 193
Turricephaly, 141t

Ulceration, decubitus, 320–325. See also *Pressure sores.*
 of lower extremity, chronic, 317–318
Ulnar club hand, 383
Ulnar dimelia (mirror-image hand), 383
Ulnar drift, correction of, 379
Ulnar nerve, 369
Ulnar tunnel syndrome, 372
Undescended testes, 337
Upper extremity. See also specific part, e.g., *Hand(s).*
 annular bands of, 384
 body contouring of, 329–330
 embryologic development of, 380–381
 entrapment neuropathies of, 373
Ureter(s), congenital malformations of, 335
Urethra, female, 336
 male, 336
Urinary incontinence, control of, 339
Urinary tract, development of, 335
Urogenital system, 335–345. See also specific part.
 development of, 335
Uvular muscle, 164

Vagina, agenesis of, 344–345
 reconstruction of, 343–345, *344*
Vascular lesions, 27–30

Vascular lesions *(Continued)*
 malignant, 30–31
Vascular malformation, arterial, 29
 capillary, 29
 syndromes of, 30
 venous, 29
Vascular mass(es), 380
Vasculitis, of lower extremity, 318
Veau-Wardill-Kilner palatoplasty, 167, *169*
Velopharyngeal insufficiency, 169
 correction of, 169–171, *170–171*
Velopharyngeal opening, narrowing of, 170
Venous insufficiency, of lower extremity, 317
Venous malformation, 29
Verrucae (warts), 379
Vertical mattress suture, 10, *11*
Vesicourethral junction, congenital valves at, 336
Virginal hypertrophy, of breast, 292
Visible light laser(s), continuous-wave, 45–46
Vision, double (diplopia), 219
Vitamin C deficiency, wound healing and, 6
Von Hippel–Lindau syndrome, 30
Von Langenbeck palatoplasty, 167, *168*
Von Mikulicz disease, 188
Vulvar carcinoma, resection of, reconstruction following, *344,* 345

Wallace rule of nines, for burns, 51, *51*
Warthin tumor, 188, *189*
Warts (verrucae), 379
Wassel's classification, of thumb duplication, 383, *384*
Weber-Fergusson incision, exposure of maxilla by, 185, *185*
Werner syndrome, associated with collagen disorders, 8
Wilke procedure, 190
"Witch's chin," 275
Wolffian duct, 335, 336
Wormian bones, 133
Wound(s), 3–17
 burn. See *Burn(s).*
 care of, 9–10
 decubitus. See also *Pressure sores.*
  recurrent breakdown of, 325
 definition of, 9
 facial, treatment of, 207–209
 healing of, collagen synthesis disorders in, 7–8
  impairment in, 6–7
  sequence in, *5,* 5–6
 management of, 3–10
 primary closure of, 9
  delayed, 12
 radiation, chest wall, treatment of, 311
 scalp, closed, 205–206
  open, 205
 scar. See *Scar(s).*
 skin sutures for, 9–10
  choice of, 10
W-plasty technique, of scar management, 17
Wrinkling, of skin, 264–265, *265*
Wrist, 349–351
 carpal bones of, *350–351*
 extension of, restoration of, 374
 injury to, lunate dislocation as, 350–351
  scaphoid fracture as, 349–350
  trans-styloid radiocarpal dislocation as, 351
 surgical anatomy of, 349, *350*

X chromosome, 343

Xanthelasma palpebrarum, 31
Xanthoma, 31
Xanthoma planum, 31
Xenograft(s), skin, 67, 72
Xeroderma pigmentosum, 32

Y chromosome, 343

Zinc, in wound healing, 7
Z-plasty repair, of cleft palate, 166, *167*
Z-plasty technique, of scar management, 15, *15–17,* 17
Zyderm collagen, 275
Zygoma, fractures of, 217–219, *217–220*
Zygomatic arch, fractures of, 218, *218*
Zygomatic body, fractures of, 218–219, *219–220*
Zygomatic buttress, 212, *213*
Zygomatic loop, for facial paralysis, 253
Zyplast collagen, 275, 276